The Nonsurgical Treatment of Fractures in Contemporary Orthopedics

The Nonsurgical Treatment of Fractures in Contemporary Orthopedics

Augusto Sarmiento MD
Former Professor and Chairman
Departments of Orthopedics, Universities of Miami and Southern California
Past President of American Academy of Orthopedic Surgeons

Loren L Latta PhD
Professor and Director of Orthopedic Research
University of Miami
Miami, Florida, USA

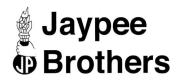

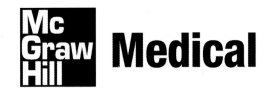

© 2011, Jaypee Brothers Medical Publishers
First published in India in 2009 by

Jaypee Brothers Medical Publishers (P) Ltd.

Corporate Office
4838/24 Ansari Road, Daryaganj, **New Delhi** - 110002, India, +91-11-43574357

Registered Office
B-3 EMCA House, 23/23B Ansari Road, Daryaganj,
New Delhi 110 002, India
Phones: +91-11-23272143, +91-11-23272703, +91-11-23282021,
+91-11-23245672, Rel: +91-11-32558559 Fax: +91-11-23276490,
+91-11-23245683
e-mail: jaypee@jaypeebrothers.com
Website: www.jaypeebrothers.com

First published in USA by The McGraw-Hill Companies, 2 Penn Plaza, New York, NY 10121. Exclusively worldwide distributor except South Asia (India, Nepal, Sri Lanka, Bhutan, Pakistan, Bangladesh, Malaysia).

ISBN-13: 978-0-07-175921-2
ISBN-10: 0-07-175921-2

To

The many orthopedic residents and colleagues who over the years provided us with their input and enthusiasm, particularly to the ones who patiently and honestly reviewed the clinical material and data that constitute the substance of the text.

■ Preface

The Nonsurgical Treatment of Fractures in Contemporary Orthopedics clearly indicates this is not a comprehensive treatise on fracture care. It deals almost exclusively with the functional nonsurgical treatment of fractures of the tibial diaphysis, the humeral shaft, the isolated fracture of the ulna and the Colles' fracture. To a lesser degree, it covers other fractures such as those of both bones of the forearm, the isolated radial shaft fracture and the femoral metaphysis fracture because the indications for nonsurgical treatment in these instances are more limited, but nonetheless are proven to be acceptable alternatives in a number of instances. While discussing tibial fractures, a separate section is devoted to the use of functional treatment in the management of delayed unions and nonunions.

The tibial, humeral shaft and Colles' fractures are the ones we have studied in greater depth over the past few decades, and to which, through clinical and research studies, we may have contributed additional knowledge and innovative management protocols. The treatment of certain fractures with functional casts and braces that allow motion of joints adjacent to the fracture and encourages physiological motion to take place at the fracture site can serve to be important lasting contributions.

The progress that modern surgical fixation of fractures has wrought has been spectacular. For example, fractures of certain long bones, such as the tibia and humerus, have long been challenging ones, but no longer as much as they were in older days. The significant progress made in recent decades has been primarily the result of advanced surgical techniques, superior metallurgy and sophisticated imaging technology. The open fracture, previously beset with frequent serious complications, has benefited the most. Intramedullary nailing and external fixators have reduced the problem to one of much lesser magnitudes. The threat of uncontrollable infection and amputation has diminished dramatically in the recent past. Unfortunately, the recent appearance of Methicillin-resistant *Staphylococcus aureus* (MRSA) has created the spectrum of an epidemic of unprecedented proportions that might have a major impact on the surgical treatment of fractures.

Surgery thus far has had a major beneficial effect in the management of fractures previously treated only by nonsurgical means requiring prolonged periods of bed confinement. The femoral shaft fractures represent the best example, since these fractures are now almost universally treated successfully by internal fixation, resulting in major reduction in costs, hospitalization and rehabilitation care. Hip and pelvic fractures, spine fractures and many others also eloquently testify to the benefits of surgical care.

While progress was being made in the surgical treatment of fractures, advances were also taking place in the nonsurgical approach to closed fractures. A better understanding of their behavior and the resulting recognition of the limitations of newer methods have allowed us to redefine the place and role of closed nonsurgical treatment of many fractures. This text is an attempt to balance the place of surgical and nonsurgical approaches in the care of several major fractures in a rational way.

Although we have published a number of books and articles in the past dealing with the functional nonsurgical care of certain fractures, additional experience mandated that major as well as minor changes needed to be made, which in some instances, constituted radical departures from the originally espoused concepts. This book addresses those issues and places the method in the best possible perspective of contemporary fracture care.

Despite the overall surgical or nonsurgical progress we have alluded to, there are not yet treatment modalities applicable to all fractures, and under all circumstances. Every modality has its indications and limitations, and may be associated with complications. Needless to say, complications from surgical treatments are usually of a greater magnitude and more difficult to overcome.

In this book, we emphasize the basic sciences of fracture repair. It encompasses both long-term clinical observations as well as results of laboratory studies performed on large and smaller animals. It is hoped that our comments would be helpful to orthopedic surgeons who must deal with all aspects of fracture management.

We look with great discomfort at the exaggerated trend where, without logic or common sense, a number of fractures which can be successfully treated by effective and less expensive treatment modalities are consistently managed by surgical means. This trend has permeated the orthopedic community to a degree where an increasing number of orthopedists and traumatologists are functioning not as surgeons/scientists but as cosmetic surgeons of the skeleton. To these people, any inconsequential deviation from the normal constitutes a complication. The obsession with anatomical reduction—as if such a reduction were always equivalent to a better clinical result—dominates the spectrum of fracture care in America and to a lesser degree in other countries. The virtual epidemic of surgical treatment of fractures of the clavicle, Colles' fractures and many others, where the indications for surgery are limited, are good representative examples. To the surgeon, the greater economic benefits inherent in the surgical treatment of fractures is significantly greater constituting an incentive to its abuse. Surgery also benefits hospitals since surgical volume increases their revenues. Probably, the most important factor in the genesis of the trend is the enormous control of education and practice of the profession by the implant manufacturing industry. Unless its pervasive influence remains unchecked, the problems associated with fracture care will continue to deteriorate.

The first chapter to this book deals with the basic sciences behind the subject of fracture healing and particularly its response to environmental factors. Although only research studies conducted in our laboratories are presented in detail, we acknowledge the contribution to the subject made by others as much as possible.

The senior author's divided academic career between the Universities of Miami and Southern California provided him the opportunity to work with other physicians and researchers at the two opposite ends of the country. Appropriate recognition and thanks are extended to them.

Augusto Sarmiento
Loren L Latta

■ Acknowledgments

We acknowledge with deep appreciation the contributions made by the dozen of Orthopedic Residents and Fellows at the Universities of Miami and Southern California and the Engineers in same institutions who actively participated in the development of the project now crystallized in this book.

■ Contents

Section V: The Isolated Ulnar Fracture

Section VI: The Colles' Fracture

Section VII: Fractures of Both Bones of the Forearm

Section VIII: Isolated Radial Shaft Fractures

Section

1

Introduction

1

Pertinent Basic Science of Fracture Healing and Biomechanics

INTRODUCTION

It is essential for the orthopedic surgeon to have a clear understanding of the differences that exist in the healing process of fractures, according to the treatment modalities currently in use.

The manner in which fractures heal is determined to a great extent on the environment surrounding the process.[1] Diaphyseal fractures treated by means of rigid immobilization do not show a peripheral callus.[2] On the contrary, those where functional activities create motion between the fragments, there is the formation of peripheral callus.[3-7] We prefer to call this callus "peripheral" rather than "periosteal" since it is very likely that the vessels that give birth to the callus come primarily from the surrounding soft tissues, and to a much lesser extent from the periosteum. We support this view which is contrary to popular opinion, with laboratory and radiographic studies, which are further detailed in subsequent pages.

Similarly, we question the role of the hematoma in fracture healing by suggesting that the hematoma rather than being a salutatory component in fracture healing, delays the reparative process. The collection of blood created by the rupture of vessels at the fracture site and its surrounding tissues needs to be reabsorbed in order to allow room for the enchondral ossification process. Though there is considerable suggestive evidence that circulating cells, such as lymphocytes, monocytes and plasma cells actively participate in the healing process, their clear role in fracture healing has not been identified. More recently, the finding of BMP (Bone morphogenic proteins) in platelets, particularly TGF Beta, has stimulated interest in the subject at hand. Nonetheless, if those cells were important in tissue healing, injection of blood into a fracture would make it heal faster. Attempts to expedite healing with such a technique has proven to be disappointing. Likewise, we should have concluded long ago that fractures accompanied with large hematomas would heal faster than those with smaller ones. This is another example of the poor understanding we still have regarding the process of ossification.

Under similar light, we refute the popular misconception of a direct relationship between the size of muscle mass surrounding the fracture site and the amount of peripheral callus. The humeral and femoral fractures are frequently used as examples to support the theory. However, it ignores the fact that many bones with none or minimal surrounding muscle masses heal equally if not faster. The clavicle, metacarpals and phalanges, which have either a minimal or no muscle envelope heal readily. It is very likely that the larger callus seen in the femur and humerus is due to the greater amount of motion that takes place at their fracture sites. Single-bone limb segments with a thick layer of surrounding muscle are inherently unstable compared to the inherently stable two-bone limb segments[1] or hand or finger fractures.[8] Such motion creates a greater degree of soft tissue irritation, and the subsequent vascular invasion responsible for the osteoblastic metaplasia of the capillary cells.

MOTION AT THE FRACTURE SITE

Two types of motion occur at the fracture site: *Elastic* and *plastic*. Elastic motion is a displacement of the bone fragments which occurs when load is applied to the limb and is completely reversed after the load is relaxed. Plastic motion is the displacement of the bone fragments which occurs when load is applied to the limb but the displacement does not recover after the load is relaxed resulting in a residual change in alignment of the fragments. Thus elastic motion effects how a fracture will heal (Figures 1.1A and B). Plastic motion effects the alignment of the bone fragments.

We have conducted a number of studies over the years aimed at determining the effects of motion at the fracture site. These studies have not only clearly shown the degrees of motion that occur during function and/or weight bearing, but also unequivocally demonstrated the greater size and strength of the callus when motion is present.

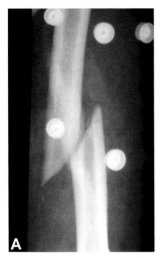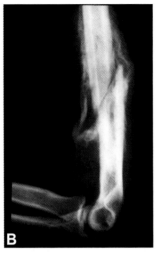

Figs 1.1A and B: (A) Radiograph of an oblique fracture of the humeral diaphysis stabilized in a brace. (B) Later radiograph showing the outline of the forming callus that clearly depicts the motion that occurred during the healing process, and the elastic nature of the motion as the fragments healed in the "relaxed" position.

HEALING WITH RIGID FIXATION OR MICROSCOPIC ELASTIC MOTION

Elastic motion with "rigid" fixation (i.e. proper plate and screw fixation) will allow motion in the order of microns at the fracture site for normal loading conditions.[9-11] With this degree of motion, the fracture will heal with direct formation of new bone on the original bone with little or no external callus (Figures 1.2A to C).[10-13] The medullary circulation will re-establish rapidly.[7] In areas of contact, cutter-heads of bone remodeling may cross the fracture site directly, (Figures 1.2A to C).[30,31,42,45]

With "rigid" fixation, the early bone forms primarily in the gaps of microscopic size between the bone ends with occasional direct "osteon-to-osteon" formation at the contact points (Figures 1.3A and B).[9,11,12,15,16] This new bone is shielded from the normal stress of functional activities because of the mechanical contribution required by the plate and screw fixation.[17-20]

HEALING WITH COMPLIANT FORMS OF FIXATION, OR MACROSCOPIC ELASTIC MOTION

With "compliant" forms of fixation (intramedullary rods, casts and braces), the elastic motion at the fracture site is at least 1 mm and can be several cms with normal loading associated with functional activities.[21-23] This elastic motion is good for fracture healing because it causes a peripheral callus to form through secondary bone formation.[3,23-29]

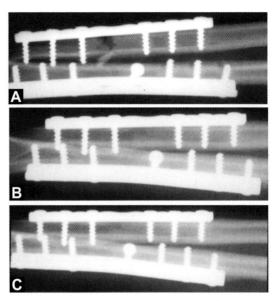

Figs 1.2A to C: (A) This both-bone forearm fracture on the day of surgery shows a small fragment of bone displaced from the gap on the ulna. (B) At 4 months post surgery, the gap is filled with bone, the fragment is no longer visible and the fractures are radiographically healed with no peripheral callus. (C) At 2 years post surgery, the radiographic picture has not changed.

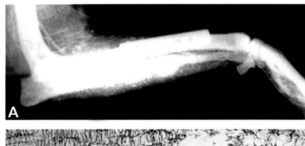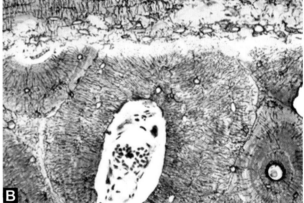

Figs 1.3A and B: (A) This both-bone fracture in the canine model had the radius plated and ulna left alone. Note the peripheral callus on the ulna, but not on the radius. (B) New bone has formed directly on the fractured surface of the osteons of this bone fragment. Note the thin layer of avascular tissue on the fracture surface where the blood supply was disrupted by the injury. The new osteocytes in the newly forming bone are larger and more active than those in the old cortical bone, and the new bone is much less organized where it fills in the small gap between the fragments.

In an attempt to further document the favorable effect of motion at the fracture site in the case of diaphyseal fractures, we conducted a serious and sophisticated laboratory study utilizing experimental rabbits.[26,30-32]

Different types of external fixators were designed that would in various degrees increase or decrease the motion that occur at the fracture site during normal walking activities. The fractures were produced by closed means in order to avoid the variables, and often misleading information that open osteotomies introduce.[33,34] Two different types of fractures were produced, transverse and oblique. The metallic frames were also divided into rigid and non-rigid ones. The animals were allowed to function without restrictions after the frames were connected to the computer that would demonstrate in a very precise manner the motion that occurred during ambulation (Figures 1.4A and B).

After completion of the biomechanical study, the animals were sacrificed and the fracture specimens were subjected to histological examination. This study demonstrated once again the fact that with increased motion at the fracture site, the size of the peripheral callus was greater and that in the more rigidly immobilized fracture, the osteogenic process was limited mostly to endosteal ossification (Figures 1.5A to D). The peripheral callus is responsible for the greater strength of the bone during the healing process as well as after completion of healing.

THE ROLE OF VASCULARITY IN FRACTURE HEALING

It is generally believed that the hematoma plays a major role in the healing of fractures.[35,36] We suspect there is no scientific evidence to support this view. It is simply a very attractive theory that has been accepted without questioning for many generations. As we will document later in this chapter, what is important is not the hematoma, but the capillaries that form around a fracture, the endothelial and perithelial cells of these new capillaries may undergo differentiation and re-differentiation into osteoblasts.

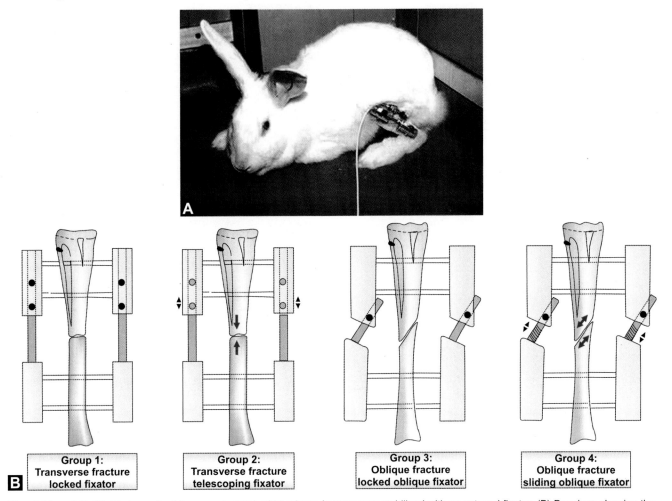

| Group 1: Transverse fracture locked fixator | Group 2: Transverse fracture telescoping fixator | Group 3: Oblique fracture locked oblique fixator | Group 4: Oblique fracture sliding oblique fixator |

Figs 1.4A and B: (A) Photograph of the experimental rabbit whose fracture was stabilized with an external fixator. (B) Drawings showing the four types of fixators used in a laboratory study. They were designed to either allow motion at the fracture or to prevent it. In the first two groups, transverse fractures were created and in the second two groups oblique, axially unstable fractures were performed.

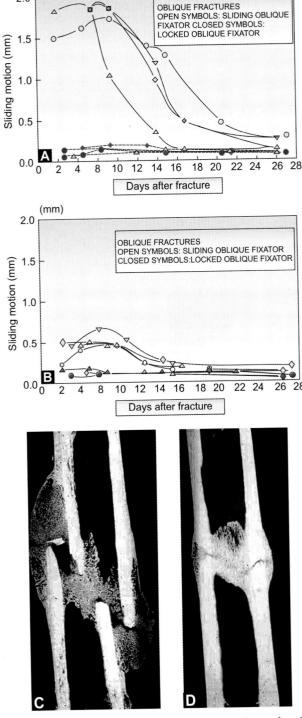

Figs 1.5A to D: The degree of motion was measured every few days in the (A) oblique fractures, both locked and unlocked, (B) and the transverse fractures, both locked and unlocked. Clearly, there was far greater motion in the unlocked oblique fractures which were associated with the largest peripheral callus, (C) than in any other group. The unlocked transverse fractures had some motion which was associated with peripheral callus, but to a much lesser degree, (D) than the unlocked oblique fractures.

With "rigid" fixation, the blood supply for fracture healing comes principally from the medullary circulation and its communications through the bone to the peripheral blood supply (Figure 1.6).[2,37] With compliant fixation systems, the surrounding soft tissues provide almost all of the blood supply to the callus bridging the fractures site (Figures 1.7A to 1.9B). Thus, early muscle activity and some localized inflammatory responses are important to bring the capillaries for early bone formation (Figures 1.10A to G.)

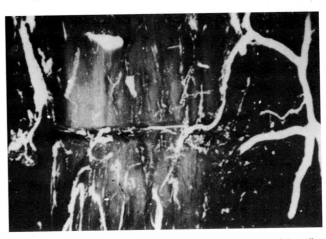

Fig. 1.6: Microradiographic illustration of the pathway of invading capillaries into the gaps between the bone fragments when the fracture is rigidly fixed.[11]

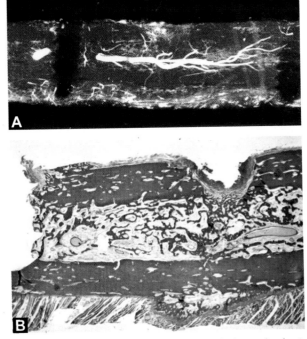

Figs 1.7A and B: Radiological and histological views of a fracture that healed in the presence of rigid fixation in the canine radius. The absence of peripheral callus is evident and the cortical healing readily seen.

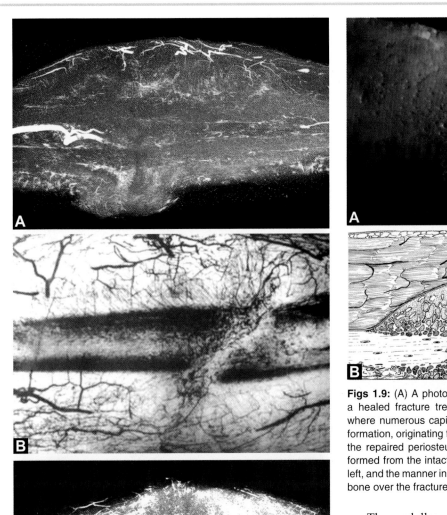

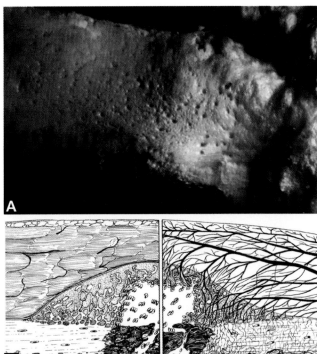

Figs 1.9: (A) A photograph of the surface of the bridging bone over a healed fracture treated without immobilization. Notice the holes where numerous capillaries penetrated the surface of the new bone formation, originating from the surrounding soft tissues, and later from the repaired periosteum. (B) Schematic drawing showing the callus formed from the intact cortical surface and the overlying soft tissues, left, and the manner in which the peripheral vessels invade the bridging bone over the fracture site, right.

The medullary blood supply is almost always disrupted even in low-energy fractures.[2,37] When there is displacement between the fracture fragments or greater degrees of motion at the fracture site, the medullary blood supply cannot cross the fracture site until the fragments can be rigidly connected by the callus.

THE STRUCTURAL MECHANICAL STAGES OF PERIPHERAL CALLUS

The following section illustrates the sequence of events through gross histological images that take place when a diaphyseal fracture heals without rigid fixation.[27] The first stage of healing at and immediately after the injury is Stage I, called "Instability." Acute symptoms accompany this stage, including swelling, pain and gross mechanical instability. This degree of instability prior to the formation of healing tissues from the body's attempt to stabilize the fracture, can be detrimental to the new forming tissues (Figures 1.12A and B). Therefore it is important to immobilize the limb segment to allow the tissues to form an early callus. Pain and swelling are the best indicators of this stage of healing.

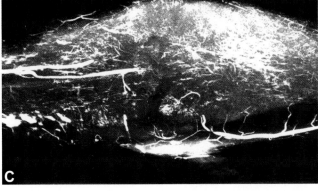

Figs 1.8A to C: Illustration of healing fractures in the experimental animal treated without rigid fracture immobilization demonstrating the vascular contributions of the peripheral tissues. Notice the continued lack of reanastomosis of the medullary artery.

This environment, supported by functional activity, is associated with more active osteoblastic activity (Figures 1.11A and B). It becomes important to understand how these types of callus form, how they can provide adequate strength to resist plastic deformation while allowing elastic motion during normal functional activities.

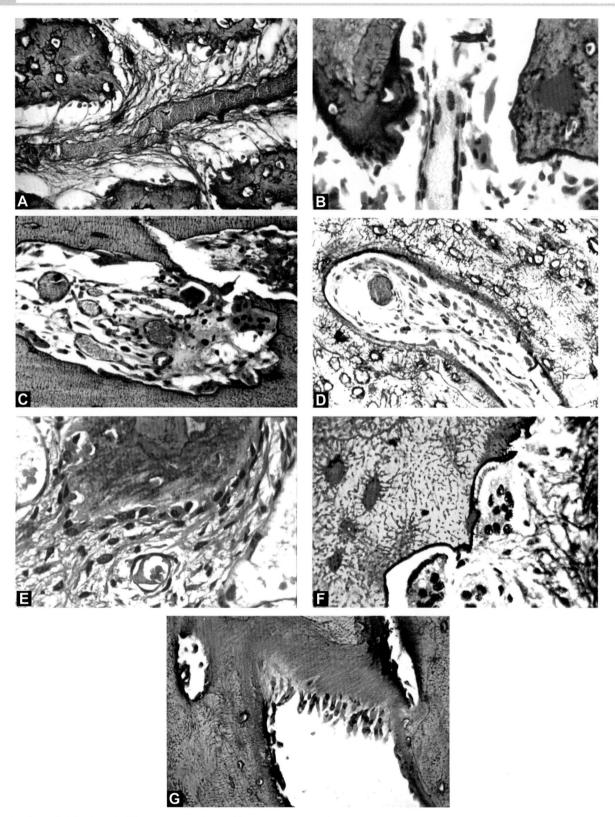

Figs 1.10A to G: Histological slides illustrating the capillary contribution to fracture healing in the presence of motion at the fracture site. The peripheral capillary invade the fracture site. The perithelial cells (and probably also the endothelial) undergo differentiation into osteoblasts, which in turn produce osteoid tissues.

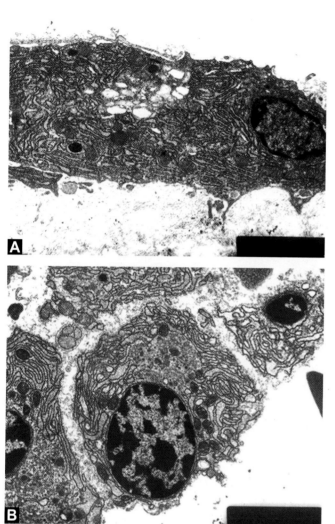

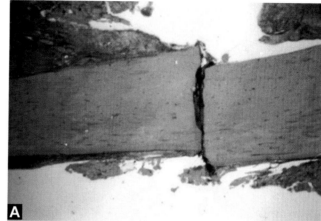

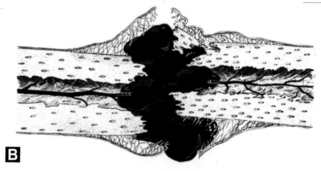

Figs 1.11A and B: (A) Transmission electron microscopy of an osteoblast in a non-immobilized healing fracture. Notice the abundant endoplasmic reticulum, indicative of activity. (B) Osteoblast from a healing fracture treated with rigid plate fixation. Notice the lesser degree of endoplasmic reticulum.

With Stage II, Soft Callus, the bone fragments can still move relative to each other because they are connected by soft tissues and cartilage, see Figures 1.1A to D. But the soft callus provides stability to the bone fragments sufficient for tissue healing, and the symptoms of pain and swelling subside. So the fracture can be moved by manual examination,[27,38] but the patient does not experience severe pain as in Stage I healing (Figures 1.13 to 1.15).

Stage III callus is called "Hard Callus" because the connection between the bone ends very rapidly becomes very rigid, and it is no longer possible to manually move the fracture fragments. The dense layer of collagen fibers covering the callus provides hundreds of small capillaries

Figs 1.12A and B: Stage I, Instability (A) Histological section illustrating the hematoma between the ends of the fracture and the absence of response to the injury at this very early stage. (B) At the time of the injury, the medullary blood supply is severed and a hematoma fills the empty space created by the fracture gap and the elevation of periosteum and soft tissues from the bony diaphysis.

to the cartilage below and this blood supply made available by the surrounding soft tissues begins to calcify the cartilage bridging the fracture site, from the outside in,[27,39-41] (Figures 1.16A and B).

Initially the calcified layer is quite thin covering the bridging cartilage. However, even as a thin layer, barely evident radiographically, the structure of the callus is quite rigid and strong (Figures 1.17A to 1.18C). This is because the resistance to bending and torsion is related to the fourth power of the diameter of the circular cross-section of the callus. So, say a callus two times the original diameter of the bone would have a 16-fold advantage mechanically over any bone at the original diameter of the diaphysis at resisting bending and torsion (Figures 1.19A to C). So the bone does not need to be as rigid and strong or as thick as the original cortex to provide rigidity and strength to the callus structure.[23,27,42]

Stage IV callus is called Fracture line Consolidation. This marks the calcification of all of the peripheral callus and obliteration of the fracture line radiographically (Figures 1.20A to C).

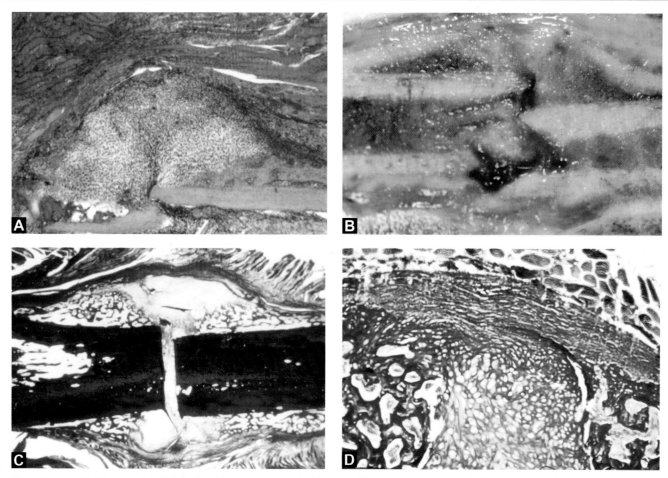

Figs 1.13A to D: Stage II, Soft Callus: (A) After a short period of time, cartilaginous tissue forms, bridging the bony fragments. There is no evidence that the hematoma becomes cartilage as the hematoma persists between the bone ends. A collagenous band forms around the cartilage replacing the torn periosteum which apparently is incorporated into the peripheral callus, and in front of new bone forms on the cortical surface where there is blood supply from the live bone fragment. (B) This same architecture of the new forming callus can be appreciated in this gross view of callus cut through the sagittal plane. (C) This illustration shows the thick peripheral band and the absence of bone at the fracture site. The cartilage is undergoing ossification from the proximal and distal fronts of new bone formation, but not from the fracture gap. (D) A closer histologic view of the bridging callus illustrates the dense band of well oriented collagenous tissue which covers the cartilage that bridges the bone fragments and separates the cartilage from the surrounding muscle.

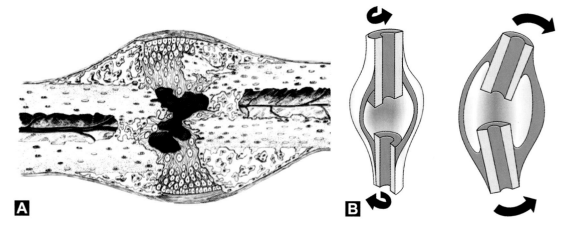

Figs 1.14A and B: With Stage II Soft Callus, the bone fragments can still move relative to each other because they are connected by soft tissues and cartilage. So the fracture can be moved by manual examination, but the patient does not experience severe pain as in Stage I healing.

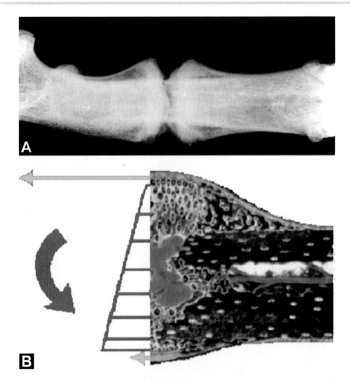

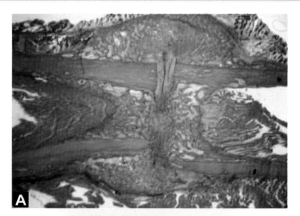

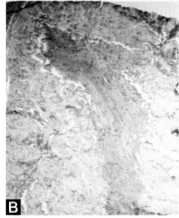

Figs 1.15A and B: (A) A radiograph of a rat femur in Stage II callus demonstrating little x-ray evidence of the bridging callus. (B) An illustration of a section through the bridging callus showing the stress profile across the fracture site when a bending movement is applied. The peripheral dense collagenous covering provides good tensile resistance while the cartilage, hematoma and fibrous tissue inside provide good compression resistance, creating a compliant, but strong coupling between the bone fragments. This mechanical structure works like an intervertebral disc with a dense layer of well-oriented collagen fibers (annulus fibrosis), covering the more fluid-like, hydraulic-like center (nucleus pulposus).

Figs 1.16A and B: Stage III, Hard Callus: (A) Histological section illustrating the further ossification of the cartilaginous mass (orange) along the collagenous peripheral band with blood supply from the surrounding soft tissues. (B) A close up view of the thin layer of new bone bridging the fracture gap in the periphery, over the thinning cartilage mass (green).

Stage V callus is called Remodeling. Once the fracture gap is calcified, and the new bone gains strength, the bone does not need the large peripheral callus to provide stiffness and strength, so the peripheral portion shrinks with the normal remodeling process, and the medullary canal is re-established along with the medullary blood supply (Figures 1.21A and B). The bone has regenerated its diaphysis.

The time and degree of maturity of each stage is varied by the age of the patient, the extent of the injury, the limb segment with a fracture and general health of the patient (Figures 1.22A to 1.23E).

THE STRENGTH OF HEALING FRACTURES

The strength of the healing bone reaches a peak apparently within a few months post-plating (about 8 weeks in the dog).[43,44] The strength of the bone beneath the plate will be approximately half its original strength immediately after surgery. This bone beneath the plate does not reach the original bone strength and even loses strength over the

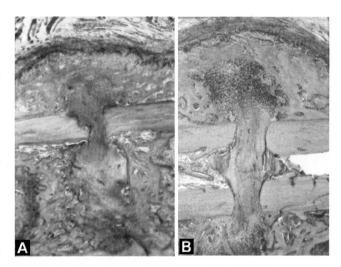

Figs 1.17A and B: Histological pictures of the progressive ossification of the cartilage from the periphery, the thickening of the peripheral bridging bone and the persistence of fibrous connective tissue between the fragments.

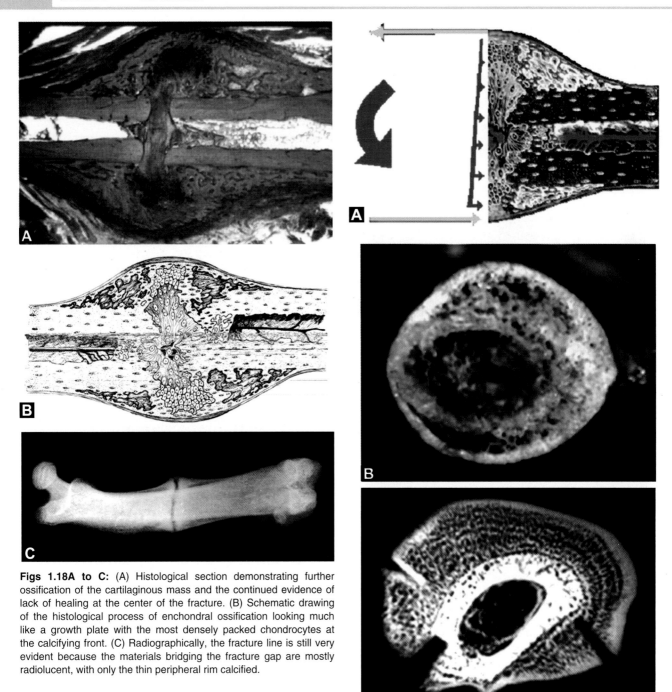

Figs 1.18A to C: (A) Histological section demonstrating further ossification of the cartilaginous mass and the continued evidence of lack of healing at the center of the fracture. (B) Schematic drawing of the histological process of enchondral ossification looking much like a growth plate with the most densely packed chondrocytes at the calcifying front. (C) Radiographically, the fracture line is still very evident because the materials bridging the fracture gap are mostly radiolucent, with only the thin peripheral rim calcified.

next few months due to cancellization of the cortical bone beneath the plate.[43-45] This change from dense cortical bone to cancellous-like bone may be due to stress protection provided by the plate or to changes in the blood supply caused by the surgical procedure.[9,12,18,19,24,43-46] New procedures and devices have been aimed at reducing the compromise to the blood supply,[12] the stress protection and improve the long-term effects on the healing bone.[47-52] Apparently the full strength of the bone is not re-established until about

Figs 1.19A to C: (A) An illustration of the stress profile in the fracture gap once the peripheral layer of cartilage has calcified, making the callus very rigid and very strong. (B and C) Cross sections of fractured bone illustrating the peripheral osseous ring that gives strong structural properties to the callus. (B) This view of the fracture surface after a bending strength test of a healing rat femur shows cartilage on the ends of the original cortex consistent with radiolucency in the fracture gap of this Stage III callus. (C) This radiograph is of a thin slice of bone being prepared for histology. The cuts in the periphery were made after dissection to mark the sagittal and frontal planes.

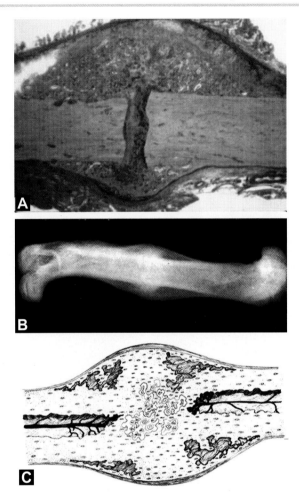

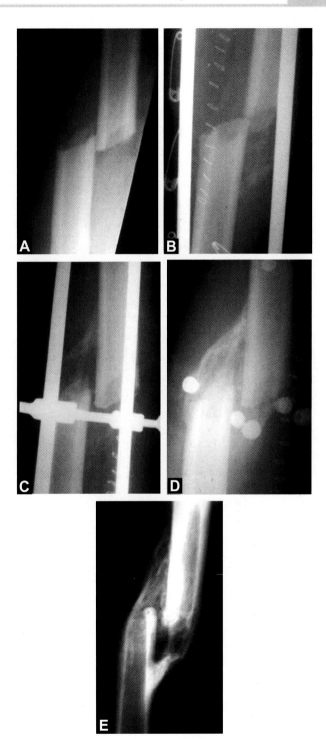

Figs 1.20A to C: Stage IV callus shows consolidation of the fracture line (A) histologically and (B) radiographically. (C) The illustration shows that in the center of the fracture, there is still fibrous connective tissues and the medullary canal is not yet re-established.

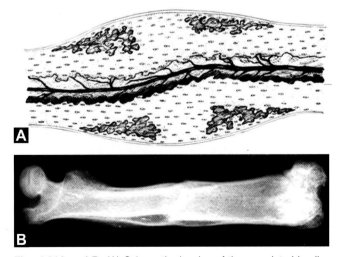

Figs 1.21A and B: (A) Schematic drawing of the completed healing process and the delayed reconstitution of medullary blood supply. (B) The remodeling phase in a rat femur.

Figs 1.22A to E: (A) This acute fracture in Stage I was taken to surgery for intramedullary nail fixation. (B) But intraoperative complications prevented the surgeon from completing the surgery, so traction was applied and soon Stage II callus developed. (C) When Stage III callus was noted, the traction was removed, and a fracture brace applied. (D) The fracture went on to consolidate at Stage IV, when the brace was removed. (E) At long-term follow-up the callus was remodeling, Stage V.

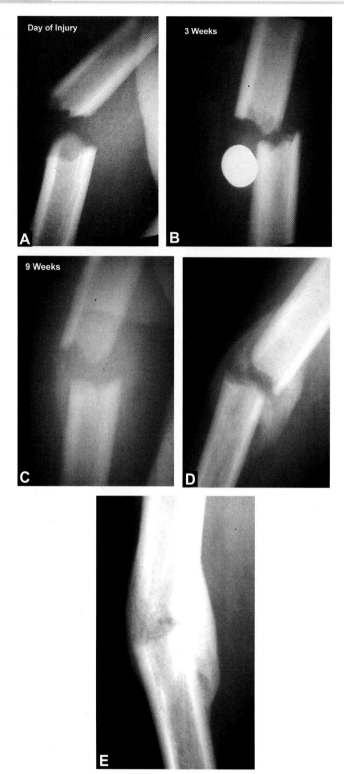

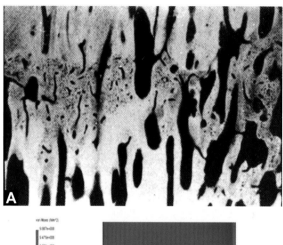

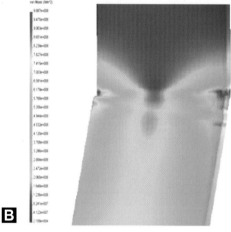

Figs 1.24A and B: (A) This microradiographic image demonstrates that even after 6 months of healing with rigid fixation, the new bone that formed in the gaps is still not completely remodeled and equal to the original cortical bone.[19] (B) A finite element model of a healing bone after rigid fixation demonstrates how the reduced modulus of elasticity and the different anisotropic orientation of the healing bone in the gap causes a stress concentration at the fracture site and makes it vulnerable to refracture.

Figs 1.23A to E: (A) Sequential radiographs of a distracted fracture of the humeral diaphysis at Stage I healing, (B) which progressed to Stage II when the brace was applied, (C) then Stage III and the brace was discontinued. (D) At later followup, the fracture line is consolidated, Stage IV, (E) and much later the remodeling is progressing, Stage V.

18-24 months while the plate is in place, although only anecdotal evidence in animal models are available to support that view.[13] Evidence from animal studies show that the bone strength from a single isolated screw can recover in about 12-16 weeks in the dog,[53] but the weakening effect of stress concentration is reactivated when the screw is removed. However, if the screws are attaching a plate to the bone, the bone never regains more than about half its original strength even up to 6 months post fracture (Figures 1.24A and B).[24]

This is why the strength of the bone at the fracture site (after plate removal) is only about half the strength of the original bone in the first few months before the new bone can remodel to orient itself to the normal direction of the osteons (Figures 1.25A to 1.26B).[9,12,17-19,54] The strength of the bone adjacent to the original fracture site also is compromised

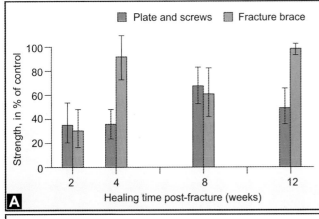

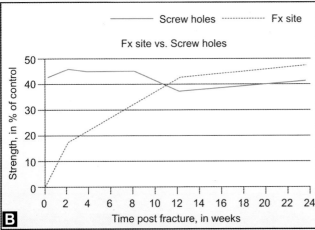

Figs 1.25A and B: (A) This graph demonstrates that in the treatment of closed fractures in the canine radius, the fracture bone that heals in the presence of motion at the fracture site is stronger than the same fracture immobilized with a plate. The bone with a plated fracture does not regain its strength even up to 6 months post-fracture in the canine radius.[24] (B) In the plated canine radius, the bending fracture strength was measured with the plates left in place in one group and after removal of the plates in the other group. With the plates intact, the failures occurred through a screw hole at the end of the plate at a failure moment of less than 50% of the intact bone bending strength of the opposite limb of the same animal. If the plates were removed prior to bending test, the failure occurred at the original fracture site up to 12 weeks post fracture, at which time the strength of the healing fracture site reached the strength of the surrounding bone with screw holes.[24]

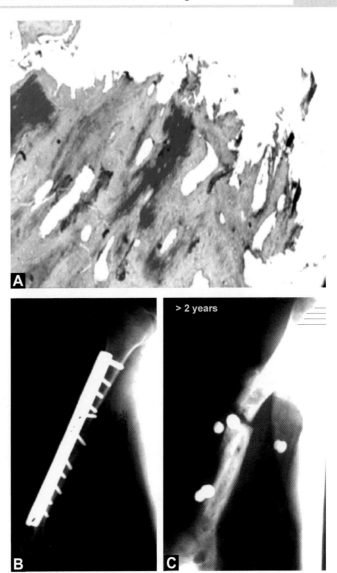

Figs 1.26A to C: (A) This closed transverse fracture of a canine radius treated with plate and screw fixation and at 8 weeks refractured in torsion by histologic evaluation of the refracture surface demonstrates a shear failure through the new bone formed at the fracture site.[6] (B) This plated humeral fracture had the plate removed over 2 years post fracture. (C) Within a week, the patient returned to clinic with a refracture through the original fracture site.

because of the stress protection of the plate which causes cancellation, cortical thinning and the screw holes cause stress concentration.[17,24] Thus refracture can occur through the adjacent weakened bone or through screw holes where there is weakened bone and no peripheral callus (Figures 1.27A to 1.28).

With "compliant" fixation within the first few days, post injury immobilization and rest are important to provide comfort until the acute symptoms subside. This is called the stage of instability.

The likelihood of refracture of long bones that heal with peripheral callus which has formed in an environment of functional activity is extremely rare. The strains of physical activity, forms the callus structure and optimizes its strength related to the mechanical demand.[23,25,27-29,42] The strength of the bone at the level of the fracture is greater than before the fracture took place (Figures 1.27A to 1.28).[5,7,18,26,27,55,56]

If a new injury occurs, a fracture would be located either above or below the original fracture. When a diaphyseal fracture is treated with methods that produce rigid

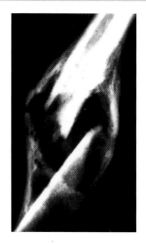

A

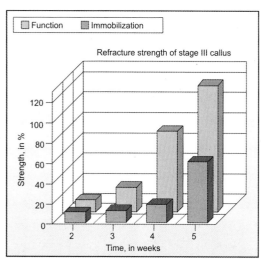

B

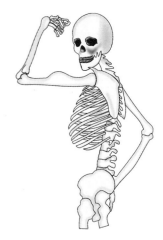

C

Figs 1.27A to C: (A) This patient was fully ambulatory with no support, walking pain free on this Stage III callus. (B) A study of rat femur fracture strength showed fractured bones that were stronger than the bone on the contralateral limb at 5 weeks post fracture if the animals were allowed to ambulate on the limbs as tolerated.[57] (C) That is why peripheral callus has been referred to as "the strength of the skeleton" (drawing courtesy of Dieter Pennig, MD).

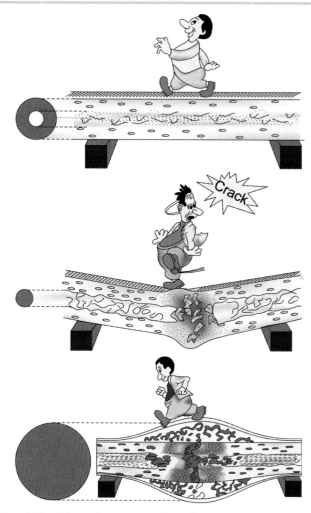

Fig. 1.28: Schematic representation of the superior mechanical strength of peripheral callus, compared to that of intramedullary callus.

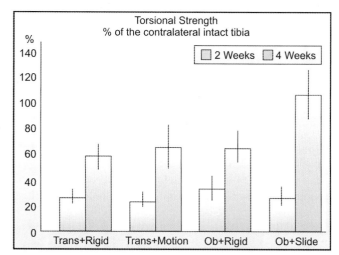

Fig. 1.29: This graph indicates that the torsional strength of the callus is greater in fractures that demonstrate greater pistoning motion at the fracture site and a larger peripheral callus.[26]

immobilization of the fragments, the strength of the bone is significantly less than the remaining of the bone (Figure 1.29). Re-fractures are therefore more likely to occur. It is possible to see a refracture of a functionally treated fracture when strenuous activities that require high levels of force are performed prior to maturation of the callus (Figures 1.30A to 1.34B).

Fracture Stability without Internal Fixation

Any study of fracture stability related to nonoperative treatments must address the role of the soft tissues in providing stability to the bone fragments. The literature addressing stability of fracture fixation is dominated by biomechanical studies of isolated bones and the hardware to internally fix them with no regard for the soft tissue support for the fragments. But any trauma surgeon knows the importance of the soft tissues for stabilizing the fractured bones. After all, patients with fractures do not present to the emergency room with a fracture of the humerus and the arm presented in two separate pieces! The arm is unstable, but the soft tissues keep the parts from separating. Recent studies of fractures in the

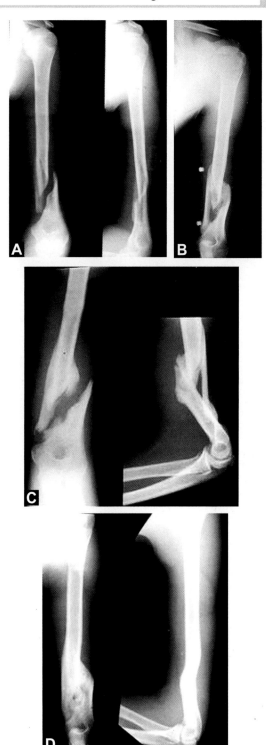

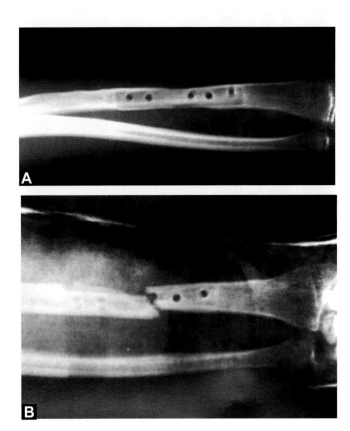

Figs 1.30A and B: (A) Radiograph of previously plated radius fracture. Notice the severe atrophy of the bone and the thinning of the cortex identified following removal of the plate. (B) The bone re-fractured following a minor injury.

Figs 1.31A to D: (A) Radiograph of oblique fracture of the distal humerus obtained through a brace applied 7 days after the initial injury. (B) Radiograph taken 2 months after the injury showing a healed fracture. The brace was discontinued at this time. (C) Radiograph demonstrating a new fracture following the hitting of a ball with a bat a few days after removal of the brace. (D) A brace was reapplied and the fracture healed solidly.

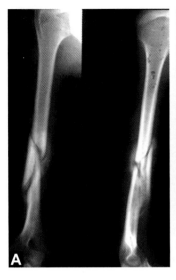
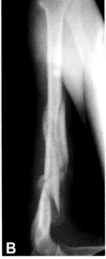
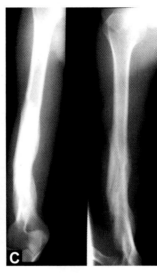

Figs 1.32A to C: (A) Radiograph of comminuted fracture obtained 5 weeks after the initial injury. (B) Patient was lost to follow-up, but returned after sustaining a new injury that produced a fracture below the old one. (C) The brace was reapplied and the fracture healed uneventfully.

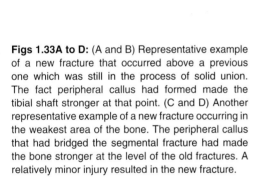
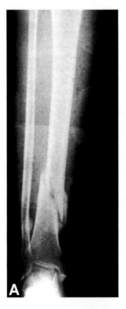
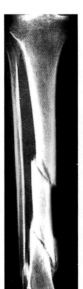
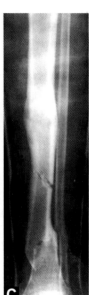
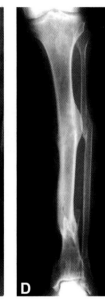

Figs 1.33A to D: (A and B) Representative example of a new fracture that occurred above a previous one which was still in the process of solid union. The fact peripheral callus had formed made the tibial shaft stronger at that point. (C and D) Another representative example of a new fracture occurring in the weakest area of the bone. The peripheral callus that had bridged the segmental fracture had made the bone stronger at the level of the old fractures. A relatively minor injury resulted in the new fracture.

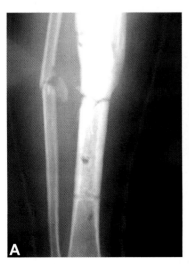
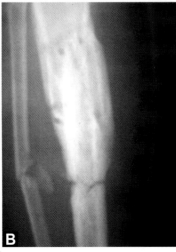

Figs 1.34A and B: Radiographs of a nondisplaced transverse fracture that occurred as the patient stepped off the curb. He had been treated with a Ilizarov frame for nearly a year for an open fracture of the proximal tibia. This is an example of the resulting strength of the bone that heals with peripheral callus.

hand have shown that the soft tissues can be a very important factor in providing stability to the fractured bones, even when internal fixation is applied to the bone fragments.[8,58,59]

SOFT TISSUE COMPRESSION

The senior author often described the "hot dog" principle of soft tissue support. If one purchases a piece of meat at the butcher, the slice of meat cannot support its own weight when held. It bends and twists out of control. But when the butcher rolls it up into a tubular shape, it becomes more rigid and can be held upright. Then the butcher wraps it tightly with brown paper and compresses the soft tissue to make a quite rigid structure. So we tested this "hot dog" principle in the laboratory by wrapping a piece of meat around a broom-stick model of a fracture. (The "broom-stick" model has often been used to test the stabilizing effects of internal fixation hardware on a "fracture" model). The resistance to load, or rigidity of the construct, was measured with the meat wrapped around the broom-stick with a simulated fracture. Then brown paper was wrapped around the meat and the compression of the soft tissue applied, the resistance to load again measured. Just the compression of the soft tissue with simple brown paper increased the rigidity of the construct by 96X! Next the meat was wrapped with Orthoplast, (the material often used to construct a fracture brace). The soft tissue again compressed and the structure loaded. The resistance to load was again increased, but only by 2X over that achieved with the brown paper (Figures 1.35A to F). The lesson from this exercise was that the rigidity and hardness of the material used to support

the soft tissues is not the most important factor in stabilizing the limb but the ability of the device to provide and maintain compression of the soft tissues that stabilizes the construct. Thus we began to use more compliant and more comfortable materials to construct fracture braces, aimed at obtaining and maintaining compression of the soft tissues in the limb segment.

Soft tissue compression protects defects or weak spots in the bone. In a study in our laboratories, a model of the bone and soft tissues was developed using a PMMA tube to simulate the bone and Zorbathane to simulate the soft tissues. We created a defect in the tube by drilling and tapping a hole the size one would make for a 3.5 mm bone screw. We then loaded the isolated bone model to failure in bending and measured the ultimate moment when the tube broke. Next we applied the soft tissue to the model and again loaded the construct to failure. Finally, we compressed the soft tissues by applying a prefabricated humeral fracture brace and loaded to failure once again. The addition of the soft tissue alone did not significantly increase the failure moment of the bone model, but compressing the soft tissue with the humeral brace did raise the ultimate moment significantly[60] (Figures 1.36A and B).

Soft tissue compression optimizes muscle function. Weight-lifters and athletes involved in intense upper limb activities which require strength often wrap their forearms and sometimes their upper arms to compress the soft tissues. They claim that it improves their performance. In a study to try to understand what mechanism may create this effect, we looked at the

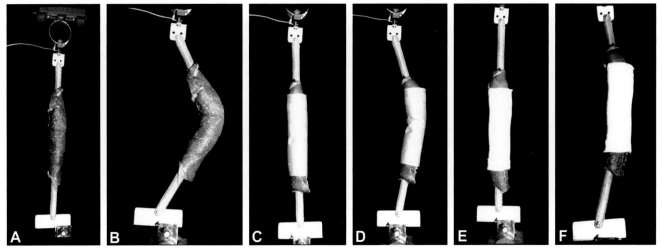

Figs 1.35A to F: (A) The model to test the "hot dog" principle was a simple piece of meat wrapped around a broom stick model of a fractured bone. (B) Under load, the construct angulated with minimal resistance. (C) Next, brown paper was wrapped around the structure, taking care to compress the soft tissues, and (D) the resistance to load was again measured. (E) Finally, the meat was compressed with a wrap of Orthoplast and, (F) the resistance to load measured. The resistance was increased by 96X when the soft tissues were compressed with brown paper, and only an additional 2X with the use of Orthoplast

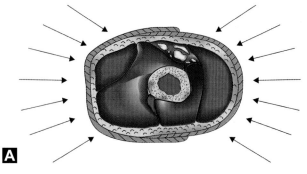

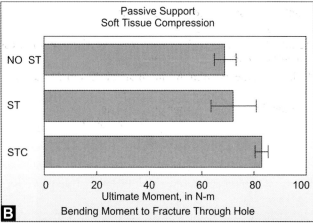

A

B

Figs 1.36A and B: (A) Soft tissue compression by the functional brace provides support to the bone to help prevent fractures through a defect, (B) by significantly increasing the strength of the construct.

EMG activity of the flexor and extensor groups of muscles in the forearm with surface electrodes on several volunteer subjects. Although one cannot estimate the actual force of the muscle groups associated with the EMG signal, it has been shown that for a given placement of the electrodes on a given subject during a short time interval, the integrated EMG signal is proportional to the force output of the underlying muscles. Using this strategy, we tried to detect any change in apparent forces produced by the muscles which might be related to compression of the soft tissues with a functional brace.[61]

Each subject was asked to actively flex the wrist as hard as they could against the measured resistance of a Cybex machine. The torque generated was measured while simultaneous EMG signals were recorded from a surface electrode placed on the flexor muscles of the forearm and another placed on the extensor side. This procedure was repeated after applying a forearm functional brace with soft tissue compression. A similar test was performed on each subject while generating maximum plantar flexion torque about the ankle, without and then with the application of a tibial fracture brace to compress the calf musculature while recording EMG signals

from the gastro-soleus muscle mass and also from the anterior compartment muscles.

From the integrated EMG signals, it was assumed that the net torque measured was a result of the torque applied by the agonist muscles minus the torque applied by the antagonist muscle group. Thus, any change in EMG signal level would represent a proportional change in torque provided by that muscle group (Figure 1.37).

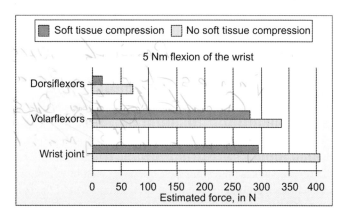

Fig. 1.37: Enhancement of muscle function was estimated by correlating integrated EMG signals with measured torque about the wrist joint on a Cybex machine set to generate 5 Nm of wrist flexion. Next a fracture brace was applied and the soft tissues compressed on the same subject with the EMG electrodes in the same place. Note the dramatic reduction in EMG signal for the antagonist muscles with soft tissue compression, reducing the force necessary for the agonists to generate the same torque.

There was a significant decrease in the peak integrated EMG signals, giving a significant reduction in the calculated peak forces generated by the muscles about the joint when the soft tissues were compressed with a fracture brace. The increased torque output appeared to be a result of a decrease of antagonist torque which resulted in an increase in net torque, without increasing the forces applied by the muscles. This gave the impression that functional activities carried out with soft tissue compression in a fracture brace could be achieved with less muscle forces in the limb segment, thus providing an additional protective effect on the healing fracture.

CONTROLLING ANGULATION

The Soft Tissue "Hinge"

Closed fractures are generally associated with minimal soft tissue damage. The soft tissues which are intact tether the bone fragments to prevent shortening beyond that allowed by the initial soft tissue damage, see Figure 1.38 A to C and section on Shortening page 30.

But with a soft tissue "coupling" between the bone fragments, there is very little inherent bending resistance since the soft tissue is more like what Charnley[16] described as a hinge than a rigid bridge (Figures 1.39A to C).

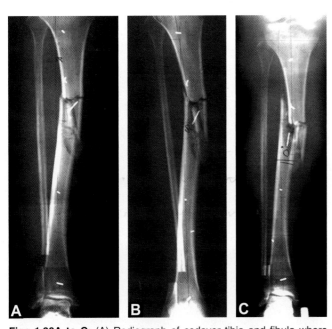

Figs 1.38A to C: (A) Radiograph of cadaver tibia and fibula where a closed comminuted fracture was mechanically produced in the laboratory. A resection ostectomy in the distal fibula was also created. When the specimen was subjected to vertical loading, the fragments did not shorten, but the fracture angulated. (B) Radiograph was obtained after the interosseus membrane was percutaneusly sectioned. Under vertical loading the extremity shortened, but angulation did not take place. (C) The experiment demonstrates the important role the soft tissue, particularly the interosseus membrane, play in determining the initial shortening of extremities with two bones.

Studies of the mechanical properties of the interosseous membrane showed that the collagen fiber bundle orientation provides a rigid and strong "ligamentous" connection between the tibia and fibula when the membrane is loaded along the direction of the fiber bundles. Also, it was clear that the "ligament" can elongate to about 100% before it loses its peak resistance to load (much like the ACL) (Figures 1.40A to C). But when the "ligament" is loaded perpendicular to the direction of the fiber bundles, the stiffness and strength are much less, and under the microscope one can see that the failure is in the interconnections between fiber bundles, but the bundles themselves are not visibly damaged (Figures 1.41A and B). So when a load is placed on the damaged "ligament," the bundles are intact. They realign to the direction of stress and still are stiff and strong in that direction and can stabilize the bones in the mode shown in Figures 1.39A to C and 1.58A and B.

Examination of the damage to the interosseous membrane in autopsy cases that had fractures of the tibia and fibula, showed that the damage to the "ligament" was primarily in the mode perpendicular to the direction of the collagen fiber bundles, and that the bundles were still intact.

The cylinder of material (the cast or brace) wrapped around the soft tissue provides a three-point support system through the soft tissues in all directions (Figures 1.42A to C). Since the cylinder is circumferential, it can support the limb in any direction that it tries to angulate. The bone fragments still are able to move within this cylinder, as evidenced by the corrective movements that typically occur within the brace when gravity alignment takes place with early functional activities for a fracture of the humerus. So the brace, though its compression of the soft tissues provides some support for the limb, provides a more comfortable and safe environment

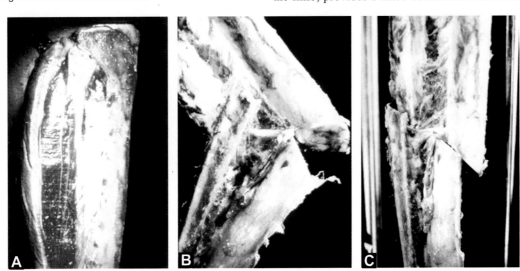

Figs 1.39A to C: (A) Illustration of tibia and fibula with all soft tissues dissected, except for the interosseous membrane. (B) A fracture of both bones had been created artificially and a deformity created by applying an axial force. Notice the "bundling of the interosseous membrane. (C) Illustration of the relative intactness of the interosseus membrane following manual reduction of the fracture.

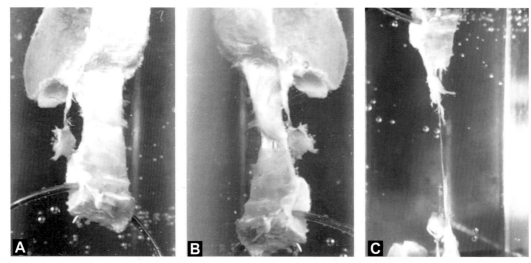

Figs 1.40A to C: (A) A section of interosseous membrane being subjected to tension along the direction of its fiber bundles. (B) As the tension increases, its fibrous structure elongates. (C) Eventually the rupture of the structure is complete. Notice the degree of separation between the two bones before rupture occurs completely.

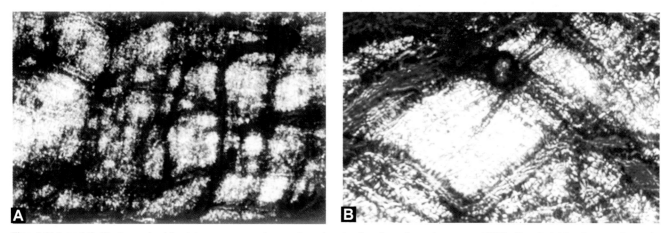

Figs 1.41A and B: Photograph of the interosseus membrane viewed under the dissection microscope (40X) after stretching the membrane in a direction perpendicular to the dominant direction of the collagen fiber bundles. When the membrane is stretched in that direction, the fibers remain intact, and only the interconnections between fiber bundles are disrupted.

for early functional activities as well as a protection from direct contact to the limb segment.[22,27,62-66]

The effectiveness of this leverage is important in Stage II callus development when patients are comfortable functioning in a brace even though the callus is soft and the fracture can be angulated if not supported.[60] It is this stage where the importance of a tight fitting, functional cast or an adjustable brace is critical. The dimensions of the limb will change throughout the day due to activities or lack thereof. So the ability to adjust the soft tissue compression is also critical. An example of a patient with Stage II callus is shown in Figures 1.43A and B. He came into clinic, weight bearing in his brace which was not kept snug on the soft tissues. His initial x-ray demonstrated gross anterior bowing in the loose brace. The brace was tightened, the soft tissues compressed, and he

walked to the x-ray department for a new x-ray. The limb was straight again, demonstrating that he was comfortable in Stage II soft callus with weightbearing, and also demonstrating that tightening the brace was very effective at re-aligning and maintaining the alignment of the limb with comfortable weightbearing. (This also demonstrated to the doctors that this patient was not capable of following instructions, so he was discharged from the clinic in a cast, and not put back into a brace until Stage III callus was evident).

Gravity Alignment

Gravity can create a natural alignment mechanism for many fractures to correct angulations. For humeral fractures, the arm naturally hangs with gravity from the shoulder. However,

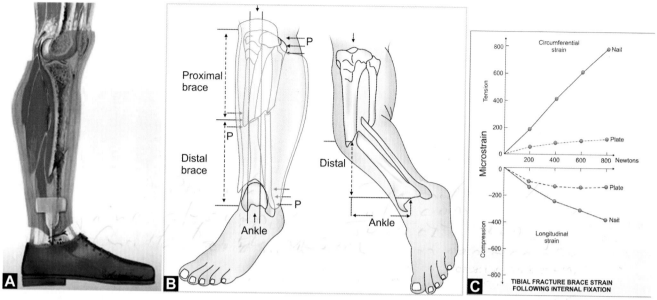

Figs 1.42A to C: Drawing depicting the containment of the bone and soft issues inside the cylinder of the brace (A). This cylinder of the fracture brace provides a 3-point support for the fractured bone which is just as effective in the sagittal plane as it is in the coronal plane, (B), because the lever arm creating a bending moment at the fracture is very small compared to the leverage of the brace compressing the soft tissues. Thus the pressure on the soft tissues is not that great even though the loads of weight bearing are substantial. Strains in the brace were measured for a mid shaft fracture in a cadaver leg that was supported only by the brace and then after internal fixation which did not allow the soft tissue "hinge" to bend, (C) For both conditions, the fracture did not angulate, but it was clear that the 3-point support system of the brace was active when the fracture was free to angulate.

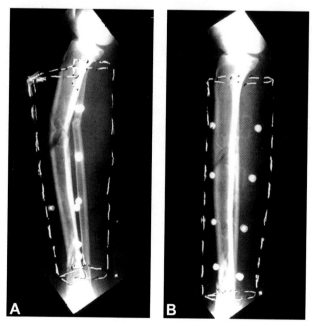

Figs 1.43A and B: This patient walked into clinic, weight bearing on the limb with the tibia brace loosely applied. (A) After tightening the brace and compressing the soft tissues (B) he walked back to x-ray and demonstrated that the brace could correct and maintain the alignment with weightbearing, and that the fracture was clearly in Stage II soft callus healing.

in the stage of acute symptoms, the patient's arm is placed in a sling or hanging cast to minimize discomfort. The arm is thus internally rotated and often pulled into varus angulation. So it is imperative that the patient be instructed to begin gentle exercises so that they can soon place the arm in its normal anatomic position and let gravity reduce the angulation and the rotation (Figures 1.44A to E). This must occur in Stage II callus before the callus fixed the arm in the position of internal rotation and varus angulation.

Tibial fractures are very different. Weight bearing can create angulation. Since the initial cast is well padded, and is applied to a limb that is often swollen at the acute stage of symptoms, the cast is not tightfitting or may become loose as swelling subsides. Since the patient is encouraged to begin some weight bearing in this cast which is not tight-fitting, it may allow for some angulation. Therefore, like with the humeral fracture, it is important to change this cast as soon as the patient is comfortable in Stage II callus and any angulation and rotational malalignment can be corrected. The easiest way to correct the angulation is to let gravity do the job (Figure 1.45). Have the patient sit in an upright position with both legs hanging over the side of the seat at a height that is comfortable for the surgeon or Orthopedic technician to apply the tight-fitting functional cast or brace while easily viewing both limbs to verify proper alignment.

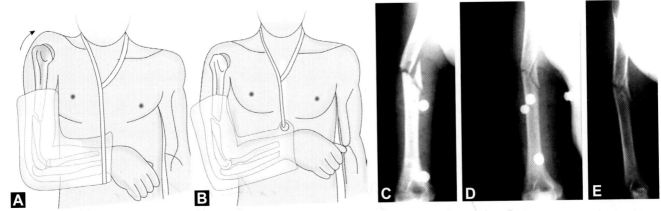

Figs 1.44A to E: (A) When the sling is applied, the arm in rotated internally, and the patient tends to shrug the shoulder to minimize pain in this acute Stage I healing. **(B)** When the patient returns to clinic and the arm is relaxed, the sling pulls the arm into varus. **(C)** So x-rays in the early stage often demonstrate varus and internal rotation at the fracture. **(D)** But with early function, the internal rotation and varus angulation, can be corrected by gravity alignment when Stage II is reached and the brace allows full range of motion of adjacent joints. **(E)** The humerus progresses through Stage III and IV naturally aligned by gravity.

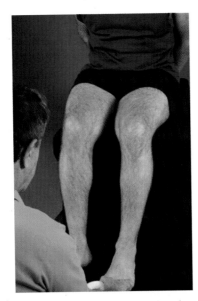

Fig. 1.45: Have the patient sit with both legs hanging over the table so gravity can help to align the bone fragments. Minor corrections in alignment can be corrected at this stage by functional cast or brace application.

Angulation and Osteoarthritis

Much fear has been voiced in the literature that minor degrees of angulation at the fracture in the diaphysis of the lower limbs will result in the development of arthritic changes in the joints above and below after many years of ambulation. However, there is no evidence of this in the literature. To the contrary, there is ample evidence that even angulations up to 15° or more do not cause long-term, adjacent joint degeneration (Figures 1.46 to 1.51).

We have ample evidence that the vast majority of closed tibial fractures managed by nonsurgical casting or bracing can be brought to heal with angular deformities of less than 8°, see Chapter 3. With few exceptions such angular deformities are physiologically and aesthetically well tolerated. Mild, cosmetically acceptable angular deformities neither lead to late osteoarthritic changes nor to early or late damage to the adjacent joints. In the very few instances where arthritic changes have been documented, initial injury of the articular cartilage was the most likely explanation. Fractures, produced from impaction forces are the ones most likely to develop arthritic changes as illustrated by many distal radial fractures, which regardless of the treatment given eventually show radiological changes, fortunately in most stances of an inconsequential nature. Therefore one must conclude that if the cartilage is irreversibly damaged, the type of treatment would not influence the fate of the cartilage and its possible eventual degeneration. Although angular deformities change the distribution of stresses on the articular cartilage, those alterations may not be sufficient to produce cartilage degeneration.

The angular deformities measured in patients in this study were in most instances acceptable from the cosmetic point of view, as 405 (90.0%) patients had less than 8 degrees of angular deformity. These figures are comparable to those reported in the literature dealing with intramedullary nailing. Deformities in this range are not likely to produce osteoarthritis later. Merchant and Dietz, based on a review of 37 patients who had tibial fractures with a follow-up of nearly 30 years, concluded that angulation of healed fractures of the distal tibia was not related to functional deficit. They additionally stated that the clinical and radiographic results were unaffected by the amount of anterior or posterior and

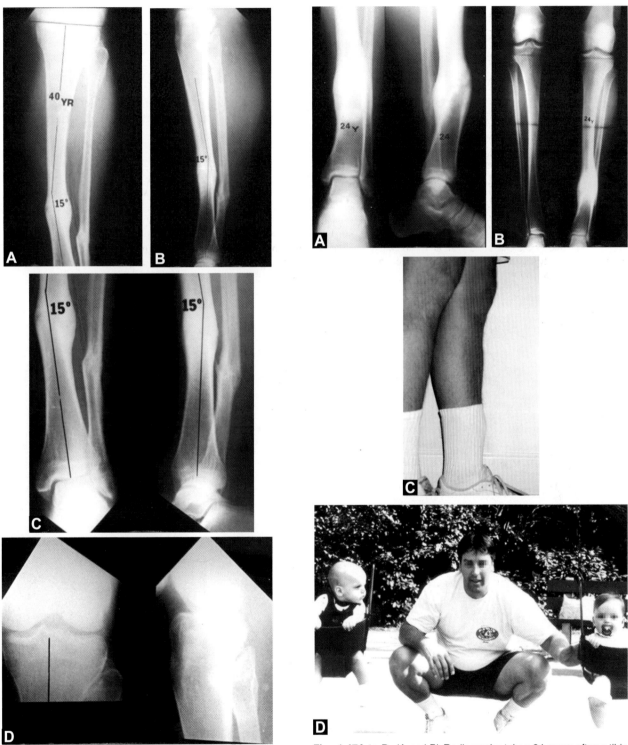

Figs 1.46A to D: (A and B) Radiographs of a tibia, taken 40 years after an open fracture sustained in an automobile accident. The fracture had healed with angular deformity of 15° in both planes. The patient was totally asymptomatic. (C and D) Closer views of the knee and ankle joints showing complete radiological absence of degenerative arthritic changes.

Figs 1.47A to D: (A and B) Radiographs taken 24 years after a tibia sustained an open fracture, allegedly treated with an above-the-knee cast. The fracture healed with a severe angular deformity. (C) Photograph of the deformity, which is readily visible under the naked eye. (D) The patient is totally asymptomatic and indulges in heavy contact sports. He is the father of the twins shown in this picture, who are the grandchildren of the senior author.

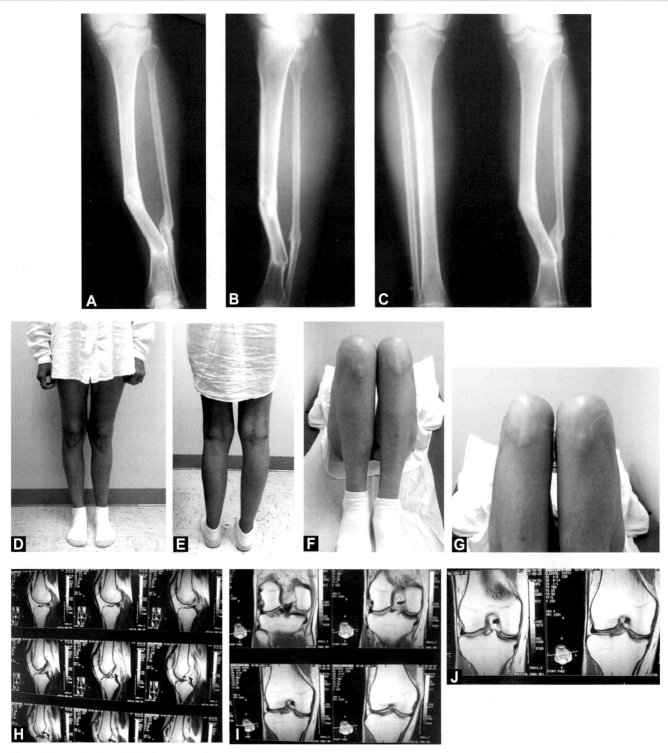

Figs 1.48A to J: (A to C) Radiographs of the tibia of a 50-year-old woman who sustained a segmental fracture 30 years earlier during the crash-landing of a small airplane. (D to G) Patient claims that prior to the accident, she had a meniscectomy performed. Her knees and ankles have remained totally asymptomatic. She was treated for an arthritic condition of her right hip with a noncemented total hip prosthesis. Close inspection of her legs does not suggest the severe deformity the x-rays show. (H to J) MRI of her knees failing to demonstrate any evidence of early osteoarthritis.

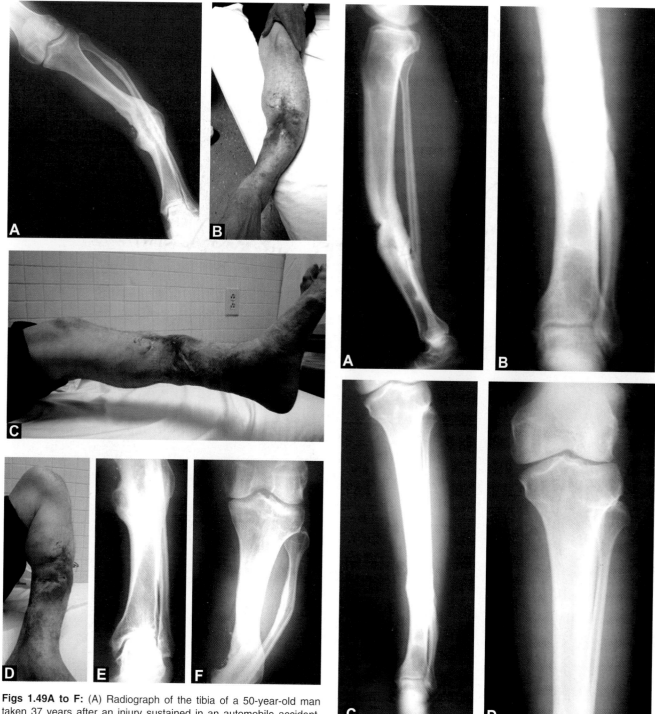

Figs 1.49A to F: (A) Radiograph of the tibia of a 50-year-old man taken 37 years after an injury sustained in an automobile accident. The patient was a poor farmer in a Central American Country. (B) The corresponding front view of the deformed leg. A gross limp was displayed but otherwise the patient was asymptomatic. (C and D) There was full range of motion of the knee, but slight limitation of motion of the ankle joint. (E and F) Radiographs of the knee and ankle joints showing no evidence of arthritic changes.

Figs 1.50A to D: (A and B) Radiographs of an open tibial fracture that healed with severe angular deformity. The fracture had been treated with an external fixator. (C and D) Radiographs obtained 5 years after the initial injury. Thus far, there is no evidence of degenerative disease in the knee or ankle joints. This might never occur.

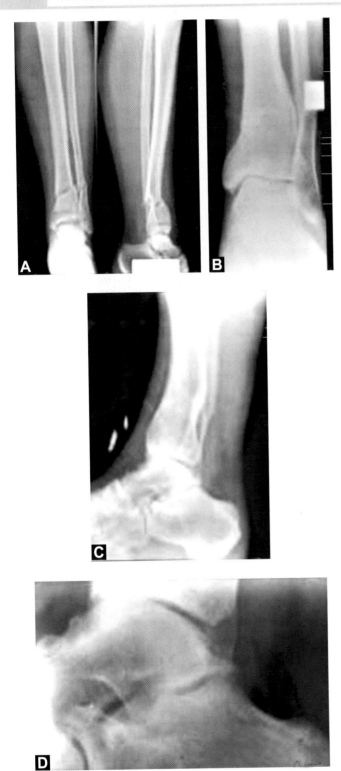

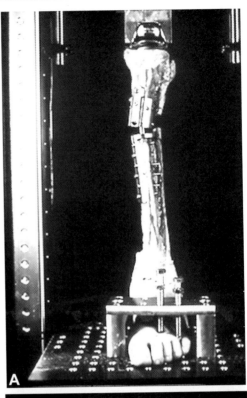

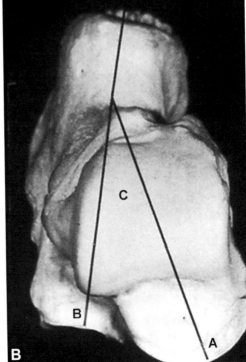

Figs 1.51A to D: Radiographs of distal diaphyseal fracture of the tibia that healed with a severe angular deformity. Thirty years later, the patient has remained asymptomatic. (Radiographs given to me by Doctor Kristensen from Denmark)

Figs 1.52A and B: (A) Photograph of the instrumentation we developed to study the manner in which various degrees of angulation at the fracture site alters the stresses at the tibio-talar joint. (B) Illustration of the relationship between the talus and calcaneus.

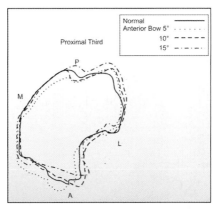 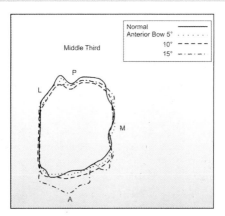 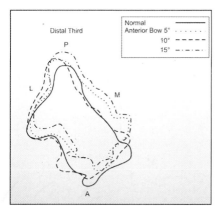

Fig. 1.53: Photographs of the alteration of weight bearing pressures at the tibio-talar joint according to the level of tibial fractures. Notice that the changes are greater in fractures in the distal-third of the bone.

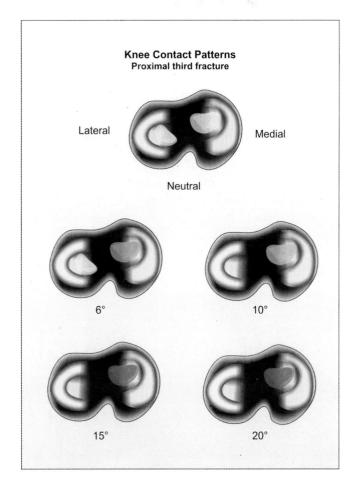

Fig. 1.54: Tracings of changes in the articular surface of the proximal tibia, according to the degrees of angular deformities in the tibial shaft.

varus or valgus angulation and the level of the fracture. Other investigators have studied the effect of angular deformities on the adjacent joints, and have found that minor deformities do not alter pressure distribution on the articular cartilage in the adjacent joints in a significant way.

The following illustrations (Figures 1.52 to 1.54) are examples of long-term angular deformities that demonstrate the healthy condition of the articular cartilage of the knee and ankle joints.

Rotational Control

Rotation of the humerus seems to correct itself with early functional activity. Part may be due to the gravity alignment and external rotation of the arm from the position in the sling. Besides the humerus also has numerous, broad muscle attachments along the diaphysis and contraction of the muscles will tend to align the muscle fibers which could produce natural corrective forces to a shaft that is rotated (Figure 1.55).

Rotational control for the forearm is achieved by molding the soft tissues into the interosseous space. Since the radius and ulna are the most widely separated and nearly parallel when the arm is in supination, rotational control can best be achieved with the arm in a supinated position[60] (Figure 1.56).

The lower leg can be stabilized in rotation by proper molding of the soft tissues in the proximal calf. The posterior tissues should be flattened and compressed against the anterior "wedge" created by the natural triangle from the tibial crest to the gastro-soleus complex. This has been shown in cadaver trials to help keep the leg from rotating within the brace[60] (Figure 1.57).

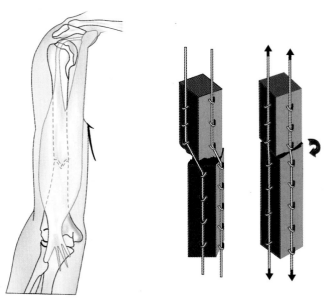

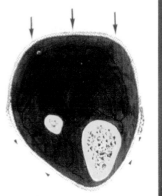

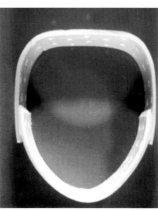

Fig. 1.57: Triangulation of the proximal calf with the molding and compression of the soft tissues helps to control rotation of the calf within the tibial brace. This molding can be accomplished with the application of a cast or custom molded brace, or by the design and closure mechanism of a prefabricated brace.

Fig. 1.55: Active motion of the elbow may also play an important role in realigning and maintaining alignmе nt in rotation because of the broad muscle attachment sites along the humerus.

SHORTENING

We have determined a "closed fracture," as an important part of the criterion for functional bracing since it is very difficult to determine, with high degree of accuracy, the initial shortening an open fracture experiences. Open fractures, particularly those with severe soft tissue damage and displacement, are often realigned and splinted with some amount of traction by transportation emergency personnel. Therefore, the initial radiograph fails to indicate the true initial shortening and displacement of the fragments. When stabilized in a cast and ambulation introduced, the fragments may shorten to unacceptable degrees, see Figures 1.38A to C and 1.58 to 1.64.

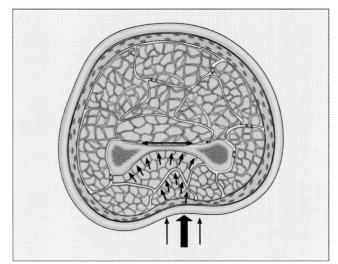

Fig. 1.56: With the arm in a relaxed attitude of supination, the radius and ulna are separated and molding of the cast or brace that compresses the soft tissue into the interosseous space tends to separate the bones and hold them apart, controlled by the interosseous membrane.

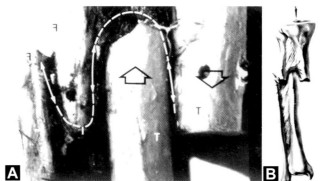

Figs 1.58A and B: Illustration of the manner in which the interosseus membrane "tethers" the bone fragments after minor disruption at the time of injury, and how it can prevent further shortening when subjected to vertical forces.

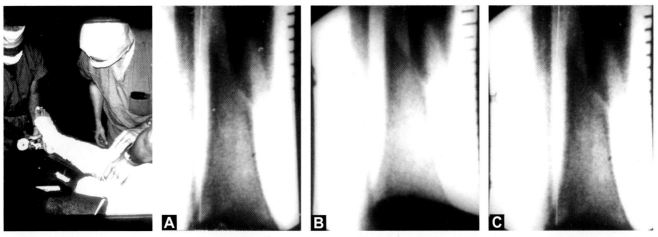

Figs 1.59A to C: Composite picture of radiographs of an oblique closed fracture of the distal tibia and proximal fibula. (A) Radiograph illustrating the shortening that occurred at the time of the injury. (B) Radiograph obtained during the application of 25 lbs. of pressure on the patient's heel. Notice the additional shortening of the limb. (C) Radiograph taken after discontinuing the pressure. The shortening of the limb returned to the original one.

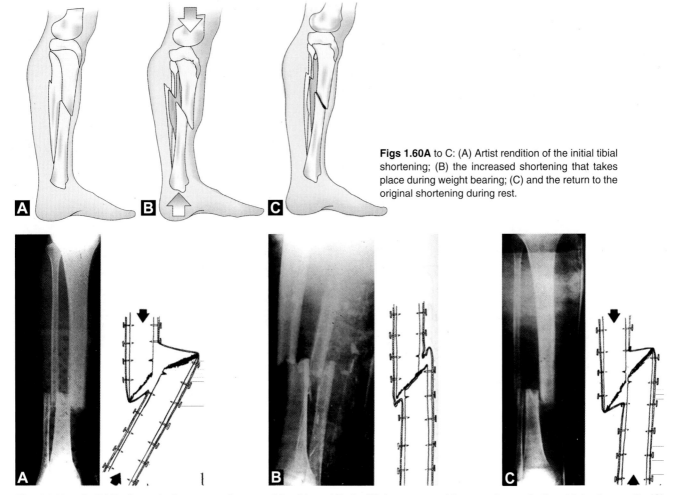

Figs 1.60A to C: (A) Artist rendition of the initial tibial shortening; (B) the increased shortening that takes place during weight bearing; (C) and the return to the original shortening during rest.

Figs 1.61A to C: (A) Radiograph of transverse fracture of the tibia and fibula. (B) Appearance of the precarious reduction obtained manually. (C) The minimal instability was lost as soon as ambulation began. Notice that the shortened limb return to the original shortening. The accompanying drawings illustrate the role the soft tissue play in the prevention of additional shortening.

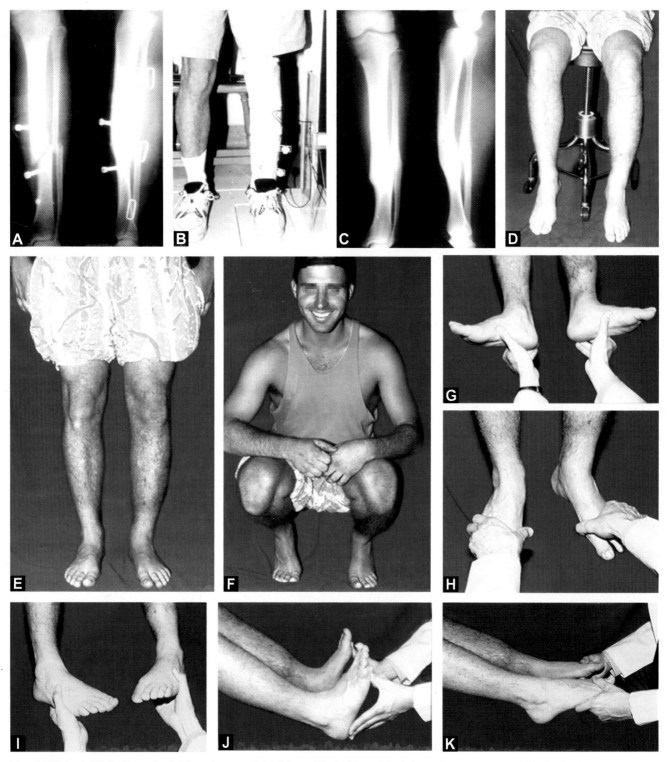

Figs 1.62A to J: (A) Radiograph of oblique fracture of the tibia and fibula. The original shortening was accepted. Under local anaesthesia two screws were inserted percutaneusly into the tibia, one above and the other one below the fracture. The heads of the screws were connected to motion sensitive devices, which in turn were attached to the computer. (B) Photograph of patient standing on a force plate, wearing a prefabricated functional brace. (C) Radiograph of the tibia after completion of healing. Notice the mild angular deformity but no additional shortening. (D) Appearance of the extremities. (E) Patient standing up after removal of the brace. (F to K) Illustrating the normal range of motion of his knee and ankle joints

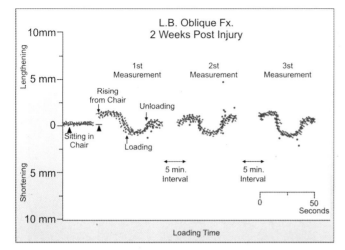

L.B. Oblique Fx.
2 Weeks Post Injury

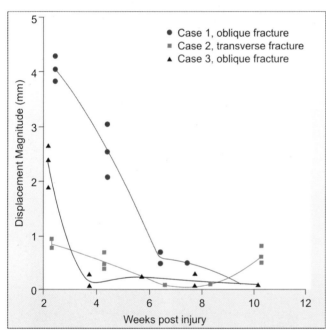

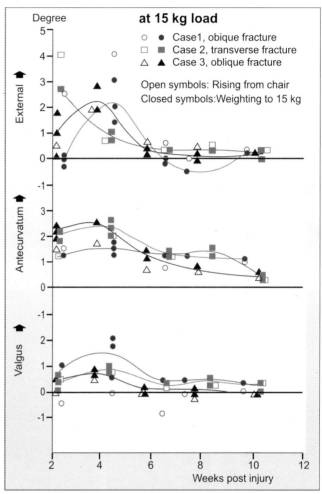

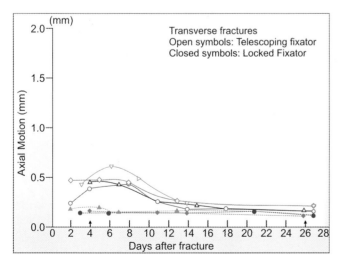

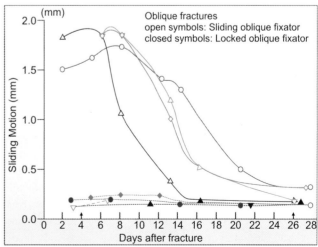

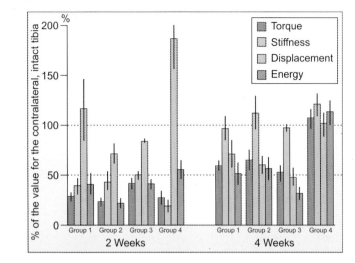

Figs 1.63A and B: (A) Recording of shortening of the tibia during the stance phase and the return to the initial shortening during the swing phase of gait. (B) Illustration of the decreasing degree of elastic shortening that occurs as the fracture gains intrinsic stability.

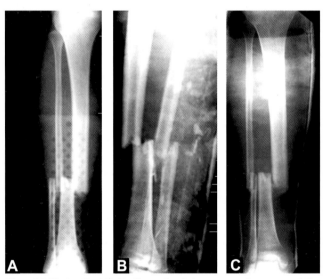

Figs 1.64A to C: (A) Radiograph of transverse fractures of the tibia and fibula illustrating the degree of the original shortening. (B) Attempts to reduce the fracture were unsuccessful, since the reduction was imperfect and unstable. (C) Shortly after the application of a cast and the initiation of weightbearing activities, *the fragments displaced to the original degree of shortening.*

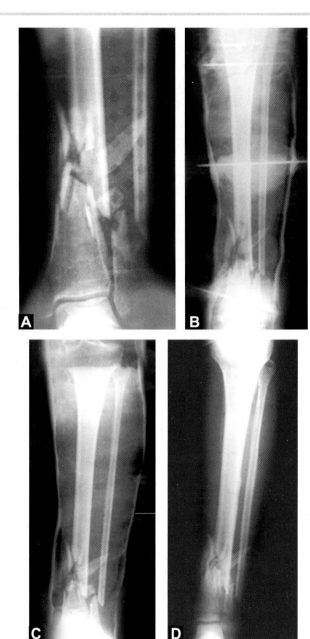

Figs 1.65A to D: See narrative in the previous page

However, it is likely that open fractures also experience final shortening at the time of injury. Figure 1.65 shows an open fracture (Type II) illustrating the shortening of the extremity when the first post-injury radiograph was taken (A). The treating physician was concerned about further shortening and elected to apply traction to the leg and insert pins above and below the fracture. In this manner, he regained length (B). However, when the pins were removed three weeks later the limb shortened again to the initial degree (C). The fracture eventually healed with acceptable shortening and alignment (D).

REFERENCES

1. Sarmiento A, Latta LL. Closed Functional Treatment of Fractures. Springer-Verlag, Berlin, GFR, 1981.
2. Rhinelander FW. The normal microcirculation of diaphyseal cortex and its response to fracture. AAOS Instructional course lecture. J. Bone Joint Surg. 1968; 50-A:784.
3. Goodship AE, Kenwright J. The Influence of Induced Micromovement Upon the Healing of Experimental Tibial Fractures. J. Bone Joint Surg., 1985 Aug; 67(4):650.
4. Kuntscher G. The Callus Problem. Warren H. Green, inc., St. Louis, MO, 1974.

5. Latta LL, Sarmiento A, Tarr R. The Rationale of Functional Bracing of Fractures. Clin Orthop. 1980; 146:28-36

6. Latta LL, Sarmiento A. Periosteal Fracture Callus Mechanics. Chapter 16. In: Symposium on Trauma to the Leg and Its Sequela. Mosby Saunders, Philadelphia, 1981.

7. Lindholm RB et al. Effect of Force Interfragmental Movements on Healing of Tibial Fractures in Rats. Acta Orthop Scand. 1970; 40:721.

8. Reyes FA, Latta LL. Conservative Management of Difficult Phalangeal Fractures. Clin Orthop. 1987; 214:23-30.

9. Olerud S, Dankwardt-Lilliestrom G. Fracture healing in compression osteosynthesis. Acta Orthop Scand Suppl. 1971; 137:1-44.

10. Perren S, Rahn B: Biomechanics of fracture healing I. Historical review and mechanical aspects of internal fixation. Orthop Surg. 1978; 2:108.

11. Rahn B et al. Primary bone healing. J Bone Joint Surg. 1971; 53A:783.

12. Perren S. Evolution of the Internal fixation of long bones fractures. J Bone Joint Jour Br. 2002; 84B:1093-110.

13. Perren S: Physical and biological aspects of fracture healing with special reference to internal fixation. Clin Orthop. 1979; 138:175.

14. Milner J, Rhinelander FW. Compression fixation in primary bone healing. Surg Forum. 1968; 19:453.

15. Claes L, Wilke HJ, Rubinacker S. Interfragmentary Strain and Bone Healing - An Experimental Study. Trans 35th Orthop Res Soc. 1989; 14:568.

16. Carter DR, Vasu R, Harris WH. The Plated Femur: Relationship Between the Changes in Bone Stresses and Bone Loss. Acta Orthop Scand. 1981; 52:241.

17. Hidaka S, Gustillo RB. Refracture of bones of the forearm after plate removal. J Bone Joint Surg. 1984; 66A:1241.

18. Jacobs R, Rahn B, Perren S. Effect of plates on cortical bone perfusion. Trans 26th Orthop Res Soc; 1980; 5:157.

19. Uhthoff HK, Dubuc FL. Bone structure changes in the dog under rigid internal fixation. Clin Orthop. 1970; 81:40-7.

20. Lippert FG, Hirsch C. The Three-Dimensional Measurement of Tibial Fracture Motion by Photogrammetry. Clin Orthop. 1974; 105:130.

21. McKellop HA, Hoffmann R, Sarmiento A, Lu B, Ebramzadeh E. Control of Motion of Tibial Fractures with Use of a Functional Brace or an External Fixator. J Bone Joint Surg. 1993; 75A:1019-25.

22. Sarmiento A, Latta LL, Zilioli A, Sinclair WF. The Role of Soft Tissues in Stabilization of Tibial Fractures. Clin Orthop. 1974; 105:116.

23. Davy DR. Model Studies of the Mechanical Behavior of Fracture Callus. Proc. 34th ACEMB. 1981; 154.

24. Kato S, Latta LL, Malinin T. The Weakest Link in the Bone-plate-fracture System: Changes with Time, Bone Plates. ASTM STP 1200. 1993.

25. Panjabi MM, White AA, Wolf JW. A Biomechanical Comparison of the Effects of Constant and Cyclic Compression on Fracture Healing in the Rabbit Long Bones. Acta Orthop Scand. 1979; 50:653.

26. Park SH, O'Connor K, McKellop H, Sarmiento A. The Influence of active Shear or Compressive Motion on Fracture Healing. J. Bone Joint Surg. 1998 Jun; 80A-6:868-78.

27. Sarmiento A, Latta L, Tarr R. Principles of fracture healing - Part II - The effects of function on fracture healing and stability. Amer Acad Orthop Sur Instr Course Lectures, XXXIII. Mosby Saunders, Philadelphia. 1984.

28. Steinberg ME, Lyet JP, Pollack SR. Stress Generated Potentials in Fracture Callus. Trans 26th Orthop Res Soc. 1980; 5:115.

29. Wolf JW et al. The Superiority of Cyclic Loading over Constant Compression in the Treatment of Long Bone Fractures: A Quantitative Biomechoanical Study in Rabbits. Trans 26 Orthop Res Soc. 1980; 5:174.

30. Gothman L. Arterial changes in experimental fractures of the rabbit's tibia treated with intramedullary nailing. Acta Orthop Scand. 1960: 120:289.

31. Kenwright J, Richardson JB, Goodship AE, Evans M, Kelly DJ, Spriggins AJ, Newman JH, Burrough SJ, Harris JD and Rowley DI. Effect of Controlled Axial Micromovement on Healing of Tibial Fractures. Lancet. 1986 Nov; 2(8517):1185.

32. Terjessen T, Johnson E. Effects of Fixation Stiffness on Fracture Healing. External Fixation of Tibial Osteotomy in the Rabbit. Acta Orthop Scand. 1986 Apr; 57(2):146.

33. Park SH, O'Connor K, Sung R, McKellop H, Sang-Hyun and Sarmiento A. Comparison of healing Process in Open Osteotomy Model and closed fracture model. Journal of Orthopedic Trauma. 1999; 13(2): 114-20.

34. Park SH, Cassim A, Llinas A, McKellop H, Sarmiento A. Technique for producing controlled closed fractures in a rabbit model. J Orthop Res, 1994 Sep; 12(5): 732-8.

35. McKibben B. The Biology of Fracture Healing in Long Bones. J Bone Joint Surg. 1978; 60B:150.

36. McKibbin B. Callus Formation. In: External Fixation and Functional Bracing. Part I - Biology of Fracture Healing. Richard Coombs, Stuart Green and Augusto Sarmiento (Eds). Orthotex, London. 1989; Ch 1: 3-7.

37. Trueta J. Blood supply and rate of healing of tibial fractures. Clin Orthop. 1974; 105:11.

38. Panjabi MM, Lindsey RW, Walter SD, White AA. The Clinician's Ability to Evaluate the Strength of Healing Fradctrues from Plain Radiographs. J Orthop Trauma. 1989; 3:29.

39. Macnab I. The role of periosteal blood supply in the healing of fractures of the tibia. Clin Orthop. 1974; 105:27.

40. Sarmiento A, Latta LL. Functional fracture bracing. Spinger-Verlag, Berlin, 1995.

41. Sarmiento A, Latta LL. Factors Controlling the Behavior of Tibial Fractures: A Correlation of Clinical and Laboratory Studies. Abst. Kappa Delta Award Paper. J Bone Joint Surg. 1976; 58A:724.

42. Davy DR, Connolly JF. The Influence of Callus Morphology on the Biomechanics of Healing Long Bones. Trans 27th Orthop Res Soc. 1981; 6:45.

43. Sarmiento A, Mullis DL, Latta LL, Alvarez RR. A Quantitative, Comparative Analysis of Fracture Healing Under the Influence of Compression Plating vs. Closed Weight-Bearing Treatment. Clin Orthop. 1980; 149:232.

44. Uhthoff HK. Prevention of bone atrophy through an early removal of internal fixation plates: An experimental study in the dog. Howmedica Trauma Workshop, New York. 1979.

45. Malinin T, Latta LL, Wagner JL, Brown MD. Healing of Freeze-dried Bone Plates - Comparison with Compression Plates. Clin Orthop. 1984; 190:281-6.

46. Woo SLY, Simon BR, Akeson WH, McCarty MP. An Interdisciplinary Approach to Evaluate the Effect of Internal Fixation Plate on Long Bone Remodeling. J. Biomech. 1977; 10:87.

47. Bradley GW, McKenna GB, Dunn HK, Daniels AU, Stratton WO. Effects of Flexural Rigidity of Plates on Bone Healing. J Bone Joint Surg. 1979; 61A:866.

48. Brown SA, Merritt K, Mayor MB. Internal Fixation with Metal and Thermoplastic Plates. In: Current Concepts of Internal Fixation of Fractures. Uhthoff HK (Ed), Berlin, Heidelberg, Springer-Verlag. 1980; 334-341.

49. Parsons JR et al. Development of a Variable Stiffness, Absorbable Bone Plate. Trans 25th Orthop Res Soc. 1979; 4:168.

50. Parsons JR, Alexander H, Corcoran SJ, Weiss AB. In Vivo Evaluation of Fiber Reinforced Absorbable Polymer Bone Plates. In: Proc of the Second Internat. Symp. on Internal Fixation of Fractures, Lyon, France. 1982; 117-20.

51. Woo S LY, Sothringer KS, Adeson WH, Coutts RD, Woo TK, Simon BR, Gomez MA. Less Rigid Internal Fixation Plates: Historical Perspcetives and New Concepts. J Orthop Res. 1984; 1:431.

52. Woo SLY, Akeson WH, Coutts RD, Rutherfore L, Doty D, Jemmott GF, Amiel D. A Comparison of Cortical Bone Atrophy Secondary to Fixation with Plates with Large Differences in Bending Stiffness. J Bone Joint Surg. 1976; 58A:190.

53. Burstein AH et al. Bone strength. J Bone Joint Surg. 1972; 54A:1143.

54. Liskova-Kiar M, Uhthoff HK. Radiologic and Histological Determination of Optimal Time for the Removal of Titanium Alloy Plates in Beagle Dogs - Results of Early Removal. In: Current Concepts of Internal Fixation of Fractures. Uhthoff HK (Ed), Berlin, Springer-Verlag. 1980: 404-10.

55. Bitz DM, Lux PS, Whiteside LA. The Effects of Early Mobilization and Casting on Blood Flow and Mechanical Properties of Fracture Healing. Trans 26th Orthop Res Soc. 1980; 5:199.

56. Chrisman OD, Snook GA. The problem of refracture of the tibia. Clin Orthop. 1982; 60:217.

57. Sarmiento A, Schaeffer J, Beckerman L, Latta LL, Enis J. Fracture Healing in Rat Femora a Affected by Functional Weight Bearing. J Bone Joint Surg. 1977; 59A:369.

58. Ouellette EA, Dennis JJ, Milne EL, Latta LL, and Makowski AL. The Role of Soft Tissues in Metacarpal Fracture Fixation. Clin Orthop. 2003; 412:169-75.

59. Ouellette EA, Dennis JJ, Latta LL, Milne EL, Makowski AL. The Role of Soft Tissues in Plate Fixation of proximal phalanx fractures. Clin Orthop. 2004; 418:213-8.

60. Latta LL, Zych GA, Zagorski JB. Design of Fracture Braces. ISPO.

61. Latta LL, Zych GA, Zagorski JB. Mechanisms by which soft tissue compression could potentially reduce the risks of fracture through stress concentrations in bone. Trans 31st Orthop Res Soc. 1985.

62. Hardy AE. Force and Pressure Recordings from Patients with Femoral Fractures Treated by Cast-Brace Application. J Med Engr Tech. 1981; 5:30.

63. Sarmiento A, Latta LL, Tarr R. The effects of Function on Fracture Healing and Stability. AAOS Instructional Course Vol. XXXIII, Mosby Saunders, Philadelphia. 1994.

64. Sarmiento A, Latta LL. Functional Fracture Bracing. J Amer Acad Orthop Surg. 1999; 7-1:66-75.

65. Sarmiento A, Latta LL. On the evolution of fracture bracing. J Bone Joint Surg. 2006; 88B-2:141-8.

66. Shannon FT, Unsworth A. Stability of Tibial Fractures in Plaster Cast: A Biomechanical Study. J Bone Joint Surg. 1978; 60B:282.

Section

2

The Tibial Fractures

2

The Closed Tibial Fracture: Introduction

Significant progress has been made in recent decades in the surgical management of tibial fractures, particularly with intramedullary nailing. The opposite has occurred with plating techniques, which have lost popularity due to realization that the method, although successful and the most appropriate in many instances, depends on the attainment of rigid immobilization, a phenomenon responsible for slower healing and inhibition of peripheral callus formation. The bone under the plate undergoes atrophy that persists for many months regardless of the design of the appliance. This atrophy predisposes to fractures after removal of the plate occurring either above or below the location of the removed plate, at the level of the old fracture, or through the screw holes left after their removal. The rigid immobilization obtained with stiff external fixators, a very appropriate and useful system, also delays healing and inhibits formation of peripheral callus on which the strength of a united fracture depends.[1-11,40,67] The wide acceptance of the concept that rigid immobilization and interfragmentary compression with a plate constitutes the ideal method of treatment is now questioned by recent generations of orthopedic surgeons who view the radiological absence of peripheral callus as an undesirable event. This is accentuated by the realization that immediate weight bearing following surgery, as it was once anticipated, is not possible. Instead, a period of stabilization in a non-weight-bearing appliance is often required until intrinsic stability takes place. In addition, a relatively low incidence of nonunions and infections has contributed to a decline in acceptance of the method. The powerful advocacy of the rigid fixation techniques by the originators of the method and the manufacturing implant industry delayed the long-needed reappraisal of the technique.[1,3] However, the recognition of the downside of plate fixation for tibial fractures of long bones fractures should not be interpreted as its condemnation, since plate fixation oftentimes is still the treatment of choice.

Contributing to the attention that surgical treatment of tibial fractures currently receives is the deeply ingrained belief that the shortening of most closed tibial fractures is usually unacceptable and more importantly, that if these fractures are treated nonsurgically, the initial shortening continues to progress with the use of the extremity. We have documented that the vast majority of closed tibial fractures with the exception of severely displaced ones resulting from very major trauma, experienced a degree of shortening at the time of the injury, which usually does not exceed three-quarters of a centimeter. This shortening, documented by clinical and laboratory studies, does not increase with the gradual introduction of early weight bearing ambulation. The mechanism through which this behavior occurs is provided by the elastic nature of the remaining intact soft tissues around the fracture, primarily the interosseus membrane.[12-17]

Axially unstable fractures (oblique, spiral, comminuted) that are manipulated in order to regain length, often return to the original shortening even in the absence of weight bearing ambulation.

The fact that in the vast majority of closed tibial fractures the initial shortening is less than one centimeter prompted us to reassess the importance of post-traumatic shortening in injured limbs. This assessment led us to conclude that as much as one centimeter of shortening does not present a "problem," since it neither produces a limp nor leads to late adverse sequelae. Such being the case, why should patients in that situation be consistently be subjected to surgery, which is more likely to be associated with complications, simply to correct a nonexistent problem?[3,14-16,19,27]

We have ample evidence that the vast majority of closed tibial fractures managed by nonsurgical casting or bracing can be brought to heal with angular deformities of less than 8°.[21-24,26-31] With few exceptions such angular deformities are physiologically and aesthetically well tolerated. Mild, cosmetically acceptable angular deformities neither lead to late osteoarthritic changes nor to early or late damage to the adjacent joints.[32-37] In the very few instances where arthritic changes have been documented, initial injury of the articular cartilage was the most likely explanation. Fractures produced from impaction forces are the ones most likely to develop arthritic changes as illustrated by many distal radial fractures, which regardless of the treatment given eventually show radiological changes, fortunately in most stances of an inconsequential nature. Therefore one must conclude that if the cartilage is irreversibly damaged, the type of treatment would not influence the fate of the cartilage and its possible eventual degeneration. Although angular deformities change the distribution of stresses on the articular cartilage, those alterations may not be sufficient to produce cartilage degeneration.[32,33,36-41]

Intramedullary nailing of femoral fractures has been the most helpful and revolutionary contribution to fracture care. It was anticipated that the great success experienced in the treatment of femoral fractures would be readily duplicated in the care of tibial, humeral and forearm fractures. In the case of the tibia the pioneering work was conducted initially by Lottes, and later by Enders. Intramedullary nailing of forearm and humeral fractures was also investigated. However, the optimism that intramedullary nailing of these fractures would be as rewarding as in the case of the tibial fracture, has not as yet met the expectations.

The anticipation that following interlocking nailing of tibial fractures, major and immediate weight bearing could be achieved did not materialize except in transverse fractures anatomically reduced and in those of nonvertical geometry rendered mechanically stable. In the instances where comminution is present, particularly in metaphyseal fractures, weight bearing results in the transfer of weight bearing stresses to the screws, and their likely breakage after repeated loading. The breakage, if it occurs before intrinsic fracture stability has developed, results in a loss of some of the regained length, and the likely creation of angular deformities. Fracture of the screws without additional angular deformity or shortening is in most instances of an inconsequential clinical nature. Other times when the resulting angular deformity is severe, surgical correction is necessary.[42-56]

Of much greater importance, however, is the fact that following intramedullary nailing, a large number of patients experience chronic knee pain which according to several studies does not improve with time. When the nails are removed in an attempt to eliminate chronic pain, only approximately 50% of patients experience relief.[60] Other investigators have shown a great frequency of chronic knee pain following intramedullary nailing as well as a number of other complications, such as compartment syndromes, infections, bone necrosis, nonunions and others.[32,36,38,43,45-48,50-72]

Frequently ignored during the treatment of tibial fractures is the cost incurred with the various treatment modalities. Though it is claimed by some that the intramedullary nailing of tibial fractures is a less costly therapeutic modality when compared with casting and bracing, there is only questionable evidence to support this claim. Quite the contrary, a few existing studies indicate that the close method of treatment is the less expensive of the two.[73] This conclusion is a logical one if one considers the many features that must be factored into the equation. Hospitalization and the surgical intervention are expensive, not only because of the cost of the implant, but the operating room charges, surgeon's fees as well as those of the anesthesiologist, laboratory, antibiotics and others. Removal of the implant at a later date also requires hospitalization and associated costs.

Needless to say, nonsurgical functional treatment is also associated with costs, but at a lower level. Plaster of Paris or plastic material used to stabilize the fracture, or even a custom-made or pre-fabricated, brace are relatively inexpensive compared with the cost of nails, plates, screws or fixators. An argument has been advanced that the closed functional treatment requires a greater number of office visits. This is incorrect. Office visits are required regardless of the treatment modality. The patient whose tibia was treated surgically must have the surgical sutures removed approximately one or two weeks after surgery in the surgeon's office. Radiographs are taken and if no problems have developed, additional instructions are given regarding weight-bearing activities.

The patient treated nonsurgically is evaluated also one or twelve days after the initial stabilization in the Emergency Room to determine if the initial stabilizing cast should be replaced with either a below-the-knee functional cast or a brace. Radiographs are obtained and instructions are also given regarding weight bearing. The latter is based on the degree of symptoms. The patient is then instructed to return again usually one week later, at which time new radiographs are obtained. When the tibia fracture is treated with a custom-made or fabricated brace, the recognition of a mild, non-anticipated angular deformity, calls for the removal of the brace and manual correction of the deformity. Then the brace is reapplied. Obviously, unacceptable deformities that cannot be corrected require surgical intervention. However, this is extremely rare, simply because severe, unacceptable deformities are corrected at the time of the initial treatment in the Emergency Room.

Contrary to popular belief, closed, axially unstable tibial fractures, i.e. oblique, spiral or comminuted, are the ones most likely to produce the best clinical results, however, this applies only to fractures with initially acceptable shortening. Fractures of the diaphyses without associated fracture of the fibula, particularly oblique ones, can rarely be treated nonsurgically, since significant angular deformity may occur. With intramedullary nails containing interlocking screws, the rigid immobilization of the fragments results in a slower healing process as depicted by the usual minimal peripheral callus. It has been our experience that transverse fractures remain painful for periods of time longer that those with more unstable geometry. This also occurs with transverse fractures treated with functional casts or braces. Furthermore, comminuted or oblique metaphyseal fractures, subjected to early weight bearing have a tendency to angulate after the screws break. The use of a plate supporting the fibula fracture has been thought to lessen the incidence of the above complication. In any event, with or without stabilization of the fibula, protected weight bearing is necessary. The opposite is true when dealing with the same fractures using functional casting or bracing. The level of the fracture plays no role in determining the onset and increased degrees of weight bearing. Symptoms are the dictating determinants of weight bearing ambulation. We have observed some patients with nailed fractures walking unassisted as early as three to four weeks. However, we also have observed patients treated conservatively ambulating in the same manner within the same period of time. Other times patients treated by either of the two methods find it difficult to walk, bearing full weight for longer periods of time.

Several decades ago, it was felt that plating of tibial fractures would not require additional casting support, and the postponement of weight bearing ambulation. It did not take long before the orthopedic community realized that a plated tibia needs in most instances additional time in a cast until radiological evidence of a union. Since peripheral callus does not form, or forms very slowly, determining bony union in a rigidly immobilized fracture is difficult. This applies to plated fractures as well as to those managed with rigid external fixators.

The following chart (Fig. 2.1), published in the early 1970s in a Dutch journal, shows that patients with tibial fractures treated with above-the-knee casts returned to employment at an earlier date when compared with those treated with plates.

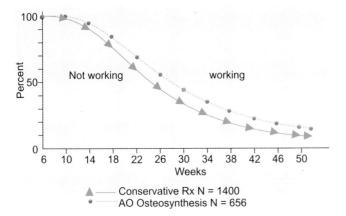

Fig. 2.1: Percentage of individuals returning to work following treatment with above-the-knee casts in comparision to those treated with plates.

It is unfortunate that a well documented comparative study has not yet been conducted regarding nailing versus contemporary conservative treatment of closed tibial fractures. It is very likely that the results would be similar to the ones reported 25 years ago. The few studies where comparisons were made were rather incomplete since the indications for bracing were either not known or simply ignored. One of those studies included open fractures and described attempts to regain length.[64]

The enthusiasm generated by the obvious success with current surgical techniques used in the treatment of open fractures has oftentimes led to heroic efforts to salvage limbs, which should have been ablated for the ultimate benefit of the patient. Open fractures of the tibia, with major bone and soft tissue damage, even if not associated with major nerve injury are often best managed by early amputation. The salvaged limbs not infrequently end up being painful and having ankylosed distal joints. Some require multiple surgical procedures over a period of many months, if not years, before the fracture is declared as being healed. By that time, many patients are unable to work. In addition, the psychological consequences of the injury and prolonged care should be taken into account, as well as the possibility of addiction to narcotics.

A common reason for the commitment to preserve limbs that should have been amputated early is unawareness of the sophistication the prosthetic field has attained in recent years. The disability created by a trans-tibial amputation is, at this time, relatively minor. A permanent prosthesis can be successfully fitted in most instances within a few weeks after the ablation procedure. If a temporary prosthesis is applied in the operating room immediately after the surgical intervention, the permanent appliance can be fitted within the next few weeks. Most below-the-knee amputees eventually walk without a limp or with a minimal or almost non-perceptible limp, and carry out virtually all activities of daily living without difficulty.

The function of below-the-knee amputees is vividly demonstrated by the ones who participate in athletic activities, particularly by the ones we observe excelling in the Para Olympic games where they indulge in activities such as football, running and basketball. It is doubtful that an individual who sustained a severe open fracture of the tibia and required multiple surgical procedures before the fracture healed ever attempted to participate in such competitive games.

Our subsequent chapters devoted to the nonsurgical treatment of tibial fractures should not be construed as an effort to minimize the very important role surgical management plays in their care. We readily recognize the need for all existing modalities and the need to be knowledgeable with all of them. Equally as important is the need for the orthopedist to be thoroughly familiar with the biology of fracture healing under different physiological environments particularly at this time when promising future developments with means to enhance healing through genetic manipulation is gaining momentum.

The fact that the popularity of surgical treatment of fractures has eclipsed nonsurgical methods in many institutions is due to a number of factors. First, great advances have been made with surgical approaches. Secondly, the orthopedic surgeon instinctively prefers surgery. After all, the performance of surgery was the primary reason why most of us chose orthopedics as a career. Thirdly, the popular perception that the surgical treatment is more prestigious and it is carried out by individuals with superior intellect. This is exemplified by the popular saying that for the solution of certain difficult situations one needs the "brain of a neurosurgeon;" no one ever said, "One needs the brain of a neurologist." Fourthly, the surgical treatments are more financially rewarding. Finally, the manufacturing industry of surgical implants presents a powerful and persuasive argument to use their equipment and instrumentation.

REFERENCES

1. Chrisman OD, Snook GA. The problem of refracture of the tibia. Clin Orthop. 1982; 60:217.
2. Moore TM, Lester DK, Sarmiento A. The Stabilizing Effect of Soft Tissue Constraints in Artificial Galeazzi Fractures. Clin Orthop Relat Res. 1985 Apr; 194:189-94.
3. Park SH, O'Connor K, McKellop H, Sarmiento A. The Influence of active Shear or Compressive Motion on Fracture Healing. J Bone Joint Surg Am. 1998 Jun; 80(6):868-78.
4. Sarmiento A, Schaeffer J, Beckerman L, Latta LL, Enis J. Fracture Healing in Rat Femora as Affected by Functional Weight Bearing. J. Bone Joint Surg Am, 1977; 59(3):369-75.
5. Sarmiento A, Mullis DL, Latta LL, Alvarez RR. A Quantitative, Comparative Analysis of Fracture Healing Under the Influence of Compression Plating vs. Closed Weight-Bearing Treatment. Clin Orthop. 1980; 149:232.
6. Schlitch T. Surgery, Science and Industry. Palgrave.-McMillan 2002
7. Trueta J. The role of vessels in osteogenesis. J Bone Joint Surg Br. 1963; 45:402-6.
8. Trueta J. Blood supply and rate of healing of tibial fractures. Clin Orthop. 1974; 105:11.
9. Uhthoff HK. Prevention of bone atrophy through an early removal of internal fixation plates. An experimental study in the dog. Howmedica Trauma Workshop, New York. 1979.
10. Uhthoff HK, Dubuc FL. Bone structure changes in the dog under rigid internal fixation. Clin Orthop. 1970; 81:40-7.
11. Wolf JW et al. The Superiority of Cyclic Loading over Constant Compression in the Treatment of Long Bone Fractures. A Quantitative Biomechanical Study in Rabbits. Trans 26 Orthop Res Soc. 1980; 5:174.
12. Latta LL, Sarmiento A. Mechanical Behavior of Tibial Fractures. Symposium on Trauma to the Leg and Its Sequela. C.V. Mosby: St. Louis, MO 1981.
13. McKellop HA, Sigholm G, Redfern FC, Doyle B, Sarmiento A, Luck J. The Effect of Simulated Fracture-Angulation of the Tibia on Cartilage Pressures in the Knee Joint. J Bone & Joint Surg. 1991; 73-A:1382-1390.
14. Merchant TC, Dietz FR. Long-term follow-up after fractures of the tibial and fibular shafts. J Bone and Joint Surg Am. 1989 Apr; 71A:599-606.
15. Orfaly R, Keating JE, O'Brien PJ. Knee pain after tibial nailing: Does the entry point matter? J Bone Joint Surg Br. 1995; 77(6):976-7.
16. Sarmiento A, Latta LL. On the evolution of fracture bracing. J Bone Joint Surg Br. 2006; 88-8(2):141-8.
17. Sarmiento A, Latta L, Zilioli A, Sinclair Wm F. The Role of Soft Tissues in the Stabilization of Tibial Fractures. Clin Orthop Relat Res. 1974; 105:116-29.
18. Austin RT. Sarmiento Tibial Plaster Prospective Study of 145 Fractures. Injury. 1981; 13:10
19. Sarmiento A, Sharpe MD, Ebramzadeh E, Normand P, Shankwiler J. Factors influencing the Outcome of Closed Tibial Fractures Treated with Functional Bracing. Clin Ortho Relat Res. 1995 Jun; (315):8-24.
20. Sarmiento A, Latta LL. Closed fractures of the middle third of the tibia treated with a functional Brace. Clin Orthop. 2008 Dec; 466:3108-15.
21. Sarmiento A, Latta LL. 450 Closed Fractures of the distal third of the tibia treated with a functional brace. Clin Orthop. 2004; 428: 261-71.
22. Sarmiento A, Latta LL. Functional treatment of Closed Segmental Fractures of the Tibia. Acta Chir Orthop Traumatol Cech. 2008; 75:325-31.
23. Sarmiento A. A Functional Below-Knee Cast for Tibial Fractures. J Bone and Joint Surg. 1967; 59:5.
24. Sarmiento A. A Functional Below-Knee Brace for Tibial Fractures. J. Bone and Joint Surg. 1970; 52(2):295-311.
25. Sarmiento A, Latta LL. Functional Fracture Bracing. The Tibia, Humerus and Ulna. Springer-Verlag 1992.
26. Sarmiento A. Functional Bracing of Tibial and Femoral Shaft Fractures. Clin Orthop. 1972; 82:2.
27. Sarmiento A. On the behavior of closed tibial fractures: clinical and radiological correlations. J Orthop Trauma, 2000; 14(3): 199-205.
28. Dehne E. Treatment of Fractures of the Tibial Shaft. Clin. Orthop. 1969; 66:159.
29. Delamarter R, Hohl M. The Cast Brace and Tibial Plateau Fractures. Clin Orthop. 1989; 242:26.
30. Sarmiento A. Functional Bracing of Tibial and Femoral Shaft Fractures. Clin Orthop Relat Res. 1972; 82:2-13.
31. Sarmiento A. The functional bracing of fractures. J Bone Joint Am. Classics Techniques 2007; 89 Suppl 2 (Part 2):157-69.
32. Court-Brown C, Keating J, McQueen M. Exchange intramedullary nailing. Its use in aseptic tibial nonunion. J. Bone and Joint Surg. 1995; 77B (3):407-11.
33. Kristensen KD, Kiaer T, Blicher J. No arthrosis of the ankle 20 years after malaligned tibial-shaft fracture. Acta Orthop Scand. 1989:208-9.
34. Lovasz G, Park SH, Ebramzadeh E, Benya PD, Llinas A, Bellyei A, Luck J, Sarmiento A. Characteristic of degeneration in an unstable knee with a coronal surface step-off. J. Bone Joint Br. 2001 Apr; 83(3):428-36.

35. Mawhinney IN, Maginn P, McCoy GF. Tibial compartment syndromes after tibial nailing. J Orthop Trauma. 1994; 8(3):212-14.

36. Kyro A. Malunion after intramedullary nailing of tibial shaft fractures. Ann Chir Gynecol. 1997; 86:56-64.

37. Wagner KS, Tarr RR, Resnick C, Sarmiento A. The Effect of Simulated Tibial Deformities on the Ankle Joint During the Gait Cycle. Foot Ankle. 1984; 5(3):131-41.

38. Freedman EL, Johnson EE. Radiographic analysis of tibial fracture malalignment following intramedullary nailing. Clin Orthop Relat Res. 1995; 315:25-33.

39. McCollough NC, Vinsant JE, Sarmiento A. Functional Fracture - Bracing of Long-bone Fractures of the Lower Extremity in Children. J Bone Joint Surg. 1978; 60A:314.

40. McKellop HA, Hoffmann R, Sarmiento A, Lu B, Ebramzadeh E. Control of Motion of Tibial Fractures with Use of a Functional Brace or an External Fixator. J Bone & Joint Surg. 1993 Jul; 75A:1019-25.

41. Tarr RR, Resnick CT, Wagner KS, Sarmiento A. Changes in Tibiotalar Joint Contact Areas Following Experimentally Induced Tibial Angular Deformities. Clin Orthop. 1985; 199:72.

42. Alho A, Ekelan A, Stromsoe K et al. Nonunion of Tibial Shaft Fractures treated with locked intramedullary nailing without bone grafting. J. Trauma. 1993; 34(1):62.

43. Bone LB, Johnson K.D. Treatment of tibial fractures by reaming and intramedullary nailing. J. Bone and Joint Surg. 1986; 68A(6):877-87.

44. Cole D, Latta LL. Fatigue failure of interlocking tibial nail implants. Orthop Trans Bone Joint Surg. 1992; 16-3A:663.

45. Court-Brown CM, Will E, Christie J, McQueen M. Reamed or unreamed nailing for closed tibial fractures. J. Bone and Joint Surg. July 1996; 78B:580-3.

46. De Smet K, Mostert AK, De Witte J, De Brauwer V, Verdonk R. Closed intramedullary tibial nailing using the Marchetti-Vicenzi nail. Injury. 2000; 31(8):597-603.

47. Finkemeier CG, Schmidt AH, Kyle RF, Templeman DC, Varecka TF. A prospective, randomized study of intramedullary nails inserted with and without reaming for the treatment of open and closed fractures of the tibial shafts. J Orthop Trauma. 2000; 14 (3):187-93.

48. Gregory P, Sanders R. The treatment of closed, unstable tibial shaft fractures with unreamed interlocking nails. Clin Orthop Relat Res. 1995; 315:48-55.

49. Gregory P, Sanders R. The Treatment of Closed, Unstable Tibial Fractures with Unreamed Interlocking Nails. Clin Orthop. 1995; 315:48-55.

50. Habernek H, Kwansy O, Schmid L, Ortner F. Complications of interlocking nailing for lower leg fractures. A three year follow-up of 102 cases. J Trauma. 1992; 33:863-9.

51. Hutson J, Zych GA, Cole JD, Johnson KD, Ostermann P, Milne EL, Latta, L. Mechanical failures of intramedullary tibia nails applied without reaming. Clinic Orthop Relat Res. 1995; 315:129-37.

52. Koval KJ, Clapper MF, Elison PS, Poka A, Bathon GH, Burgess AR. Complications of reamed intramedullary nailing of the tibia. J Ortop Trauma. 1991; 5:184-9.

53. Lang GJ, Cohen BE, Bosse MJ, Kellam JF. Proximal third tibial shaft fractures. Should they be nailed? Clin. Orthop. 1995; 315:64-74.

54. Templeman D, Varecka T, Kyle R. Exchanged reamed intramedullary nailing for delayed union and nonunion of the tibia. Clin Orthop. 1995; (315):169-75.

55. Williams J, Gibbons M, Trundle H, Murray D, Worlock P. Complications of nailing in closed tibial fractures. J Orthop Trauma. 1995; 9(6):476-81.

56. Wiss DA, Stetson WB. Unstable fractures of the tibia treated with reamed intramedullary nails. Clin Orthop Relat Res. 1995;315: 56-63.

57. Alho A, Eckeland A, Stromsoe K, Folleras G, Thorensen B. Locked intramedullary nailing of tibial fractures. J Bone Joint Surg. 1990; 72B:805-11.

58. Bonnevialle P, Bellumore Y, Foucras L, Hezard L, Mansat M. Tibial fractures with intact fibula treated by reamed nailing. Rev Chir Orthop Reparatrice Appar Mot. 2000; 86(1):29-37.

59. Buehler KC, Green J, Woll TS, Duwelius PJ. A technique for intramedullary nailing of proximal third tibia fractures. J Orthop Trauma. 1997; 11(3):218-223.

60. Court-Brown CM, Gustilo T, Shaw AD. Knee pain after intramedullary nailing of proximal third tibia fractures. J Orthop Trauma. 1997; 11:103-5.

61. Court-Brown CM, Keating JF, McQueen MM. Infection after intramedullary nailing of the tibia. Incidence and protocol for management. J Bone Joint Surg Br. 1992; 74-B (5):770-16

62. Court-Brown CM, Christie J, McQueen MM. Closed intramedullary tibial nailing. Its use in closed and Type I open fractures. J Bone Joint Surg Br. 1990; 72B (4):605-11.

63. Guilar J, Vazquez P, Ortega M. False aneurysm of the posterior tibial artery complicating fracture of the tibia and fibula. Rev Chir Orthop Reparatrice Appar Mot. 1995; 81(6):546-8.

64. Hooper GJ, Keddell RG, Penny ID. Conservative management or closed nailing for tibial shaft fractures. A randomized prospective trial. J. Bone and Joint Surg. 1991 Jan; 73B:83-5.

65. 13, Keating GJ, Orfaly R, O'Brien PJ: Knee pain after tibial nailing. J Orthop Trauma. 1997; 11:10-3.

66. McKellop HA, Llinas A, Sarmiento A. Effects of Tibial Malalignment on the Knee and Ankle. Ortho. Clin. N. Amer. 1994 Jul; 25:3.

67. Olerud S, Dankwardt-Lilliestrom G. Fracture healing in compression osteosynthesis. Acta Orthop Scand Suppl. 1971; 137:1-44.

68. Peter RE, Bachelin P, Fritschy D. Skiers' Lower Leg Shaft Fracture. Outcome in 91 Cases Treated Conservatively with Sarmiento's Brace. Am J Sports Med. 1988 Sep-Oct; 16(5):486-91.

69. Ricciardi-Pollini PT, Falez F. The Treatment of Diaphyseal Fractures by Functional Bracing. Results in 36 Cases. Ital J Orthop Traumatol. 1985 Jun; 11(2):199-205.

70. Toivanen JA, Vaisto D, Kannus P. Anterior knee pain after intramedullary nailing of fractures of the tibial shaft. A prospective, randomized study comparing two different nail-insertion techniques. J Bone and Joint Surg. 2002; 84A:580-5.

71. Toivanen JA, Vaisto O, Kannus P, Latvala K, Honkonen SE, Jarvinen MJ. Anterior knee pain after intramedullary nailing of fractures of the tibial shaft. A prospective, randomized study comparing two different nail-insertion techniques. J Bone Joint Surg Am. 2002; 84-A(4):580-5.

72. Vaist O, Toivanen J, Kannus P, Jarvinen M. Anterior knee pain and thigh muscle strength after Intramedullary nailing of a tibial shaft fracture. An 8-year follow-up of 28 consecutive cases. J Orthop Trauma; 2007 Mar; 21:165-171.

73. Downing ND, Griffin DR, Davis TR. A Comparison of the relative costs of cast treatment and intramedullary nailing for tibial diaphyseal fractures in the UK. Injury. 1997; 28(5-6):373-5.

3

Overall Management Protocol

As indicated in the above section, closed fractures of the tibia essentially experience, at the time of the injury, the final and total amount of shortening. Attempts to regain length by manipulation alone are likely to result in loss of the gained length upon the introduction of weight-bearing stresses. Even the active contraction of the ankle and toes flexors and extensors may produce the same result. This information suggests that axially unstable fracture of the tibial diaphysis that experience unacceptable shortening at the time of the initial injury and cannot be rendered stable by manipulation, should not be treated with early casting or bracing techniques. In some instances if activity can be postponed until intrinsic stability develops at the fracture site, bracing can be carried out. Another option is the use of skeletal traction to the extremity until such stability is attained. External fixators can accomplish the same goal but should not be kept in place for too long a period of time. The rigid immobilization of the tibial fragments delays the healing of this bone while allowing the fibular fracture to progress to healing in a rapid fashion. When the fixator is removed and weight bearing is introduced, the fibula is usually healed. However, the tibia not yet sufficiently stable, may develop a varus deformity.

Transverse fractures with associated fibula fracture that can be manipulated and rendered stable can be treated with functional braces, providing the reduction is a secure one.

Open fractures are usually accompanied with an initially greater degree of shortening. Therefore, functional bracing has a very limited role to play in their management. In general, only type I open fractures produced by lower energy forces can be considered appropriate subjects for nonsurgical functional treatment. Among them are fractures resulting from low velocity gunshot wounds when the initial shortening is acceptable. However, if the shortening is accepted because of attenuating circumstances, it can easily be compensated with a shoe lift.

4

Acute Care: Compartment Syndrome

Closed diaphyseal tibial fractures resulting from low energy forces do not, as a rule, require hospitalization. However, even if produced from rather mild trauma, hospitalization is recommended if the extremity is very swollen and painful after initial stabilization. Any signs or symptoms that suggest the possibility of a muscle compartment syndrome developing, require careful consideration. Hospitalization for an overnight observation is strongly recommended. Otherwise, a period of observation in an emergency room area is sufficient.

There is considerably reliable data to indicate that following the presence of a compartment syndrome, irreversible damage to the affected musculature takes place after eight hours. This suggests that surgery performed many hours beyond that offers no functional benefits; quite the contrary it may result in creating fertile ground for infection and the need for subsequent unsightly scars. Surgically exposing irreversibly damaged muscles requires their excision resulting in more serious aesthetic deformities (Figure 4.1).

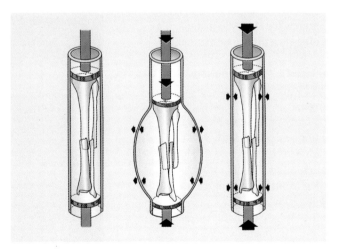

Fig. 4.1: Schematic drawing attempting to explain the ill-effects that forceful restoration of length to a fractured tibia may have. In the intact limb, the soft tissues are contained by the skin and fascia. Once a fracture occurs, the skin and fascia expand laterally in order to accommodate the bleeding and swelling without increasing too much the pressure on the soft tissues. Once traction to regain length and stabilization in a cylinder cast is obtained, the pressure in the soft tissues may be high enough to create a compartment syndrome. This is a likely mechanism for some compartment syndromes.

5

The Initial Above-the-Knee Cast

All closed tibial diaphyseal fractures require a period of stabilization in an above-the-knee cast. Since the initial stabilizing cast is applied at a time when the patient is experiencing the pain and fear that necessarily accompanies acute fractures, some type of sedation is necessary. If the symptoms are of an unusual high degree, it is important to ascertain that a muscle compartment syndrome is not developing, in which case the pressure in the various compartments of the leg should be measured. If the clinical and laboratory tests are negative, but the out-of-proportion pain persists it is better not to apply a cylindrical cast. A posterior splint of Plaster of Paris is recommended and the patient should be admitted to the hospital for closer observation and monitoring of the compartments pressures.

Under usual circumstances, when pain is acute, the above-the-knee cast should be preceded by the administration of strong sedation and analgesic agents.

It is desirable, but not necessarily indispensable, that the patient sits on a high table with his hips and knee at 90° of flexion, and the non-injured limb readily exposed. The exposure of both lower extremities allows to identify the overall appearance of the normal leg, so its alignment can be reproduced in the broken one (Figure 5.1).

Under no circumstances should the leg be held by the foot or toes or the knee in extension. This maneuver readily encourages a recurvatum deformity at the level of the fracture (Figure 5.2).

Padding is rolled over the extremity. The amount of padding should be determined based on the expectation of additional enlargement of the leg, in which cases, it would be best to be generous with it. Otherwise, a thinner layer is best, since the alignment of the fractures is better maintained.

The following details concerning the application of the cast apply to those fractures which are expected to be managed with nonsurgical functional methods. These fractures, as we

have repeatedly emphasized, are the axially unstable ones (oblique, spiral, comminute or segmental) where the initial shortening prior to any treatment is acceptable in anticipation that such shortening will not increase with the functional use of the extremity. Transverse fractures, if not displaced, are mechanically stable and obviously cannot shorten and the described technique also applies in these cases. For the transverse displaced fractures, a manual reduction is necessary, and it should be carried out under supervised anesthesia in a hospital environment.

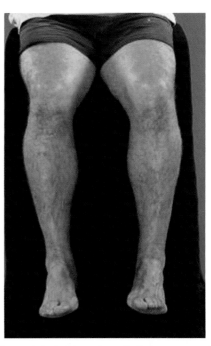

Fig. 5.1: It is most desirable to have both legs exposed during the application of the original and subsequent casts and brace. It allows the surgeon the opportunity to reproduce the alignment of the normal leg into the injured one.

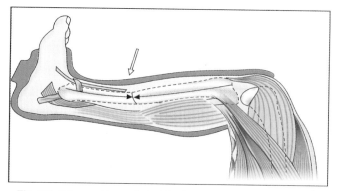

Fig. 5.2: If the cast is applied while the leg is held from the toes, a recurvatum deformity can readily occur.

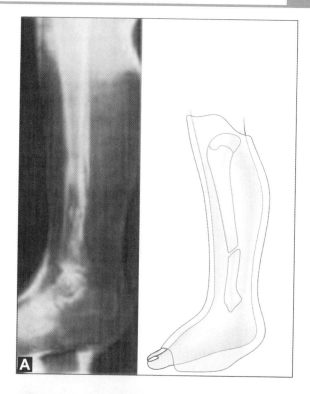

The above-the-knee cast is best applied in three stages.

Stage 1: An assistant holds the foot at 90° of flexion. This must be done very gingerly, for otherwise a recurvatum deformity can be produced. During this stage, no attention to the fracture is needed. However, care should be given to eliminate any rotational deformity that is likely to be present. An external rotation is the most common one when both bones are fractured. The same is not necessarily true when the fibula is intact (Figures 5.3 and 5.4).

The longitudinal and transverse arches of the foot should be carefully molded.

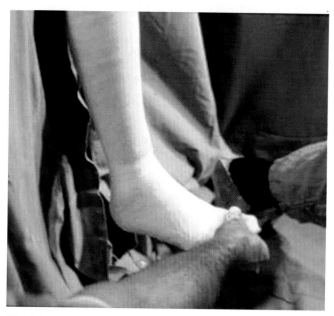

Fig. 5.3: An assistant gingerly holds the foot in a neutral position, avoiding an equinus attitude, which at a later date will make ambulation difficult and likely to produce a recurvatum deformity when the ankle joint is freed.

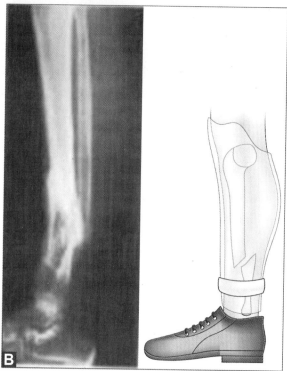

Figs 5.4A and B: (A) Radiograph and accompanying drawing of a tibia well aligned but with the foot in an equinus position. (B) Radiograph and accompanying drawing showing how a recurvatum deformity readily occurs upon freedom of the ankle joint and weightbearing on the "ball" of the foot.

Stage 2: Once the Plaster of Paris has dried, additional rolls are wrapped overlying the previously applied plaster to the level of the tibial tubercle. It is during this time that the best possible alignment of the fractured fragments is attempted. Since traction is not necessary in the case of the unstable fractures that meet the criteria outlined above, the alignment of the fragments must be done gingerly without forceful maneuvers. Angular deformities are corrected and the best possible alignment is sought (Figures 5.6A to C).

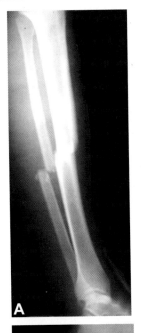
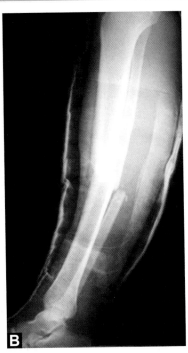
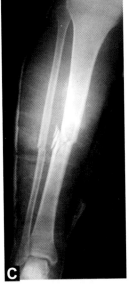

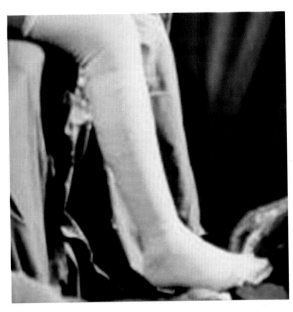

Fig. 5.5: During the second stage, and while the leg hangs freely over the side of the table, the cast is extended from just above the ankle to the tibial tubercle. It is during this time that correction of angular deformities is done. The wrapping material is firmly done without worrying about excessive pressure over bony prominences.

Figs 5.6A to C: (A) Radiograph of tibial fracture demonstrating the recurvatum deformity produced by the holding of the knee in extension during the initial stabilization. (B) Radiograph taken through the below-the-knee functional cast showing correction of the deformity. This was accomplished simply by keeping the hip and knee at 90° of flexion during casting, and the application of steady pressure over the posterior apex of the deformity and compensatory pressure over the anterior aspect of the distal tibia. (C) Radiograph showing the good alignment of the fragments.

It is important to avoid extension of the knee during this stage, since a recurvatum deformity may be produced (Figures 5.7A to C).

Stage 3: Once the plaster has dried, the knee is extended and additional plaster is wrapped overlapping the leg portion of the cast to the proximal thigh. There is no reason to flex the knee since, as stated earlier, no additional shortening is expected. Ambulation with the knee immobilized in flexion is impossible if weight bearing is to be introduced (Figure 5.8).

Upon completion of the casting procedure, if it had not been monitored with fluoroscopy, two radiographs are obtained to determine the acceptability of the reduction. If the position of the fragments is unacceptable, it becomes necessary to either wedge the cast or replace it. A less than ideal alignment is often allowed in anticipation that at the time of application of the subsequent below-the-knee functional cast or brace within the next one or two weeks, a better alignment will be achieved (Figure 5.9).

After the application of the above-the-knee cast, the patient should be allowed to ambulate bearing as much weight as he or she wishes to apply. Needless to say, pain dictates the degree of weight borne by the fractured limb. It is advisable to instruct the patient to keep the leg elevated during the sitting position and to carry out frequent active motion of the toes and isometric exercises of the calf and thigh musculature. These exercises produce motion at the fractures site which are conducive to osteogenesis.

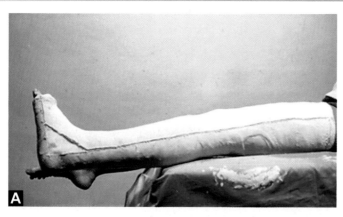
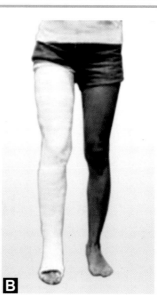

Figs 5.7A and B: The completed above-the-knee cast should not hold the knee in flexion. Since the final shortening of closed tibial fractures is the same one as experienced initially, there is no need to flex the knee; a position that tends to perpetuate itself if the cast is in place for a long period of time.

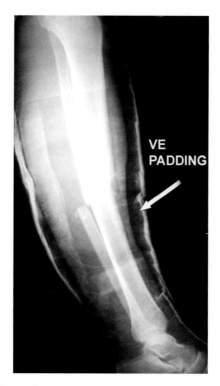

Fig. 5.8: Excessive padding under the cast or plastic material is unnecessary and even harmful when the cast is applied after the initial swelling and pain have subsided. With this degree of padding, angular deformities can develop.

6

The Below-the-Knee Functional Cast

The functional cast should be applied as soon as the acute symptoms subside. To apply it before that happens, is a painful and unnecessary experience. On the other hand, postponing its application until "early callus" is seen on radiographs, is also a misguided and erroneous practice. First, it deprives the patient of the opportunity to benefit from the convenience of a free knee joint and the advantage of graduated weight bearing ambulation. Secondly, it might create an undesirable environment due to the fact that when the tibia and fibula are fractured, the fibula, usually, heals faster. By the time callus is seen on the tibia, the fibula is likely to be solidly united, creating a situation similar to that of an acute tibial fracture with an intact fibula leading to the development of an angular varus deformity. The benefit of motion at the fracture site should be granted to both bones (Figures 6.1 to 6.6).

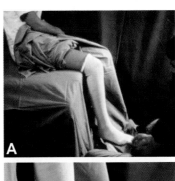

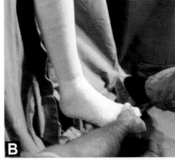

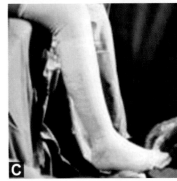

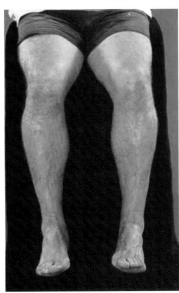

Fig. 6.1: For the application of the functional cast, the patient should sit on a high table with the hip and knee at 90°.

Figs 6.2A and B: (A) First, stockinette is rolled over the leg, extending to a couple of inches above the knee. (B) Over a thin layer of cotton padding, and while gingerly holding the ankle at 90°, Plaster of Paris or fiberglass material is rolled from the toes to approximately two inches above the ankle joint. (C) Rolling over has been done completely

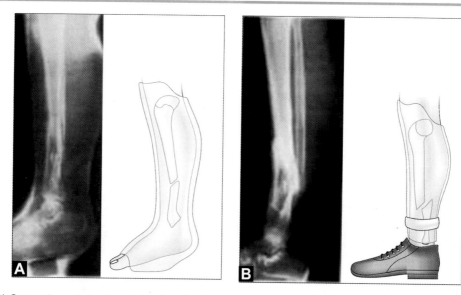

Figs 6.3A and B: (A) Composite radiograph and drawing showing a well-aligned tibial fracture in a cast, but with the ankle in equinus. (B) Composite radiograph and drawing illustrating the development of a recurvatum deformity after the cast is replaced with a brace that allows motion of the ankle. Weight bearing, under this circumstance takes place on the "ball of the foot."

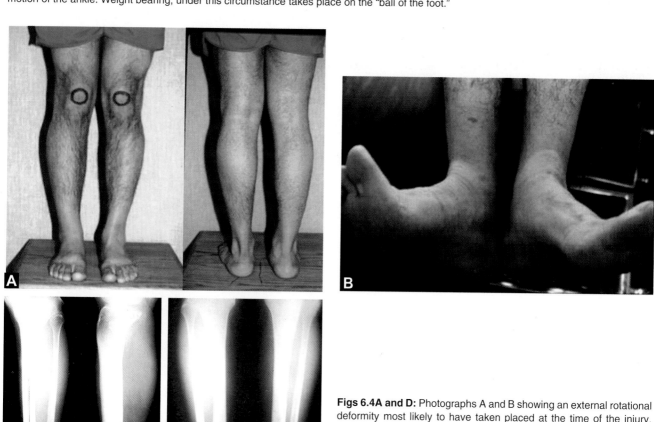

Figs 6.4A and D: Photographs A and B showing an external rotational deformity most likely to have taken placed at the time of the injury, but failed to receive correction at the time of application of the original stabilizing above-the-knee cast. C and D are radiographs of the injured and normal legs showing that when a rotary deformity exists, the visual relationship between the tibia and fibula change. Since the fibula is located in posterolateral position in reference to the tibia, additional external rotation further hides the fibula behind the tibia. If the malrotation is of the nature of an internal rotation, the space between the two bones increases.

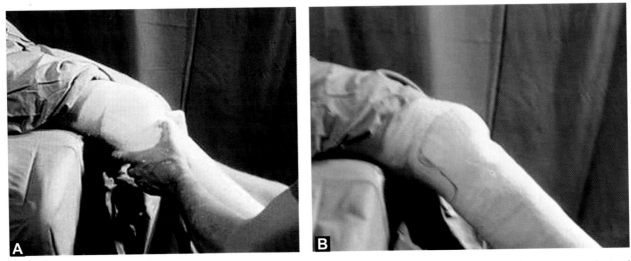

Figs 6.5A and B: (A) The molding of the patellar tendon is done while the wrapping material is still in a soft stage. The pressure on the tendon is minimal and requires that the patient's quadriceps be relaxed. This is why the patient's heel, at this time, should rest on the surgeons lap. (B) The trim line in the proximal cast should be done in such a manner as to eventually permit full flexion and extension of the knee joint; Superiorly, to just above the proximal pole of the patella: Laterally, as far posteriorly as possible, without interfering with the hamstring tendons; Posteriorly, at a level opposite to the tibial tubercle.

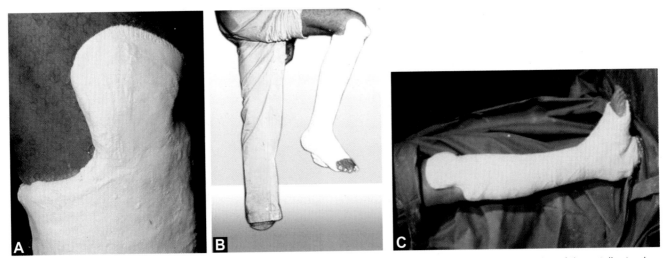

Figs 6.6A to C: (A) Illustration of the proximal end of the below-the-knee functional cast showing the mild indentation of the patellar tendon, the long posterior wings of the cast, and the proximal trim opposite to the tibial tubercle. The firm contact between the wings of the cast and the femoral condyles assist in providing angular and rotary stability. (B and C) Illustration of the degree of flexion of the knee the cast permits.

7

The Pre-fabricated Functional Brace

As we mentioned in the introduction to the book, shortly after we reported on the significant success we had achieved with prefabricated braces, some surgeons engaged in financial ventures with manufactures of braces who began to market appliances that disregarded basic features of importance.

For example, they dismissed the importance of the proximal wings of the brace, during the weight bearing phase of gait-assist in the prevention of angular and rotatory stability.

The brace can be made of either Plaster of Paris of the hard or soft type or of plastic materials. These plastic materials may

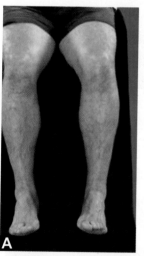
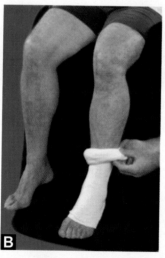
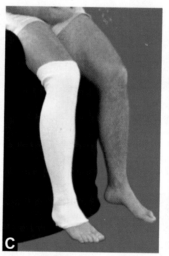
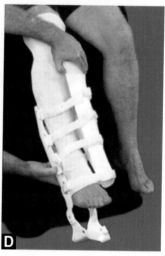
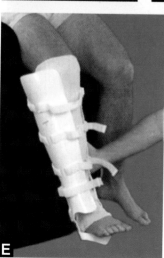
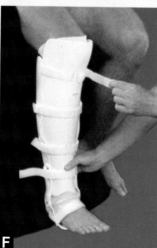
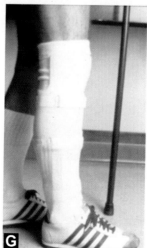

Figs 7.1A to G: Sequential photographs of the application of the pre-fabricated brace. The patient sits on a high table with the hips and knees at 90°. Both extremes are exposed. The straps of the brace are not released during its application and are adjusted once the fit of the appliance appears to be satisfactory.

be of a custom-made type or pre-fabricated. In any event, it is important to recognize that the brace must be made adjustable in order to maintain the desirable snugness of the appliance. The adjustability of the brace makes it possible to compress the soft tissues at all times and, in that manner which perpetuates the hydraulic environment that controls angulation (Figures 7.1A to 7.2C).

BRACE APPLICATION

There are a number of pre-fabricated tibial braces in the market. What is most important in choosing a brace is the understanding of the philosophy and rationale of the technique and the method of implementation of the treatment (Figures 7.3A to 7.4).

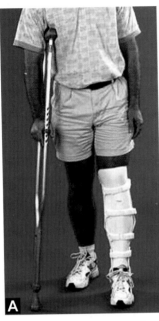
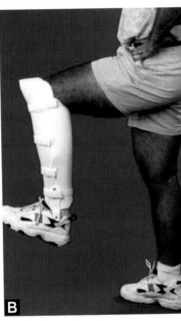
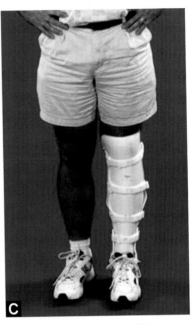

Figs 7.2A to C: The brace once properly applied provides firm contact with the proximal tibial and femoral condyles. This contact assists in reducing angular and rotary forces, particularly in fractures in the proximal third of the tibia. The patellar tendon indentation does not contribute to concentration of forces, but helps in obtaining better contact between the brace and the condyles. (A) Partial weight bearing ambulation always begins with the assistance of two crutches or a walker. The degree of weight bearing is dictated by the symptoms experienced. Under no circumstances should full-weight bearing be encouraged if pain is experienced. (B) The brace should permit full flexion and extension of the knee without impingement of the hamstrings. (C) Full weight bearing is permissible when painful symptoms have completely disappeared.

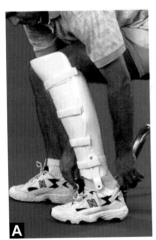
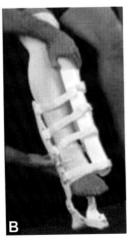
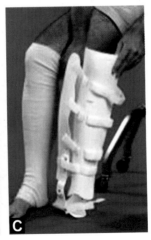
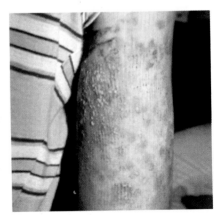

Figs 7.3A to C: Patient demonstrates the donning and doffing of the brace for hygienic purposes.

Fig. 7.4: Representative example of maceration of the skin in a patient with a braced fracture of the humerus. This is an extremely rare complication, and almost always secondary to failure to remove the brace every day, or every few days, for hygienic purposes.

8

The Custom-made Brace

Contrary to the technique of brace construction with wrapping products, the Orthoplast method calls for the use of a thermoplastic material. The Orthoplast sheet is a synthetic rubber that when been dipped in hot water for a couple of minutes becomes soft and malleable. Once outside the hot water, it begins to harden to its original rigidity. It is during this time that the sheet is wrapped over the limb and molded to accommodate the requirements of the frictional brace.

BRACE APPLICATION

There are situations when the components of a brace are not available to the treating physician. In such situations, a below-the-knee functional cast can be used in anticipation of obtaining comparable results. If the cast is to be used in preference to the brace, it is often best to postpone its application until the swelling has decreased to a greater degree, simply because the circular cast lacks the adjustability features to accommodate the reduction of swelling and limb atrophy.

The use of crutches is essential and weight bearing should be determined by the degree of symptoms. It should be increased gradually and not be permitted to become full unless it is not accompanied with pain.

The following photos illustrate the step-by-step application of the Orthoplast brace (Figures 8.1 to 8.8).

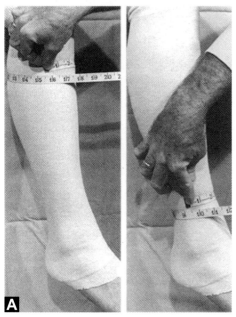

Fig. 8.1: The girth of the leg is measured from the level of the tibial tubercle to just above the ankle.

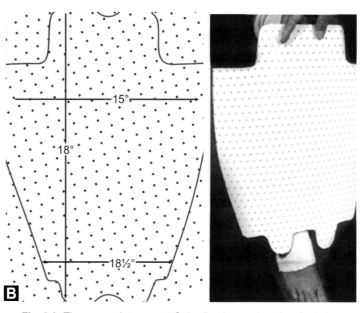

Fig. 8.2: The appropriate pre-cut Orthoplast brace sheet is selected.

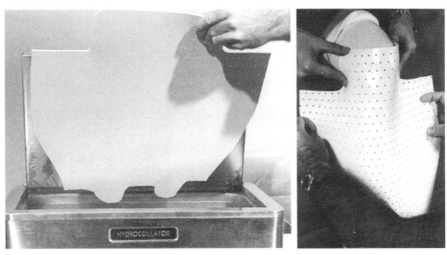

Fig. 8.3: The Orthoplast sheet is dipped in hot water for a few minutes until it becomes soft and pliable.

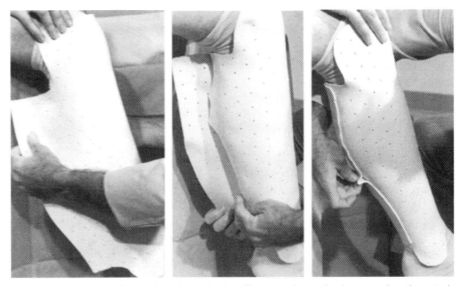

Fig. 8.4: The Orthoplast sheet is then folded over the leg. The posterior portion is pressed on the anterior one, avoiding as much as possible wrinkles in the material.

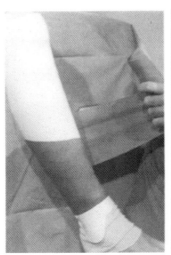
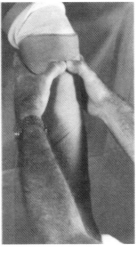

Fig. 8.5: An elastic bandage previously dipped in cold water is firmly wrapped over the still soft plastic material. It is at this time when angular correction can be made. The patellar tendon is molded, while the lateral condylar wings of the Orthoplast and the sub-popliteal space are firmly compressed. Though the patellar tendon is not a weight bearing structure, its compression makes the proximal fit to the brace more effective. The molded condylar wings assist in obtaining the greatest degree of angular stability.

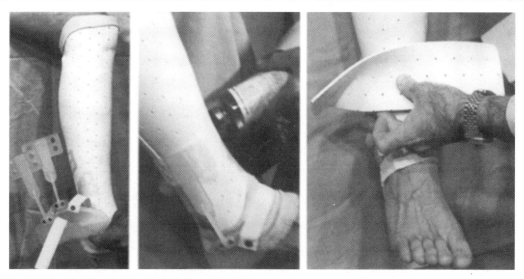

Fig. 8.6: The plastic ankle joint is tried. Then the surface of the brace where the wings of the ankle insert contacts with the brace is moistened with carbon tetrachloride in order to ensure firm bonding of the material.

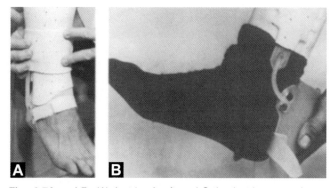

Figs 8.7A and B: (A) A strip of softened Orthoplast is wrapped over the wings of the ankle insert. The dorsal band that ensures stability of the brace when the shoe is not in place is fasted over the dorsum of the foot. (B) The flexible joint allows for the easy donning of a sock.

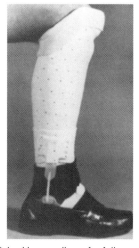

Fig. 8.8: The finished brace allows for full range of motion of the knee and ankle joints.

9

The Role of the Fibula

The presence or absence of a fibular fracture accompanying a tibial fracture plays a major role in determining healing as well as angulation. This is more important than the location and geometry of the tibial fracture.

It is commonly accepted that the fibula heals faster than the tibia. This premise is correct, but the explanation given for this fact may not be correct. The prevalent explanation is based on the mistaken belief that long bones that are surrounded by large muscles heal at a faster rate (Figure 9.1). This assumption is readily contradicted by the fact that most of the fibular diaphysis is deprived of muscle coverage, and many bones with minimal or no muscle coverage heal rapidly and almost consistently. The clavicle, metacarpals and metatarsals, the ulna and phalanges, the fractures less likely to experience nonunion are eloquent examples.

Demonstrating the faster healing of the fibula when associated with a tibial fracture, is best exemplified by the situation when an external fixator is used. The fixator immobilizes the tibial fracture but leaves the fibula fracture non-immobilized and free to experience healthy motion between the fragments (Figures 9.2A to D).

There is ample evidence, which we have reinforced throughout this text, that closed axially unstable fractures e.g. oblique, spiral, comminuted, do not shorten above and beyond the initial shortening, regardless of the presence or absence of weight bearing stresses. This we have explained by the fact that the remaining intact soft tissues, particularly the interosseous membrane, provide a tethering mechanism that prevents further shortening (See Chapter 1).

The still pervasive perception that closed fractures shorten when subjected to weight bearing forces is responsible for the practice of applying above-the-knee cast with the knee in flexion, in order to avoid the "additional" shortening.

The fear that stresses at the fracture site results in an additional shortening prompts many surgeons to delay the introduction of weight bearing ambulation until "some callus" is visible on radiographs. This erroneous practice does more harm than good, since during this period of time the fibula solidly heals, creating the unhealthy situation of a tibial fracture with an intact fibula, and the resulting common complication of a varus deformity (Figures 9.3 and 9.4). Active, intermittent forces applied to the fractured tibia and fibula should be introduced early.

Fractures of the tibia with intact fibula are prone to develop varus angulation (Figures 9.5 to 9.7). Usually, the shortest tibial fragment experiences the greatest deviation. Fractures located in the proximal and distal third of the tibial diaphyses are the ones likely to angulate the most (Figures 9.8 and 9.9). However, the degree of final angulation is determined by the geometry of the tibial fracture. An oblique tibial fracture where the direction of the fracture is from proximal to distal and from medial to lateral angulates more severely than a similar fracture that runs from lateral to medial. In the latter instance the proximal fragment abuts against the distal fragment which is made relatively stable by the interosseous membrane (Figures 9.8 to 9.12).

Not all tibial fractures with an intact fibula develop a varus deformity. We have concluded that if the initial radiograph does not show a deformity it is very likely that the fracture will heal without a deformity or with a very mild one (Figures 9.6, 9.13 to 9.18). This is the case in transverse fractures, however, in oblique ones the chances of development of a varus deformity grow exponentially (Figures 9.10, 9.11, 9.20 to 9.22). These latter fractures, therefore, should not be treated with closed functional methods. Intramedullary nailing is at this time the treatment of choice.

Whenever a tibial fracture with an intact fibula shows a valgus angulation, it is most likely due to a dislocation of the proximal tibio-fibular joint (Figures 9.4 and 9.15A and B). Likewise, shortening in the absence of a fibula fracture is usually due to a similar dislocation. Common sense indicates that with an intact fibula a tibial fracture cannot produce shortening. Appropriate treatment to the joint is necessary to avoid a recurrent dislocation or chronic pain a that level.

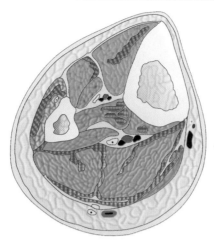

Fig. 9.1: Cross section of the leg at the middle-third level showing the large muscle mass that fills the interosseus space. These muscles are an obstacle to severe deformity.

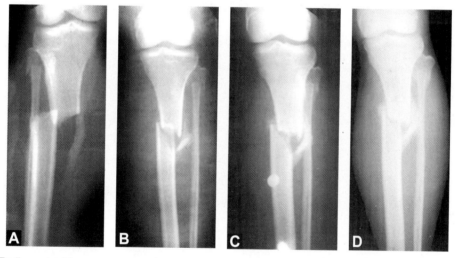

Figs 9.2A to D: (A) Radiograph of transverse, severely displaced fracture of the proximal tibia with an associated nondisplaced-transverse fibular fracture. (B) The fracture was reduced under anesthesia. (C) The fracture was treated with a below-the-knee functional cast. (D) Notice early callus formation and the moderately severe varus angular deformity.

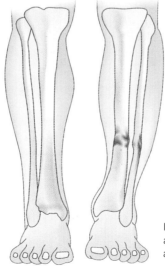

Fig. 9.3: Schematic drawing illustrating the fact that a varus deformity of the tibia is not as noticeable as a valgus one.

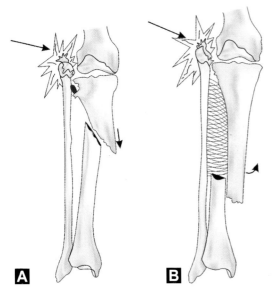

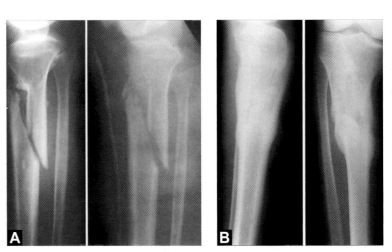

Figs 9.4A and B: (A) Drawings depicting tibia fractures with an intact fibula showing a valgus deformity (B) or significant shortening of the tibia. Such shortening is impossible unless the fibula is dislocated proximally.

Figs 9.5A and B: (A) Radiograph of long, oblique fracture of the proximal tibia with an intact fibula. (B) The fracture was treated with a below-the-knee functional brace, but weight bearing was delayed due to the intactness of the fibula. The fracture healed with a few degrees of varus angulation of a very acceptable degree.

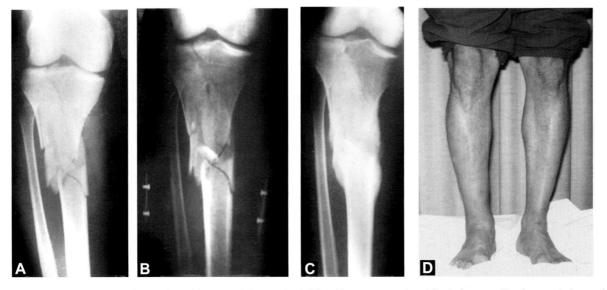

Figs 9.6A to D: (A) Radiograph of comminuted fracture of the proximal tibia without an associated fibula fracture. The fracture is intraarticular as it enters the lateral condyle. (B) The fracture was treated with a below-the-knee functional brace. (C and D) The fracture healed with excellent alignment. Full weight bearing was not permitted till evidence of early callus was documented in order to prevent the angular deformity that frequently occurs when the fibula is intact.

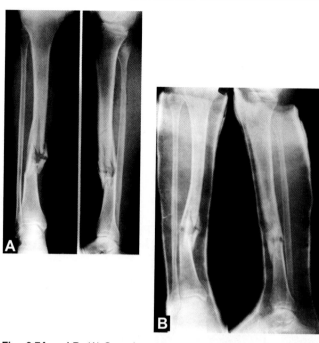

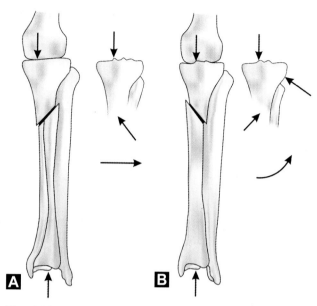

Figs 9.7A and B: (A) Open fracture at the junction of the middle and distal thirds of the tibia, produced by a low-velocity bullet. The fibula is intact. (B) The fracture was treated with a below-the-knee functional cast. A severe varus deformity readily occurred. Open fractures of this type should never be treated in a weight-bearing environment.

Figs 9.9A and B: Drawings depict the mechanism through which deformities may develop with fractures in the proximal-third of the tibia when the fibula is intact. (A) The fracture runs proximally to distal, and from lateral to medial direction, the distal fragment -stabilized by the interosseous membrane- prevents major angular deformity. (B) If the fracture runs proximal to distal from medial to lateral direction, a varus deformity may occur, since the proximal fragment can displace without opposition.

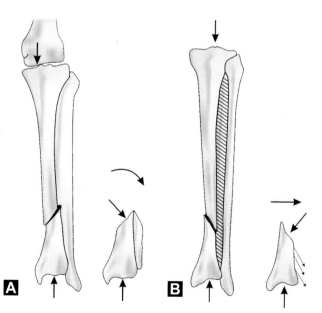

Figs 9.8A and B: (A) Drawing depicting an oblique fracture of the distal tibia running from a proximally to distally and from lateral to medial directions. The distal and shorter fragment angulates toward the fibula without meeting resistance. (B) The fracture, running from proximally to distally, and from a medial to lateral direction cannot angulate severely, because the distal fragment abuts against the long-proximal fragment.

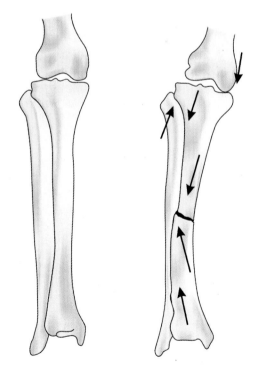

Fig. 9.10: Artist rendition illustrating the mechanism through which a tibial fracture with an intact fibula may develop a varus deformity.

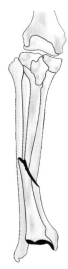

Fig. 9.11: Example of severe deformity that may be seen when the tibial fracture is at a higher level than the metaphyseal region. Since at this level the fibula is significantly more posterior than the tibia at a lower level, the displacement is usually greater.

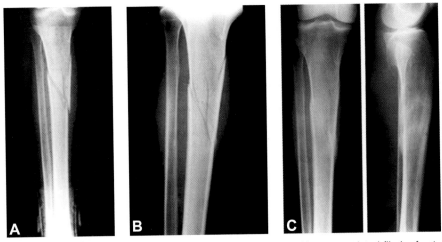

Figs 9.12A to C: a) Radiographs of minimally displaced oblique fracture of the tibia without associated fibular fracture. The direction of the fracture is from lateral to medial, rendering stable against varus angular deformity. (B) Radiograph taken in the below-the-knee functional brace. (C) The fracture healed without angular deformity.

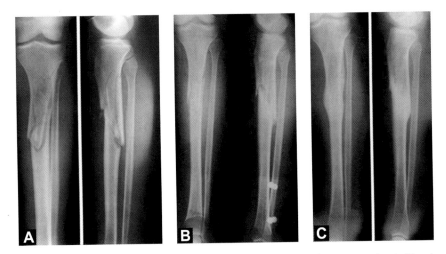

Figs 9.13A to C: Oblique fracture in the proximal-third of the tibia with an intact fibula. The fracture was treated in a brace because there was no angular deformity of any degree following the initial insult. The fracture healed uneventfully.

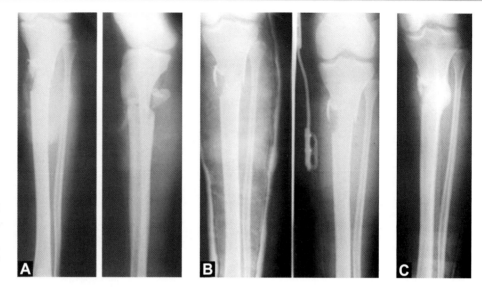

Figs 9.14A to C: Slightly comminuted fracture in the proximal-third of the tibia without an associated fibula fracture, treated with a functional brace. The fracture healed with a few degrees of varus deformity.

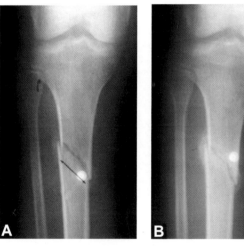

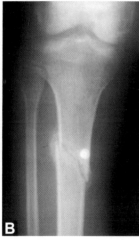

Figs 9.15A and B: (A) Radiograph of oblique fracture of the proximal-third of the tibia with an intact fibula. The obliquity of the fracture from lateral to medial precludes the varus deformity that may occur when the fracture has the opposite direction. (B) The fracture was treated in a below-the-knee functional brace, and healed with excellent alignment.

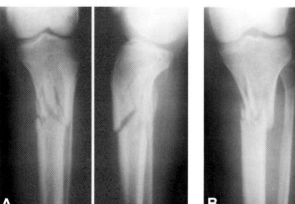

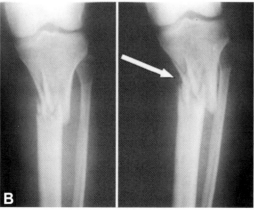

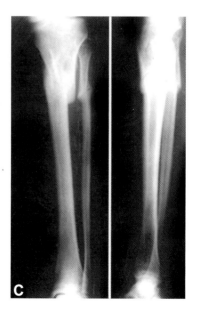

Figs 9.16A to C: (A) Antero-posterior and lateral radiograph of comminuted fracture of the proximal tibia. The absence of a fibular fracture was not recognized at that time. (B) A below-the-knee brace was applied after failing to recognize the absence of a fibular fracture. The fracture immediately angulated into varus. (C) The deformity was corrected manually after a fibular osteotomy was performed. The extremity was once again stabilized in a brace. The fracture healed uneventfully.

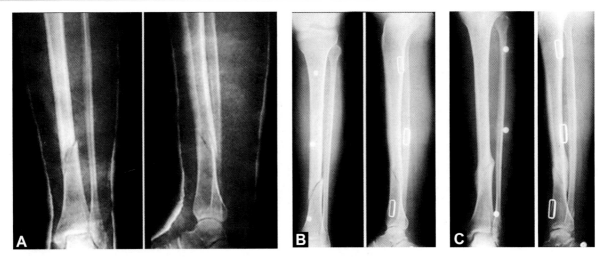

Figs 9.17A to C: (A) Radiograph obtained through a cast of an oblique fracture of the tibia at the junction of the middle and distal fragments, without an associated fibula fracture. (B) Radiograph obtained through the functional brace. (C) Final radiograph showing the fracture solidly united with an almost imperceptible varus deformity.

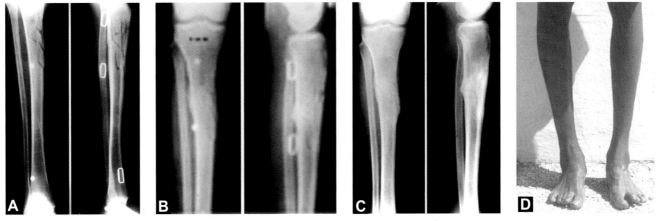

Figs 9.18A to D: (A) Radiograph of comminuted, non-displaced fracture of the proximal tibia with an intact fibula. (B) Radiograph obtained through the functional brace. (C) Radiograph taken upon completion of healing. (D) Appearance of the lower extremities.

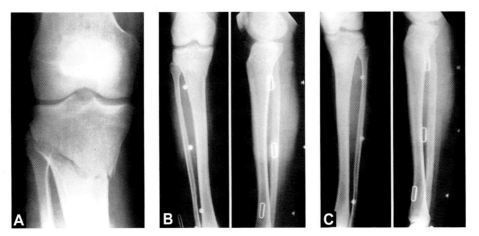

Figs 9.19A to C: (A) Radiograph of fracture of the proximal tibia with an intact fibula. The direction of the fracture, from lateral to medial and from proximal to distally ensures that a varus deformity does not develop under weight bearing. (B) Radiograph obtained through the functional below-the-knee brace. (C) Radiograph taken after completion of healing. Notice the absence of angular deformity.

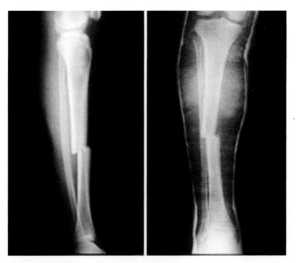

Fig. 9.20: Lateral and antero-posterior views of a transverse tibial fracture with an intact fibula. The final varus deformity is unacceptable. Fractures of this type are best managed with closed intramedullary nailing, recognizing however, that chronic knee pain might develop.

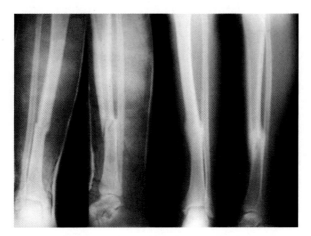

Fig. 9.21: Illustration of a transverse tibial fracture with an intact fibula, demonstrating a mild varus deformity that did not increase with the introduction of graduated weight bearing ambulation.

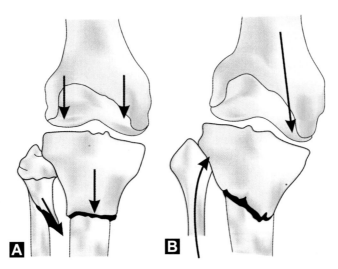

Figs 9.22A and B: Drawings depicting the importance of the fibula in The behavior of tibial fractures. (A) the fractured fibula prevents the development of an angular deformity, (B) The intact fibula creates a mechanical environment leading to a varus angulation.

10

Overall Clinical Experiences

We had an opportunity to carefully review our experiences with the treatment of 1000 closed fractures of the tibia during the senior author's (A.S.) tenure at the University of Southern California/Los Angeles County Medical Center—1979, 1992 – This review was published in a peer review journal.[1] The following is an abbreviated version of the original document. Prior to the University of Southern California experience, the senior author had treated an additional 800 tibial fractures with functional braces, some of which were open fractures.[2-5]

Two thousand three hundred and eighty four closed tibial fractures were treated with functional braces. Follow-up was possible for 1000 patients to completion of treatment with adequate radiographs and clinical records. From this group, 40 patients (4%) were excluded, 32 patients for whom data was incomplete and eight patients who had been treated with external fixation prior to treatment in a fracture brace.

Of the remaining 960 patients, there were 218 females and 742 males, aged between 14 to 85 years (mean = 33 $\pm$ 13 years). The mechanism of injury was related to vehicular accident in 45% of injuries (motor vehicle accident, auto versus pedestrian, and auto versus bicycle). The remaining 55% of injuries were either from falls (37%) or direct blow to the leg (8%).

At follow-up, if length and alignment were considered acceptable and pain and swelling had subsided, a pre-fabricated functional brace was applied. This was done between 1.4 and 23 weeks (mean = 3.7 weeks) following injury. In most cases, it was possible to apply the brace before the end of the second week. However, if the extremity was still significantly swollen and painful, the bracing was postponed for an additional week or two.

METHODS AND ANALYSIS RESULTS

For the group of 960 patients, healing time ranged from 6.7 to 75 weeks, with a mean of 18.1 weeks and a mode of 13.4 weeks. Delayed union (healing time greater than 30 weeks) was seen in 58 patients (6%); nonunion in 10 tibias (1.04%); final shortening more than 20 mm was measured in 13 tibias (1.4%). Angulation greater than 7° of varus was measured in 87 tibias (9.05%); and more than 7° of valgus in 17 tibias (1.77%); anterior apex angulation greater than 10° was seen in 17 tibias (1.77%); with posterior apex more than 10° in 29 tibias (3.2%). From the original group of 1000 patients, the brace was discontinued due to inability to control angulation in 13 (1.35%) patients.

Student's t-test and chi-square analyses were used to compare the effect of patient and fracture characteristics on final outcome.

FACTORS INFLUENCING HEALING TIME

Healing times longer than 30 weeks were observed in 58 (6%) of 960 patients. A higher percentage of patients with high energy fractures had delayed union as compared with low energy fractures. Specifically, the probability of delayed union in high-energy injuries was 10%, more than double that in low-energy fractures (4%), (P = 0.01). Additionally, delayed union was observed more commonly in comminuted and segmental fractures than in oblique or spiral fractures. Specifically, the probability of delayed union was 9% and 21% in comminuted and segmental fractures respectively, compared with 5% and 2% with oblique and spiral fractures respectively (P = 0.001). The probability of delayed union in transverse fractures was 6% (Figures 10.1 and 10.2).

No statistical correlation was observed between delayed union and gender (P = 0.96), fibular condition (P = 0.36), and angulation in any plane (P = 0.55). While not statistically significant (P = 0.29), the probability of delayed union in mid-shaft fractures was 7% compared with 5% in distal fractures.

Student's t-test comparing patients with less than 30 weeks healing time to patients with more than 30 weeks healing time demonstrated no statistically significant differences in mean age, initial displacement, initial shortening, or initial angulation. However, time to bracing was significantly less in patients with healing time less than 30 weeks. That is, mean time to bracing was 3.5 weeks ?2.6 in patients with healing times less than 30 weeks, compared with 7.0 weeks ?9.2 in patients with healing times more than 30 weeks.

Factors Influencing Nonunion

There were 10 nonunions (1.04%). Perhaps because of the small group size, it was difficult to statistically assess the relative influence of factors affecting the incidence of non union. Of the 10 non-unions, seven were in males, three in females. There were five high energy, one medium energy, and four low energy injuries. There were three comminuted, four oblique and three transverse fractures. Four were in the distal-third of the tibia, five in the middle-third, and one in the proximal-third. The fibula was fractured in nine and intact in one. None of the above correlations were found to be statistically significant (P > 0.3). In addition t-testing demonstrated no significant correlations (P > 0.13).

Factors Influencing Final Shortening ≥ 20 mm

There were 13 patients with final shortening ≥ to 20 mm (1.35%). By chi-square analysis, there were no statistical correlations between final shortening and gender, energy of injury, fracture type, fracture location, or initial angulation (P > 0.18). All fractures with final shortening ≥ 20 mm had an associated fibular fracture (Figure 10.3).

Student t-test demonstrated correlations between increased final shortening and age, time to bracing, initial displacement, and initial shortening.

As shown in our previous study,[6] in 95% of the 960 fractures, the final shortening was less than 12 mm. The overall mean final shortening was 4.28 mm, compared with mean initial shortening of 4.25 mm. This confirmed our long-held hypothesis that in closed diaphyseal tibial fractures treated with functional bracing, final shortening does not increase beyond initial shortening with graduated weight-bearing activities.[3,4,7-9]

Factors Influencing Brace Discontinuance

From the initial group of 1000 patients, the fracture brace was discontinued for 13 (1.3%) of the patients for inability to control angulation. The brace was discontinued in 12 males and one female. There were six high energy, one medium energy, and six low energy injuries. Six were comminuted fractures, three were oblique, one was segmental, and three were transverse. Five fractures were located in the distal-third, six in the middle-third, and two in the proximal-third. The fibula was intact in two and fractured in the remainder. None of the above correlation were statistically significant, (P > 0.14). In addition, student's t-test demonstrated no correlations between the incidence of brace discontinuation and age, time to bracing, initial displacement, initial shortening, and initial angulation (P > 0.22).

Factors Influencing Final Coronal Angulation (Varus/Valgus)

There were 367 fractures (33%) that healed with no angulation in the coronal plane. Final varus angulation was observed in 322 (48%) fractures. There were 87 (9.06%) patients with varus ≥ 7°, and 17 (1.77%) patients with final valgus angulation ≥ 7°. Final varus ≥ 7° occurred more commonly in patients who had initial varus angulation or initial posterior angulation (P < 0.001), and in those who had initial displacement (P = 0.005). Mean displacement in the group with < 7° was 27% ? 25%, compared with 36% ? 25% in the group with ≥ 7° final varus angulation.

Similarly, final valgus angulation ≥ 7° occurred more frequently with initial valgus angulation and those with initial anterior angulation, (P = 0.01) (Figures 10.4A to C).

It should be noted that in fractures of the tibia with intact fibula, particularly those with initial varus deformity, the deformity may increase further into varus.[10,11] Because of our awareness of this risk, a number of such fractures were initially treated by means of closed intramedullary nailing, and were therefore neither braced nor included in this study.

Factors Influencing Sagittal Angulattion (Anterior/Posterior)

There were 17 (1.77%) tibias with final anterior angulation ≥ 10°, and 29 (3.02%) tibias with final posterior angulation ≥ 10°. Final anterior angulation ≥ 10° occurred more commonly in middle-third fractures (P = 0.004) and in those with initial anterior angulation as well as those with initial horizontal displacement. (P = 0.03). Final posterior angulation ≥ 10° occurred more commonly in high energy fractures (P = 0.02), as well as those with initial posterior angulation (P = 0.001).

DISCUSSION

The results of this study demonstrate that appropriate patient selection is critical to satisfactory outcome with functional bracing (Figures 10.5A to F). Both patient characteristics and fracture attributes were found to correlate with outcome.

While some correlations were found between fracture and patient characteristics and final outcome, it should be emphasized that these were correlations and not absolute predictors of ultimate anatomic deviation.

For the different outcome variables, the rate of outcome outside of the arbitrarily determined parameters ranged from 1 to 9.1%. The two most frequent categories in the outside group were final varus ≥ 7° and healing time greater than 30 weeks. High energy injuries were correlated with healing times greater than 30 weeks, as were segmental and comminuted fractures, consistent with the energy required to produce this fracture pattern. As these fractures did go on to eventual healing, perhaps the definition of delayed union should be extended for this fracture type.

Our studies have shown that, in closed diaphyseal tibial fractures, the initial shortening remains unchanged. This indicates that only transverse fractures that are reduced and stabilized, or axially unstable fractures with initially acceptable shortening should be braced. Traction applied to regain length in axially unstable fractures results in recurrence to the original shortening upon the introduction of early weight bearing forces.[9,12-14]

Sagittal posterior angular deformities may often be a result of immobilization of the ankle in equinus in the original cast. In such a case, upon removal of the cast and the subsequent application of the brace, the patient first bears weight on the ball of the foot rather than on the heel, resulting in bending stresses that tend to produce a posterior deformity at the fracture site. Therefore, when the cast is applied, care must be taken to hold the foot in neutral position.

We have arbitrarily determined, based on ours and other people's observation, that 12 to 15 mm of initial shortening in closed, axially unstable fractures, should not be an indication that other treatment modality is more appropriate based on the perception that such degree of shortening rarely produces a limp or is associated with late adverse sequela. The same applies to angular deformities where 5 to 8° of varus angulation are cosmetically and physiologically acceptable. It is difficult to detect a 5° varus angulation during clinical observation of the extremities. Valgus deformity is more readily recognized, particularly in individuals with slender legs who in addition have a greater than usual valgus knees. People with large, particularly flabby legs, camouflage angular deformities better.

Fractures of the tibia with intact fibula are prone to develop varus angulation.[4,5,15-20] The shortest tibial fragment usually experiences the greatest deviation. Fractures located in the proximal and distal-third of the tibial diaphysis are the ones that usually angulate the most. However, the degree of final angulation is determined by the geometry of the tibial fracture. An oblique tibial fracture where the direction of the fracture is from proximal to distal and from medial to lateral angulates more severely than a similar fracture that runs from lateral to medial. In the latter instance, the proximal fragment abuts against the distal fragment which is made relatively stable by the interosseous membrane.[14,22]

There is no evidence that a few degrees of angular deformity following an extra-articular diaphyseal tibial fracture produces osteoarthritis at a later date. Several comprehensive studies dealing with long-term follow-up of patients, who healed their tibial fractures with residual angulation, failed to demonstrate clinical osteoarthritis.[23,24] Our own experience supports the findings and views reported in that study. We have never seen a patient with knee or ankle degenerative arthritis where the etiology of the condition was traced to an extra-articular diaphyseal fracture of the tibia that healed with less than 10° of angulation. It is not known either how much angular deformity results in late osteoarthritis.

Our own laboratory studies concerning the effect of angulation on the articular cartilage of the knee and ankle joints have shown that angulation of less than 10° produce minimal alteration in force distribution.[25-28]

It is inappropriate to consider any anatomical deviation, a complication, if such a deviation is aesthetically acceptable, does not produce a limp and does not have adverse late pathophysiological sequela. Therefore, tibial angulation of less than 8° and shortening of less than 12 mm should be called ?anatomic deviations rather than complications.

Functional bracing has been used for the treatment of a large number of fractures. However, as it is true for all other treatment modalities, it is not a panacea. Complications and permanent anatomical deviations are encountered with plate osteosynthesis, external fixation, and intramedullary nailing. Current concerns regarding the cost of medical care emphasize the role fracture bracing plays in the management of certain long bone fractures. The system and philosophy of functional bracing must be clearly understood as well as its limitations and contraindications. Proper selection of patients and attentive follow up are an important part of this therapeutic approach. When acceptable fracture shortening or alignment cannot be maintained, a different treatment method should be pursued.

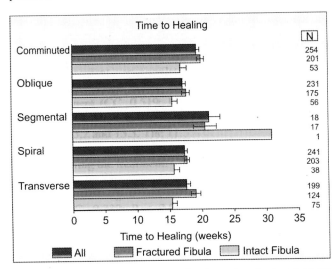

Fig. 10.1: Mean values of time to healing for various fracture type are shown separately for those with fractured and those with intact fibulae, along with standard error of the mean.

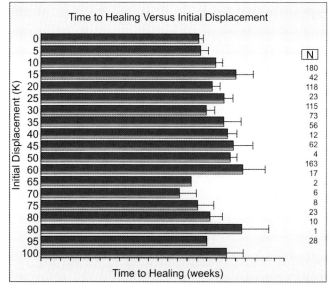

Fig. 10.2: Mean values of time to healing for fractures with different amounts of displacement are shown, along with standard error of the mean.

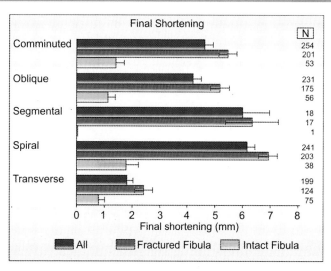

Fig. 10.3: Mean values of final shortening for different fracture types are shown separately for those with fractured and those with intact fibulae, long with standard error of the mean.

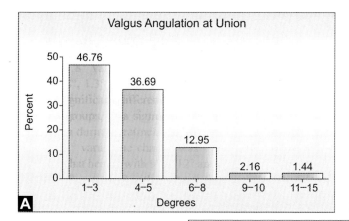

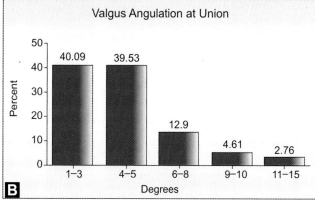

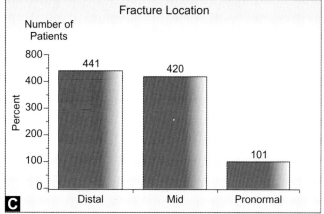

Figs 10.4A to C: Percentage of individual experiencing angulation at union (B) An union angulation at union
(C) Angulation depending on the fracture location

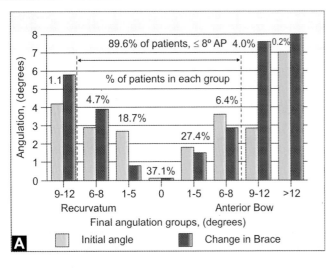

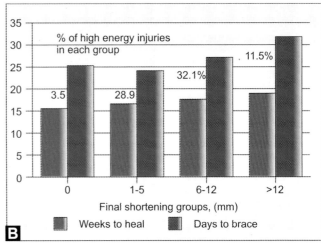

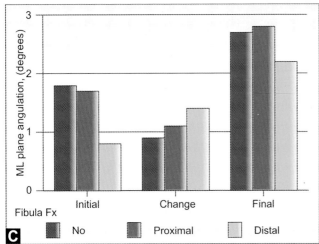

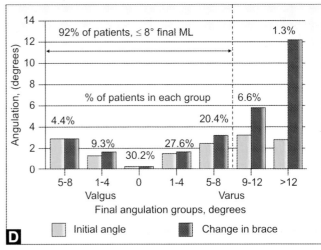

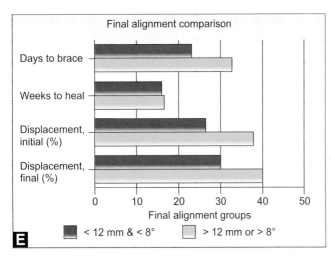

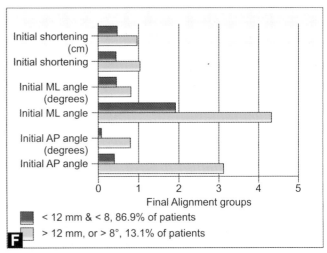

Figs 10.5A to F: Final results of the study based on the amount of shortening and angulation produced

REFERENCES

1. Sarmiento A, Sharpe MD, Ebramzadeh E, Normand P, Shankwiler J. Factors influencing the Outcome of Closed Tibial Fractures Treated with Functional Bracing. Clin Ortho Relat Res. 1995 Jun; (315):8-24.

2. Sarmiento A, Latta LL. Closed Functional Treatment of Fractures. Springer-Verlag: Berlin 1981.

3. Sarmiento A. A Functional Below-Knee Cast for Tibial Fractures. J Bone and Joint Surg. 1967; 59:5.

4. Sarmiento A. A Functional Below-Knee Brace for Tibial Fractures. J. Bone and Joint Surg. 1970; 52(2):295-311.

5. Sarmiento A. Functional Bracing of Tibial and Femoral Shaft Fractures. Clin Orthop Relat Res. 1972; 82:2-13.

6. Court-Brown CM, Will E, Christie J, McQueen M. Reamed or unreamed nailing for closed tibial fractures. J. Bone and Joint Surg. July 1996; 78B:580-3.

7. Sarmiento A, Schaeffer J, Beckerman L, Latta LL, Enis J. Fracture Healing in Rat Femora as Affected by Functional Weight Bearing. J. Bone Joint Surg Am, 1977; 59(3):369-75.

8. Sarmiento A, Mullis DL, Latta LL, Alvarez RR. A Quantitative, Comparative Analysis of Fracture Healing Under the Influence of Compression Plating vs. Closed Weight-Bearing Treatment. Clin Orthop. 1980; 149:232.

9. Sarmiento A, Latta L, Zilioli A, Sinclair WM F. The Role of Soft Tissues in the Stabilization of Tibial Fractures. Clin Orthop Relat Res. 1974; 105:116-29.

10. Cole D, Latta LL. Fatigue failure of interlocking tibial nail implants. Orthop Trans Bone Joint Surg. 1992; 16-3A:663.

11. Court-Brown CM, Gustilo T, Shaw AD. Knee pain after intramedullary nailing of proximal third tibia fractures. J Orthop Trauma. 1997; 11:103-105.

12. Latta LL, Sarmiento A. Mechanical Behavior of Tibial Fractures. Symposium on Trauma to the Leg and Its Sequela. C.V. Mosby: St. Louis, MO 1981.

13. Orfaly R, Keating JE, O'Brien PJ. Knee pain after tibial nailing: Does the entry point matter? J Bone Joint Surg Br. 1995; 77(6):976-7.

14. Sarmiento A, Latta LL. On the evolution of fracture bracing. J Bone Joint Surg Br. 2006; 88-8(2):141-8.

15. Bonnevialle P, Bellumore Y, Foucras L, Hezard L, Mansat M. Tibial fractures with intact fibula treated by reamed nailing. Rev Chir Orthop Reparatrice Appar Mot. 2000; 86(1):29-37.

16. Dehne E. Treatment of Fractures of the Tibial Shaft. Clin Orthop. 1969; 66:159.

17. Rosa G, Savarese A, Chianca I, Coppola D. Treatment of Fractures of the Lower Limbs with Functional Braces. Et al J Orthop Traumatol. 1982 Sep; 8(3):301-8.

18. Sarmiento A, Latta LL. Functional Bracing in Management of Tibial Fractures. The Intact Fibula. AAOS Symposium on Trauma of the Leg and Its Sequela. Moore TM (Ed). The C.V. Mosby Company. 1981; 278-98.

19. Sarmiento A, Latta LL. Closed fractures of the middle third of the tibia treated with a functional Brace. Clin Orthop. 2008 Dec; 466:3108-15.

20. Sarmiento A, Latta LL. 450 Closed Fractures of the distal third of the tibia treated with a functional brace. Clin Orthop. 2004; 428: 261-71.

21. Sarmiento A, Latta LL. Functional Fracture Bracing. The Tibia, Humerus and Ulna. Springer-Verlag 1992.

22. Sarmiento A. On the behavior of closed tibial fractures: clinical and radiological correlations. J Orthop Trauma, 2000; 14(3):199-205.

23. Ricciardi-Pollini PT, Falez F. The Treatment of Diaphyseal Fractures by Functional Bracing. Results in 36 Cases. Ital J Orthop Traumatol. 1985 Jun; 11(2):199-205.

24. Mawhinney IN, Maginn P, McCoy GF. Tibial compartment syndromes after tibial nailing. J Orthop Trauma. 1994; 8(3):212-14.

25. McCollough NC, Vinsant JE, Sarmiento A. Functional Fracture - Bracing of Long-bone Fractures of the Lower Extremity in Children. J Bone Joint Surg. 1978; 60A:314.

26. McKellop HA, Hoffmann R, Sarmiento A, Lu B, Ebramzadeh E. Control of Motion of Tibial Fractures with Use of a Functional Brace or an External Fixator. J Bone & Joint Surg. 1993 Jul; 75A:1019-25.

27. Rankin, EA, Metz CW Jr. Management of delayed union in early weight-bearing treatment of the fractured tibia. J. Trauma. 1970 Sep; 10(9):751-9.

28. Tarr RR, Resnick CT, Wagner KS, Sarmiento A. Changes in Tibiotalar Joint Contact Areas Following Experimentally Induced Tibial Angular Deformities. Clin Orthop. 1985; 199:72.

11

Fractures in the Proximal-third and Representative Examples

It is well known that fractures of the tibia, located in its proximal-third are the ones most likely to present difficulties during intramedullary nailing.[1-13] With closed functional treatment, we have also encountered some difference in the ultimate angular deformity, but of a minimal degree. The difficulties increase when the fibula is intact. The realization that the intact fibula plays a major role in determining the angular behavior of tibial fractures, we have concluded that in the absence of a fibular fracture, functional bracing should not be carried out unless the initial radiograph shows no angular deformity of any degree.

We treated 110 skeletally mature patients with proximal-third diaphyseal fractures of the tibia with functional bracing from June 1983 to June 1992. The following is an abbreviated version of published article dealing with the subject at hand.[14]

The age of the patients ranged from 16 to 82 years with a mean of 36.3 years. Associated injuries occurred in 18 patients. Nineteen patients (17.6%) were females and 89 (82.4%) were males.

Fractures were classified according to configuration, association to fibular fracture and mechanism of injury (high or low energy trauma). Multivariate analysis was used to determine association between variables.

The time of application of the brace ranged from 4 days to 19.1 weeks, with an average of 31.3 days and a mode of 11 days. Eighty-four of the patients (80%) had the brace applied within the first 6 weeks. X-rays were taken after the application of the brace to confirm maintenance of acceptable alignment.

The left side was involved in 45 patients (42%) and the right in 63 patients (58%). The energy of trauma was defined as high in 71 patients (65.7%), and low in 37 patients (34.3%). The mechanism of injury was defined as low energy of trauma when a direct blow or fall caused the fracture. High-energy trauma was defined when the injury resulted from a motor vehicle accident, motorcycle accident or pedestrian-vehicle accident.

Forty-five fractures (42%) were comminuted; 35 (31%) were oblique; 20 (19%) were transverse; 4% were segmental and 4% were spiral. An associated fibular fracture was present in 73 patients (68%): 66 fractures were located in the proximal third, four in the middle third and three in the distal third. Shortening was measured in the initial x-rays in millimeters between the edges of clearly defined fragments. Displacement was defined as a percentage of the amount of translation of the fragments with respect to the width of the bone at the level of the fracture and was measured in antero-posterior and lateral x-rays. Angulation was measured in degrees following the longitudinal axis of the main fragments.

The initial displacement of the fragments ranged from 0 to 100% with an average of 20.08%. Seventeen fractures (16%) had an initial displacement of greater or equal to 50%. Initial shortening ranged from 0 to 15 mm with an average of 3.86 mm. Nineteen fractures (18%) had initial shortening equal to or greater than 10 mm. Thirty-two fractures (30%) had an initial valgus angulation that ranged from 0 to 25° with an average of 5.58°; 24 fractures (22%) had an initial varus angulation that ranged from 0 to 10° with an average of 5.61°. There were 21 fractures (19%) with a posterior angulation that ranged from 0 to 12° with an average of 4.4°; 30 fractures (28%) had an initial anterior angulation that ranged from 0 to 15° with an average of 5.63°.

Fracture union was determined when the patient was pain-free while bearing full weight, no motion could be clinically demonstrated at the fracture site and peripheral callus bridging was confirmed on x-rays; nonetheless, patients were encouraged to continue wearing the brace until callus maturation was evidenced. We defined time to union as the number of weeks that transpired from the day of the fracture to the day of discontinuation of the brace.

PATIENT AND FRACTURE VARIABLES

One hundred and eight patients (98%) were followed to completion of treatment.

Patient and fracture variables included in the study were age, side of injury, type of fracture (transverse, oblique, comminuted, spiral or segmental), initial displacement, initial shortening, initial angulation (both frontal and sagittal planes), and associated injuries.

Energy of trauma was correlated with the type of fracture. In high-energy trauma, the most frequent type of fracture was comminuted (34 fractures, 48%), while in low-energy trauma, the most frequent type was an oblique fracture in 17 patients (48%). Three patients (3%) required change from the brace to a cast temporarily in order to ensure adequate reduction, and subsequently were placed in the brace to completion of the treatment. Two other patients (2%) presented skin breakdown as a complication caused by pressure from the brace; they were treated by padding of the brace around the injured skin and with dressing changes until they healed. There were no compartment syndromes found in the patients included in the study.

FRACTURE OUTCOMES

Outcome variables were defined as healing time, final shortening, and final angulation and displacement both in the frontal and sagittal planes. The differences among mean values of outcome variables were compared using analysis of variance followed by the least significant difference method in order to determine which groups demonstrated differences in outcome. Associations between variables were assessed with Chi-square and Student's t-test. Statistical significance was determined through the P value.

Healing of the fractures took place from 6.6 weeks to 40.5 weeks, with an average of 17.1 weeks, and a mode of 11.6 weeks. Three fractures (2.8%) required discontinuation of the conservative treatment and had some form of surgery. One of these was treated with a fibular ostectomy and then was treated with functional bracing. Another patient was treated with interfragmentary screw fixation because of loss of reduction, which could not be manipulated; and the third patient was treated with bone grafting followed by functional bracing. All three fractures healed following these interventions.

Final shortening of the fractures ranged from 0 to 20 mm with an average of 3.6 mm. Ninety-seven fractures (92%) healed with shortening of 10 mm or less.

Twenty-eight fractures (26.7%) healed with no displacement in any of the planes. The average final displacement was 19.4%.

No angulation in the frontal plane was seen in 46 fractures (43.8%). Twenty-two patients (21%) had a valgus angulation with a range from 0 to 11° and an average of 3.9°. Thirty-seven (35.2%) fractures healed with varus angulation averaging 5.61°, ranging from 0 to 15°. Thirteen fractures (12.3%) had angulation of more than 6° in the coronal plane; most of these were in varus (10 fractures).

In the sagittal plane, no final angulation was seen in 58 fractures (55.2%). Final posterior angulation or recurvatum was seen in 17 fractures (16.2%) with a range from 0 to 10° and an average of 4.6°. Final anterior angulation or antecurvatum was encountered in 30 fractures (28.6%) with a range from 0 to 11° and an average of 4.5°.

CLINICAL RESULTS

Healing Time

Fracture type was associated with time to union. Comminuted and transverse fractures had an increased time to healing with 18.1 and 17.1 weeks respectively. The shortest average time to union was found in oblique fractures with 15.6 weeks.

Energy of trauma was also associated to the time to union. Low-energy trauma resulted in union of the fracture in an average of 15.2 weeks while high-energy trauma led to union at an average time of 18.1 weeks. This difference was statistically significant (P = 0.03).

The presence of a fibular fracture was significantly associated to delayed healing with an average of 18.3 weeks while patients without it healed their fractures in an average of 14.9 weeks (P = 0.02).

The age of the patients was not associated to the time to union. When 30 years of age was used as a cutting point, we found that average time of healing below that age was 16.6 weeks compared to 17.4 weeks for patients above 30 (P = 0.755).

The time transpired from the fracture to the day of bracing had a direct association to the number of weeks to union, and this difference was statistically significant with P < 0.0005.

Final Shortening

Final shortening was associated with the energy of trauma, fracture type, initial displacement and association to a fibular fracture. The average final shortening in patients with high-energy trauma was 4.8 mm while that of those patients with low-energy trauma was 1 mm (P < 0.001). Those patients with an associated fibular fracture presented a mean final shortening of 4.9 mm while those without it had an average final shortening of 0.9 mm (P < 0.001). The patients with a distal fibular fracture (three patients) did not have any shortening on the final radiological evaluation; there was no statistically significant difference in shortening between patients who had a concomitant fibular fracture in the middle or upper thirds of the bone. Patients who had an initial displacement of less than 50% had an average final shortening of 2.5 mm, while those patients with greater than 50% of initial displacement resulted in an average shortening of 9.1 mm (P < 0.001). Finally, shortening was greater with segmental fractures, followed by spiral and comminuted fractures.

Final Angulation

There were no associations between final anterior and posterior angulation and final varus-valgus angulation, displacement or shortening. Final angulation varied according to the presence of fibular fracture. On average, final angulation with a concomitant fibular fracture was 1° of varus; without a fibular fracture, it was 1.4°. Analyzing patients with a fibular fracture, we found that those patients that initially had varus or valgus angulation had a tendency to correct the degree of initial angulation. Of the 26 patients that had a neutral initial alignment, nine progressed to a varus angulation of an average of 6.1°, while the others maintained their neutral alignment.

There was no association between presence of a fibular fracture and a greater incidence of anterior or posterior angulation.

Final Displacement

Associations were found between the amount of initial displacement and final displacement as well as between energy of trauma and final displacement. Patients with an initial displacement of less than 50% healed with a final displacement of 14.4% in average, while those with an initial displacement of more than 50% healed with an average of 45.2%; this difference was statistically significant (P < 0.001). Patients with a high energy of trauma had a final displacement of 23.6% and those with low-energy of 10.9% (P < 0.001).

DISCUSSION

In our study, complications were limited to superficial skin breakdown, which was readily treated by padding of the brace and observation, and nonunion, which was low (2.8%), and the patients were then treated surgically with a subsequent course to union. We did not find compartment syndromes in the patients treated with the brace. If a patient developed a compartment syndrome at the time of presentation, fasciotomy was performed and the patient was not included in the study. Only 12% of the fractures healed with an angulation of more than 6° in the frontal plane, and most of these cases had a varus angulation.

Recent report by Downing et al concludes that there is no difference in the overall cost to the community between patients treated with casting and those with intramedullary nailing. The study is based on a small series of patients and even though it includes calculations on the impact of lost work days with the primary treatment, it does not include the costs that could be raised by complications like infection, need for hardware removal or nail exchange. We have calculated

previously the difference in cost between functional bracing and intramedullary nailing, revealing a significantly lower cost with the former. Age did not affect the healing time; this concept is frequently misunderstood. In children, there is no doubt that healing of fractures takes place quicker when comparing them to adults, but at least as far as the tibia is concerned, age does not seem to affect the healing time in a population of adults.

The time of application of the brace also affected the time to healing. This emphasizes the importance of early motion and weight bearing in the healing of fractures.

It is important to mention that the patients included in this study were not consecutive patients. Some patients might have escaped conservative management due to the fact that they were not suitable for conservative treatment from the beginning, mainly because of initial unacceptable shortening or in polytrauma patients with a clear initial surgical indication. Otherwise the studied population is comparable to the more frequent isolated closed tibial fractures with minimally associated injuries.

REPRESENTATIVE EXAMPLES

Some of the representative examples illustrating the fractures in proximal-third of tibia are shown in Figures 11.1 to 11.18.

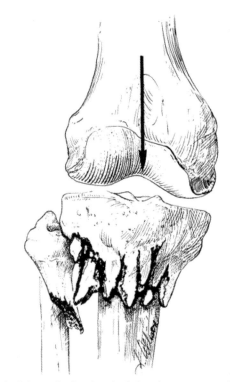

Fig. 11.1: Schematic drawing depicting the presence of a proximal tibial fracture associated with a fracture of the fibula. The fibula fracture prevents the varus deformity frequently seen when the fibula is intact.

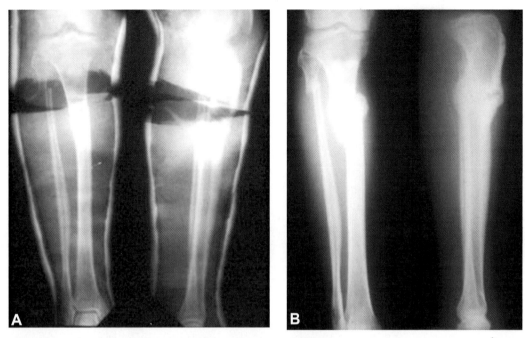

Figs 11.2A and B: (A) Radiograph of slightly oblique fracture of the proximal tibia and an associated fibular fracture. Initially obtained alignment was improved by wedging above-the-knee cast. (B) Following correction of angular deformity, a below-the-knee functional cast was applied. The fracture healed with excellent alignment and produced very acceptable shortening.

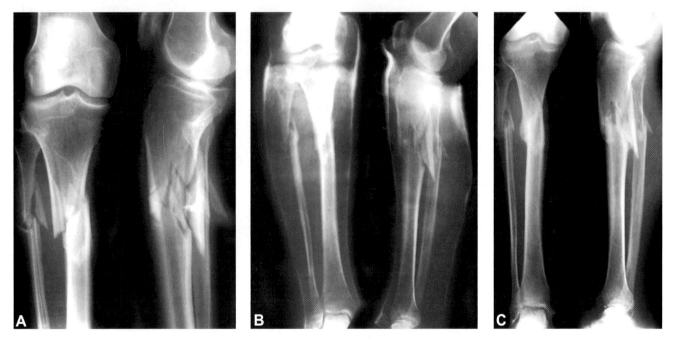

Fig. 11.3A to C: (A) Radiograph of a comminuted fracture of the proximal-third of the tibia and an associated fibula fracture. The patient was a 57-year-old blind man. (B) The fracture was treated with a below-the-knee functional cast. The fracture healed with excellent alignment and with the minimal shortening that developed at the time of the initial injury. (C) Appearance of the extremities. Notice the mild shortening of the injured extremity.

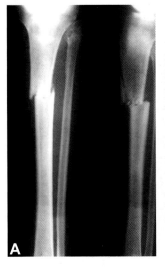
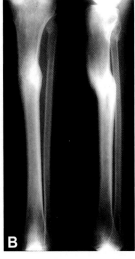
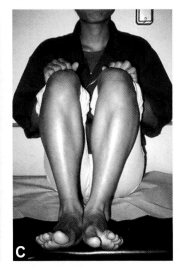

Figs 11.4A to C: (A) Antero-posterior and lateral radiographs of transverse fracture of the proximal-third of the tibia without an associated fracture of the fibula. The fracture translatory deformity was manually corrected and stabilized in an above-the-knee cast. (B) As soon as the acute symptoms improved, the cast was replaced with a below-the-knee functional brace. (C) The fracture healed in excellent alignment.

Figs 11.5A to F: (A) Antero-posterior and lateral radiographs of comminuted fracture of the proximal tibia with an associated fibular fracture. Notice the translatory deformity but the minimal amount of shortening. (B) The fracture was treated in a below-the-knee functional brace after the translatory deformity was partially corrected at the time of application of the initial above-the-knee cast. (C) Radiographs taken after solid union of the fracture had developed. Notice the satisfactory alignment of the fragments and the maintenance of the initial shortening. (D to F) Photographs of the patient's lower extremity demonstrating excellent cosmetic and functional appearance of the fractured extremity.

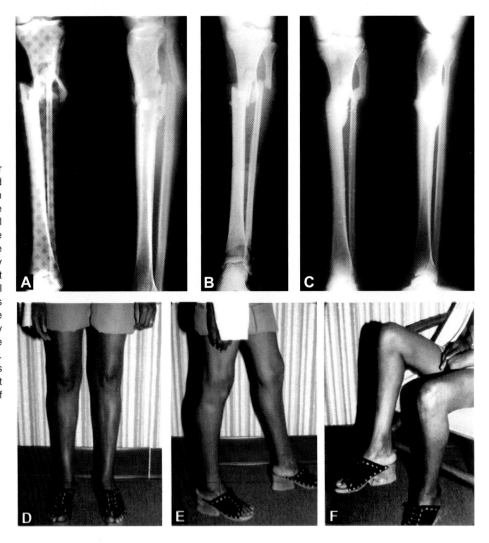

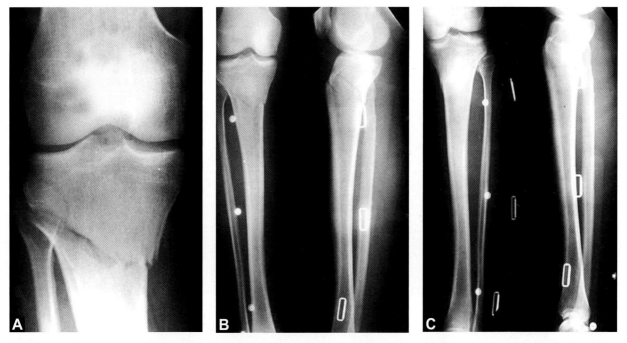

Figs 11.6A to C: (A) Fracture of the tibia running from lateral to medial—a direction that precludes or reduces the possibility of varus angulation. (B) Radiograph obtained 3 weeks later. (C) Radiograph showing the healed fracture without angular deformity.

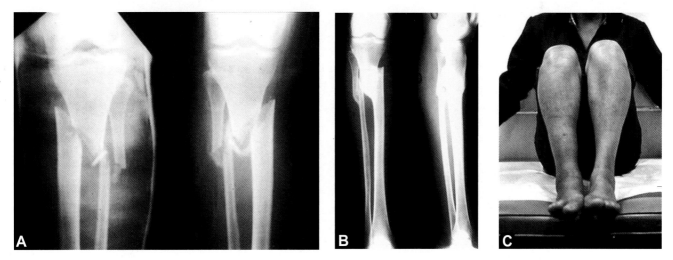

Figs 11.7A to C: (A) Radiograph illustrating a fracture in the proximal-third of the tibia and fibula. The significant shortening as expected because the patient was first seen by us 3 weeks after the initial insult. (B) The fracture healed without additional shortening. Notice the difference in the length of the lower extremities, which the patient initially compensated with a lift in the shoe. (C) At a later date, the lift was discarded as he felt the length discrepancy did not make him limp.

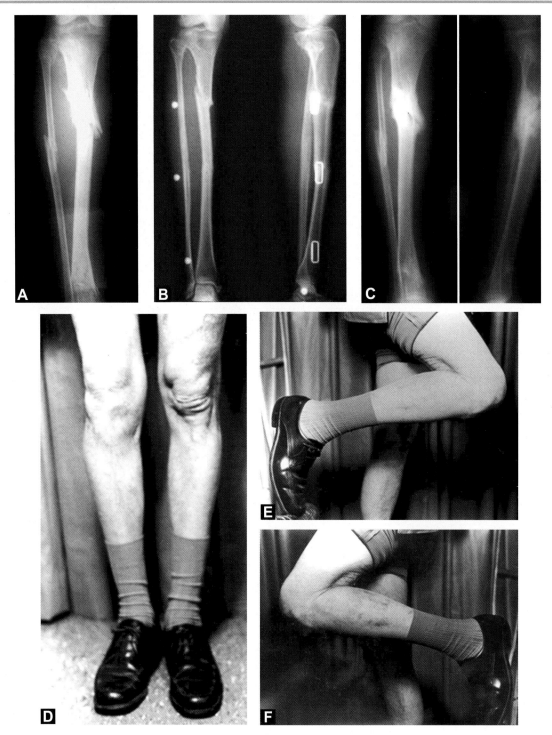

Figs 11.8A to F: (A) Radiograph of comminuted fracture of the proximal-third of the tibia with an associated fracture of the fibula. (B) Radiographs obtained after the application of a below-the-knee functional brace. (C) The fracture healed with excellent alignment and showed no additional shortening. (D to F) Photos of both lower extremities.

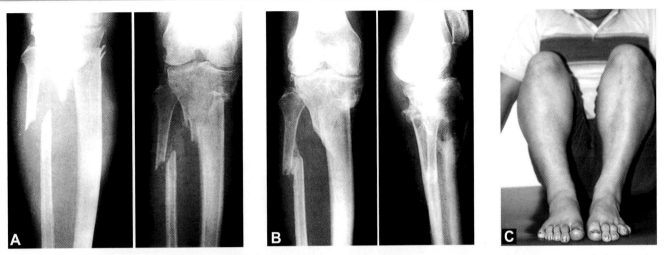

Figs 11.9A to C: (A) Radiograph of oblique fracture of the proximal tibia with associated fibular fracture. (B) The fracture was manipulated under heavy sedation and reduced in a stable manner. The limb was first stabilized in an above-the-knee cast for 2 weeks and then replaced with a below-the-knee brace. (C) The fracture healed with excellent alignment and function.

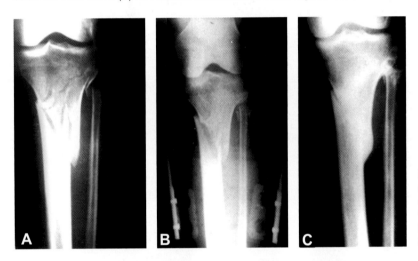

Figs 11.10A to C: (A) Radiograph of slightly comminuted fracture of the proximal tibia with an associated fracture of the neck of the fibula. (B) The fracture was treated in a below-the-knee functional brace. (C) The fracture healed with an excellent alignment.

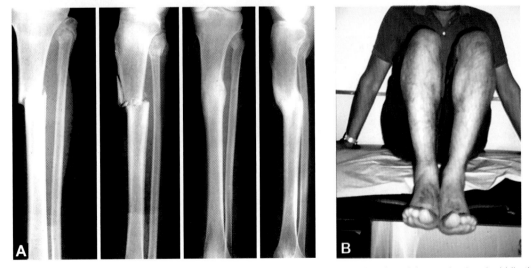

Figs 11.11A and B: (A) Composite of radiograph of transverse fracture of the tibia at the junction of the proximal and middle-thirds. The proximal fibula sustained an impacted fracture. (B) Patient shows the acceptable cosmesis of his injured extremity.

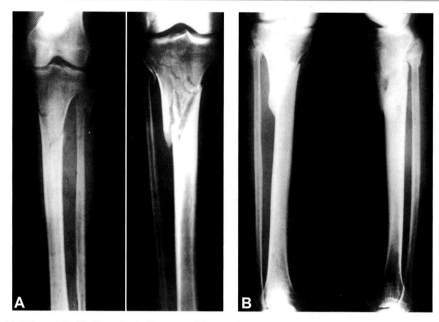

Figs 11.12A and B: (A) Comminuted fracture of the proximal tibia with an associated fracture of the fibula. (B) The fracture healed with good alignment.

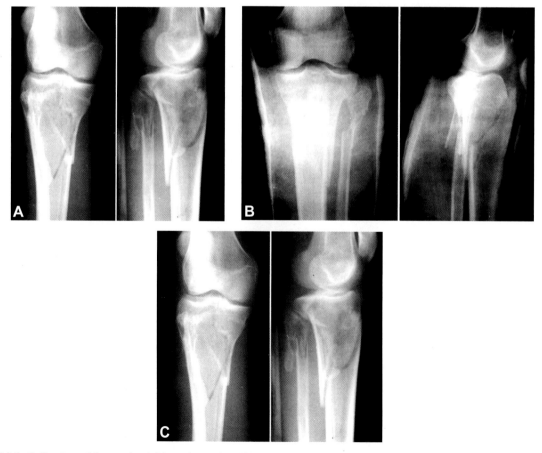

Figs 11.13A to C: Fracture of the proximal tibia and associated fibular fracture treated with a below-the-knee functional cast. The last films were taken 6 weeks after the initial injury. No further follow-up was possible.

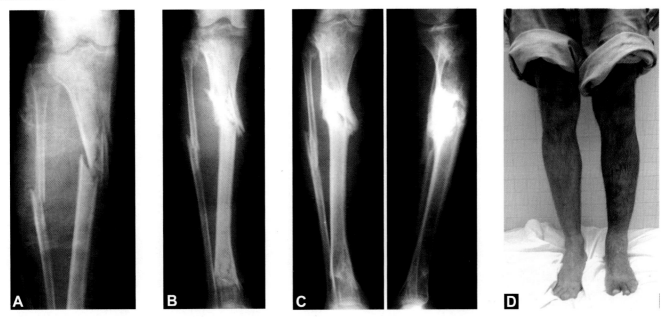

Figs 11.14A to D: (A) Radiograph of comminuted fracture in the proximal-third of the tibia with an associated fibula fracture. (B) The fracture was treated in a functional brace. (C) Radiograph illustrating the final appearance of the healed fracture. (D) Appearance of the patient's lower extremities. Notice the still swollen right leg.

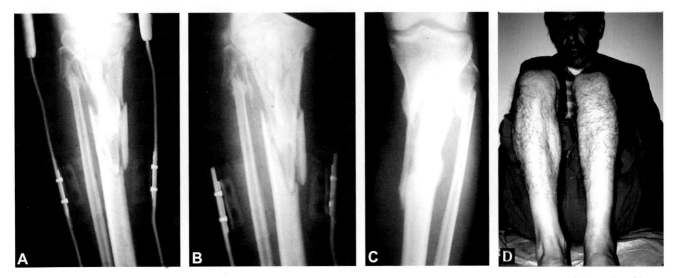

Figs 11.15A to D: (A) radiograph of open (Grade 1) comminuted fracture of the left tibia with approximately less than 1 cm of shortening. Picture was taken through the brace, which was initially constructed with a thigh corset. (B) The corset was removed 4 weeks after its addition. (C) The fracture healed with approximately 1.5 cm of shortening. (D) Patient demonstrates the cosmetic appearance of the extremity and the resulting inconsequential shortening.

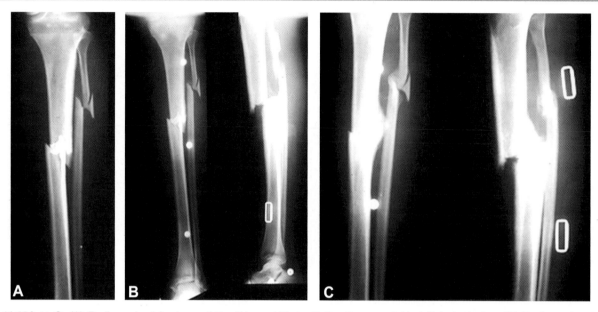

Figs 11.16A to C: (A) Radiograph of fractures of the tibia and fibula. Notice the acceptable initial shortening. (B) Radiographs obtained after application of the functional brace. (C) Final radiographs obtained after completion of healing. Notice that the initial shortening did not increase.

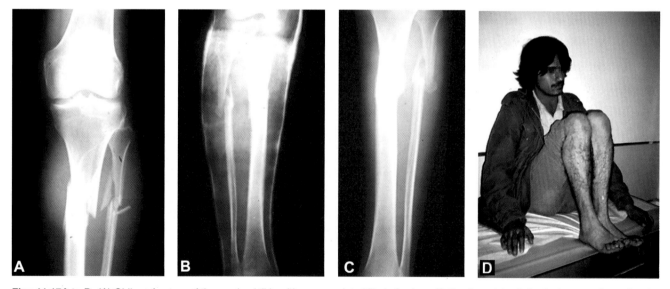

Figs 11.17A to D: (A) Oblique fracture of the proximal tibia with an associated fibula fracture. Notice the minimal shortening experienced at the time of the initial insult. (B) Radiograph obtained after the application of the below-the-knee functional cast. (C) Radiograph showing the healed fractures without additional shortening or angulation. (D) Patient demonstrating the apparent equal length of his lower extremities.

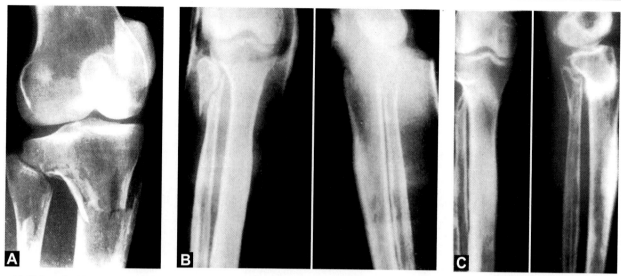

Figs 11.18A to C: (A) Radiograph of slightly comminuted fracture of the proximal tibia associated with an oblique fracture of the fibula. (B) Radiograph obtained after the application of the below-the-knee functional cast. (C) Radiograph illustrating the healed fractures without additional shortening or angulation.

REFERENCES

1. Alho A, Eckeland A, Stromsoe K, Folleras G, Thorensen B. Locked intramedullary nailing of tibial fractures. J Bone Joint Surg. 1990; 72B:805-11.
2. Buehler KC, Green J, Woll TS, Duwelius PJ. A technique for intramedullary nailing of proximal third tibia fractures. J Orthop Trauma. 1997; 11(3):218-23.
3. De Smet K, Mostert AK, De Witte J, De Brauwer V, Verdonk R. Closed intramedullary tibial nailing using the Marchetti-Vicenzi nail. Injury. 2000; 31(8):597-603.
4. Finkemeier CG, Schmidt AH, Kyle RF, Templeman DC, Varecka TF. A prospective, randomized study of intramedullary nails inserted with and without reaming for the treatment of open and closed fractures of the tibial shafts. J Orthop Trauma. 2000; 14 (3):187-93.
5. Freedman EL, Johnson EE. Radiographic analysis of tibial fracture malalignment following intramedullary nailing. Clin Orthop Relat Res. 1995; 315:25-33.
6. Gregory P, Sanders R. The treatment of closed, unstable tibial shaft fractures with unreamed interlocking nails. Clin Orthop Relat Res. 1995; 315:48-55.
7. Habernek H, Kwansy O, Schmid L, Ortner F. Complications of interlocking nailing for lower leg fractures. A three year follow-up of 102 cases. J Trauma. 1992; 33:863-9.
8. Koval KJ, Clapper MF, Elison PS, Poka A, Bathon GH, Burgess AR. Complications of reamed intramedullary nailing of the tibia. J Ortop Trauma. 1991; 5:184-9.
9. Kyro A. Malunion after intramedullary nailing of tibial shaft fractures. Ann Chir Gynecol. 1997; 86:56-64.
10. Lang GJ, Cohen BE, Bosse MJ, Kellam JF. Proximal third tibial shaft fractures. Should they be nailed? Clin. Orthop. 1995; 315: 64-74.
11. Olerud S, Dankwardt-Lilliestrom G. Fracture healing in compression osteosynthesis. Acta Orthop Scand Suppl. 1971; 137:1-44.
12. Toivanen JA, Vaisto D, Kannus P. Anterior knee pain after intramedullary nailing of fractures of the tibial shaft. A prospective, randomized study comparing two different nail-insertion techniques. J Bone and Joint Surg. 2002; 84A:580-5.
13. Williams J, Gibbons M, Trundle H, Murray D, Worlock P. Complications of nailing in closed tibial fractures. J Orthop Trauma. 1995; 9(6):476-81.
14. Martinez A, Latta LL, Sarmiento A. Functional Bracing of Fractures of the Proximal Tibia. Clin Orthop. 2003; 417:293-302.

12

Fractures in the Middle-Third, Clinical Results and Representative Examples

In one of our studies, we reported on 434 patients with closed fractures of the middle-third of the tibia with complete follow-up. The following is an abbreviated version of that document.[1]

MATERIAL

One hundred and twenty six (28%) patients were female, and 324 (72%) were male. Their ages ranged from 16 to 86 years (average, 31.5 ± 12.7 years; median of 27 years and mode of 26 years). One hundred and forty three (32.9%) fractures were comminuted, 112 (25.8%) were oblique, 38 (8.7%) were spiral, 125 (28.8%) were transverse, and 16 (3.7%) were segmental. Three hundred and twelve fractures (71.9%) had associated fibular fractures and 122 (28.1%) had intact fibulae. From the group of 312 tibial fractures with associated fibular fractures, 239 (76.6%) fibula, fractures were located in the middle-third, 51 (16.3%) in the proximal-third, and 22 (7.1%) in the distal-third.

Fractures were considered low-energy produced if they were the result of direct blows, falls to the ground, falls from a bicycle or a kick on the leg. Fractures were considered high-energy produced if they occurred in an accident involving a bicycle and an automobile, a motorcycle accident, a motor vehicle accident, or a pedestrian being hit by a motor vehicle. Two hundred (46.1%) were considered low-energy produced fractures, and 232 (53.4%) high-energy produced fractures. One hundred (23.0%) were produced in motor vehicle accidents (MVA), 88 (20.2%) in pedestrian/vehicle accidents (PVA), 43 (9.9%) in motorcycle accidents (MCA), 121 (27.8%) in falls (F), 61 (14.1%) by a direct blow, 18 (4.1%) from a kick, and three (0.7%) through an unknown mechanism.

METHODS

The application of the brace, accomplished when the acute symptoms have subsided, took place at an average of 26.3 ± 20.2 days after the injury with a median of 20 days and a mode of 17 days. Ambulation was to continue with the use of external support, bearing weight on the extremity according to symptoms. Frequent tightening of the straps was encouraged in order to maintain the desirable snugness of the brace as swelling subsided. Neither the shoe nor the brace was to be initially removed. At the second follow-up one week later, the brace was temporarily removed and the leg was inspected. If discomfort and swelling were minimal, the patient was instructed on the appropriate way of donning and doffing the brace for hygienic purposes. A next appointment usually was made for 4 weeks later. Data were recorded for initial angulation, displacement, and shortening as observed on radiographs obtained before treatment. From the clinical charts, the age, gender, date of injury, date of bracing, date of healing, and complications were recorded. Statistical analysis was done with the Systat (Systat Inc., Point Richmond, CA USA) program to analyze by linear regression the correlation of parameters with age, time to healing, time to bracing, initial displacement, final displacement, change of displacement, initial shortening, final shortening, initial medial-lateral plane angulation, final medial-lateral plane angulation, change of angulation in that plane between the initial bracing and final follow-up, and the same for the antero-posterior (AP) plane. All other continuous variable analysis was done with the Student's t test, adjusted for multiple comparisons.

CLINICAL RESULTS

Healing Time

A fracture was considered united when radiographs showed callus bridging of the major fragments, and the patient was able to ambulate without pain or external support. The average healing time was 16.4 ± 5.9 weeks, with a median of 15.3 weeks, and a mode of 14.4 weeks (Figure 12.1). Patients' age correlated mildly with healing time, correlation coefficient

(CC) = 0.092, P = 0.056. Patients younger than 35 years achieved healing on an average time 16.1 ± 5.9 weeks, with a median of 15.1 weeks, and a mode at 13.4 weeks. Patients older than 35 years achieved healing at an average of 17.2 ± 5.8 weeks, with a median of 15.7 weeks and at a mode of 11.6 weeks. The earlier mode in the group of 122 patients older than 35 years may be a result of the slightly lower incidence of high-energy injuries (48.4%) versus 55.5% in the group of 311 patients younger than 35 years. There was a difference in time to achieve healing according to the time of application of the brace.

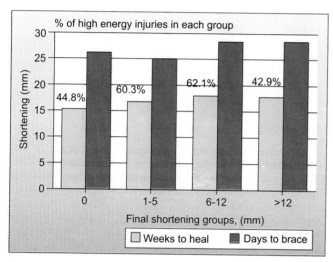

Fig. 12.1: A graph showing the degree of shortening in relation to time to bracing. For the 365 patients who had a brace applied in less than 6 weeks (15.8 ± 5.8 weeks), compared with the 68 patients who had a brace applied after 6 weeks (19.5 ± 6.2 weeks; P < 0.0005.

The healing time of the 312 fractures associated with a fibular fracture (71.9%) was 17.0 ± 5.9 weeks, median 16.1 and mode 14.4 weeks. For the 122 fractures (28.1%) with an intact fibula, the healing time averaged 14.8 ± 5.6 weeks, median 13.7 and mode 9.4 weeks (P < 0.0005).

Fifty one fractures of the fibula were proximal, 239 were mid-third and 22 were distal. The tibias healed in 16.2 ± 5.6 weeks if the fibular fracture was proximal; 17.2 ± 5.9, if it was mid-third; and 17.2 ± 7.1 if it was distal.

Shortening

The average shortening was 3.5 ± 4.3 mm (range, 0 to 25 mm; 2 mm median, and 0 mm a dominant mode. Initial shortening was highly correlated with initial displacement (CC=0.650, P < 0.001) as well as final shortening, and final displacement, (CC=0.654, P < 0.001). The 420 (96.7%) patients who achieved healing with ≤12 mm shortening had a higher %age of high-energy injuries, 56.9%, than the 14 (3.3%) patients who achieved healing with >12 mm shortening, 50.0% high energy. The patients who achieved healing with >12 mm shortening had greater initial shortening (11.4 ± 6.2 mm) than patients who

achieved healing with ≤12 mm shortening (3.6 ± 4.6 mm; P < 0.005). The amount of shortening change during treatment was related to the initial shortening (Figure 12.2).

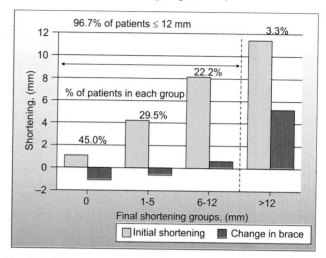

Fig. 12.2: The amount of shortening change during treatment was greater in the small group of patients who achieved healing with > 12 mm shortening compared to those who ended up with ≤ 12 mm (Change=5.2 ± 6.1 mm, versus -0.6 ± 3.8 mm; p < 0.0005).

Angulation

In the ML plane, 414 (97.0%) fractures healed with ≤ 8° angulation. Three (0.7%) fractures had varus angulation > 12? and 10 (2.3%) fractures had 9° to 12° varus (Figure 12.3).

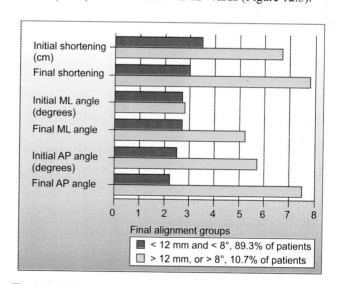

Fig. 12.3: High-energy injuries accounted for 61.5% of all the fractures with > 8° varus or valgus, whereas the 53.3% of the 414 patients with < 8° varus or valgus had high-energy injuries. The initial angulation in the 13 fractures that healed with > 8° varus or valgus was 3.2° ± 3.2 compared with those fractures that healed in the < 8° group, which was 2.7° ± 2. There was no significant difference in the initial angulation in these groups, but there was a significant difference in the change in angulation during treatment: 2.7° ± 2.8 versus. 11.8° ± 7.5 (P < 0.0005).

In the AP plane, 399 (93.4%) fractures healed with ≤ 8° angulation. Ten (2.3%) fractures had > 8° anterior bowing and 18 (4.3%) fractures had > 8° of recurvatum. High-energy injuries accounted for 53.8% of all the fractures with > 8° AP angulation, whereas the 50.0 % of the 399 patients with < 8° AP angulation had high-energy injuries. The initial angulation in the 28 fractures that healed with > 8° AP angulation was 7.3° ± 4.5 compared with those fractures that healed in the < 8° which was 2.5° ± 3.1, (P < 0.00005). There was also a significant difference in the change in angulation during treatment: 2.5° ± 2.9 versus 6.5° ± 5.8 (P < 0.0005).

The initial and final shortening was significantly greater for those patients that had final angulation > 8° in the AP plane (final shortening: 3.4 mm ± 4.2 versus 5.5 mm ± 5.9, P < 0.05) but not for those > 8° in the ML plane. The healing time was also greater for those patients that had final angulation > 8°: 16.3 weeks ± 5.8 versus 20.7 weeks ± 7.2, P < 0.02, for ML plane angulation; and 16.2 weeks ± 5.7 versus 19.6 weeks ± 7.7, P < 0.02, for AP plane angulation.

There was no significant difference in angulation of the tibia in the ML plane whether the fibula was fractured or not, 2.9° ± 3.9 versus 3.0° ± 2.6. There was a statistically significant difference in angulation of the tibia in the AP plane if the fibula was fractured or not, 2.1° ± 2.8 versus 3.0° ± 3.4. There was no significant difference in angulation of the tibia in the ML or AP plane for fractures of the fibula in the proximal, mid or distal third.

Anatomical Alignment

A most desirable final anatomic alignment of the tibia was considered if angulation was ≤ 8° in any plane, and shortening ≤ 12 mm (Figures 12.4 and 12.5). Using these arbitrary criteria, patients were divided into two groups: Group I in the most desirable final anatomic position and Group II outside the most desirable final anatomic position. There were 46

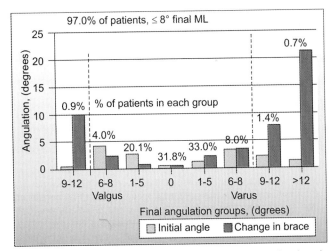

Fig. 12.4: Graph showing coronal angular deformity that developed during functional treatment.

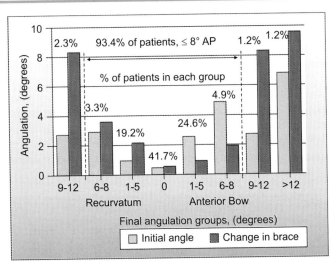

Fig. 12.5: Graph illustrating the initial and final recurvatum and anterior bowing of the fractures in the study.

(10.8%) patients in Group II. The mechanism of injury did not have a major impact regarding final alignment as 53.5% of the patients in Group II had fractures resulting from high-energy injuries, and 57.1% of the patients in Group I had high-energy injuries. The parameters that were significantly different between Group I and II were: time to heal (16.1 ± 5.7) weeks versus 19.0 ± 7.1 weeks; P < 0.02, initial displacement (26.0% ± 25.1% versus 42.4% ± 31.0%; P < 0.005), and final displacement (20.7% ± 20.1 versus 41.8% ± 33.0%; P < 0.005). As expected, initial shortening had a significant influence (3.5 ± 4.6 mm, versus 6.7 ± 6.2 mm; P < 0.02) along with the change in shortening during treatment (-0.6 ± 3.7 mm, versus 1.2 ± 5.8 mm; P < 0.03). The initial angulation in the ML plane was not significantly different between Groups I and II, but in the AP plane it was, 2.2 ± 2.5 versus 7.5 ± 5.0, P < 0.0005. The change in angulation during treatment was significantly different for both planes: 2.6° ± 2.9 versus 5.6° ± 5.8; P < 0.0005, for the ML plane; and, 2.4° ± 2.9 versus 4.9° ± 5.1, P < 0.001.

Joint Motion and Length of Follow-Up

No attempt was made to record range of motion (ROM) of the knee and ankle. We had previously observed that the short time these joints are immobilized in the initial cast is not sufficient to create permanent limitation of motion. Long-term follow-up was not obtained. Previous experience had shown that in our teaching at county hospital once the brace is discontinued a large percentage of patients do not return for additional follow up.

Comparison to Proximal and Distal-Third Fractures

In two previous occasions, the authors reported on 105 fractures of the proximal-third of the tibia.[2] and 450 closed fractures of the distal-third.[3] Comparing the final shortening between groups, the middle-third fractures had significantly less shortening than the distal-third group, 3.5 mm ± 4.3 versus 5.1 mm ± 4.8, P < 0.0001, but was not significantly different from the proximal-third group at 3.6 mm ± 4.5. Comparing final angulation in the AP plane showed no significant differences between the groups, but in the ML plane 97.0% of the mid-third fractures had 8° angulation compared to 90.6% of the proximal-third fractures and only 90.0% of the distal third fractures. By Chi-square analysis, the difference was significant.

REPRESENTATIVE EXAMPLES

Representative examples illustrating fractures in the middle-third of tibia are shown in Figures 12.6 to 12.39.

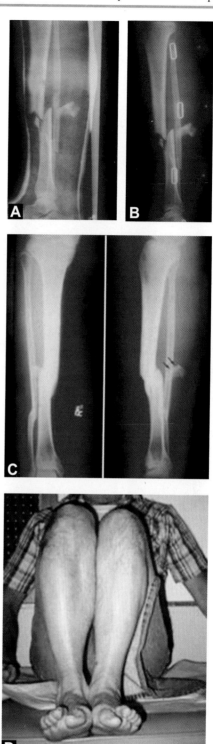

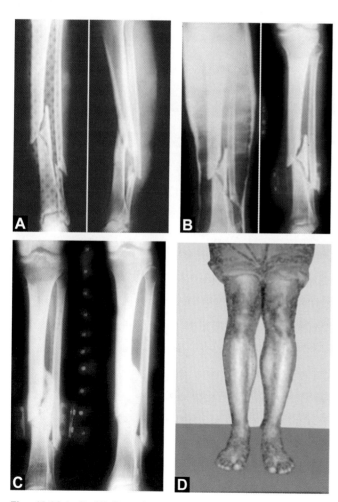

Figs 12.6A to D: (A) Comminuted fracture of the middle-third of the tibia with an associated fibular fracture. Notice the mild shortening of the tibia and the recurvatum deformity. (B) First radiographs obtained following the initial insult. No attempt was made to regain length. The second radiograph was obtained shortly after the application of the below-the-knee functional brace. Notice the absence of change in the length of the tibia. (C) Radiographs showing progressive healing of the fracture without change from the original shortening. (D) Photograph of the patient's legs.

Figs 12.7A to D: (A) Radiograph of comminuted fracture in the middle-third of the tibia and associated fibular fracture. Notice the shortening. (B) Radiograph obtained in the initial above-the-knee cast. Notice the accepted shortening. (C) Radiographs taken after completion of healing. Notice the absence of change in the length of the fractured leg. (D) Clinical photograph showing the mild, though inconsequential shortening of the left leg. The patient was a diabetic.

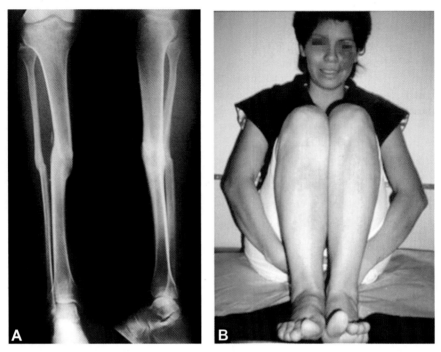

Figs 12.8A and B: (A) Radiograph of healed fracture of the middle-third of the tibia and fibula in a few degrees of valgus. (B) The clinical appearance of the extremities. It is virtually impossible to detect the deformity.

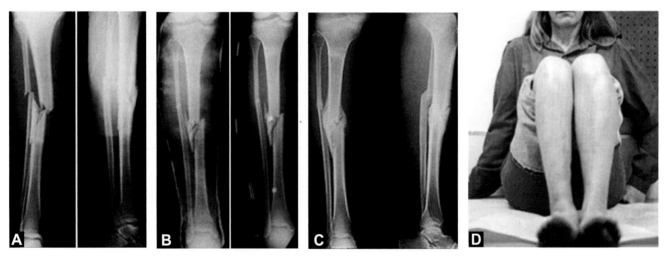

Figs 12.9A to C: (A) Radiograph of comminuted fractures of the tibia and fibula in the middle-third of the tibia. (B) Radiographs taken in the original above-the-knee cast and then in the brace. (C) Radiographs obtained after completion of healing. (C) Clinical appearance of the lower extremities. Notice the still atrophied right lower extremity.

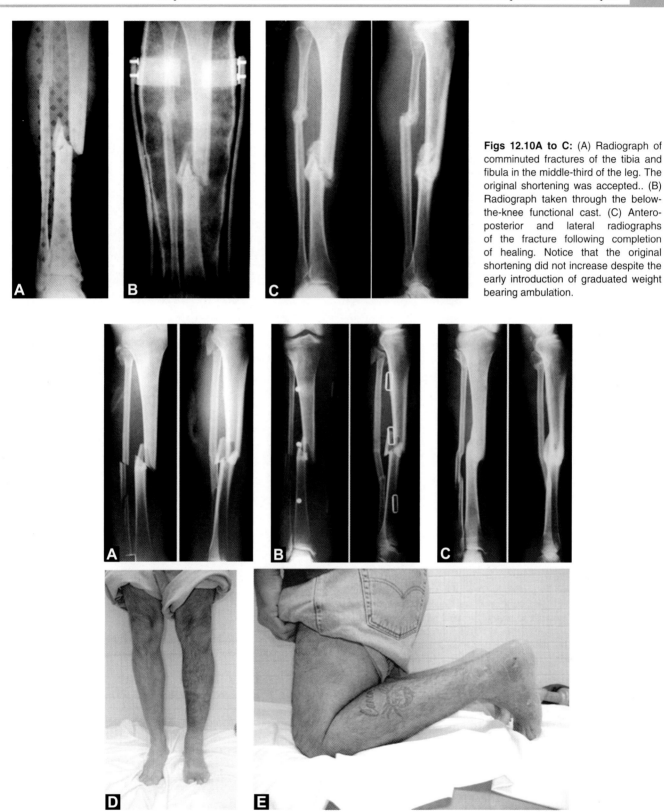

Figs 12.10A to C: (A) Radiograph of comminuted fractures of the tibia and fibula in the middle-third of the leg. The original shortening was accepted.. (B) Radiograph taken through the below-the-knee functional cast. (C) Antero-posterior and lateral radiographs of the fracture following completion of healing. Notice that the original shortening did not increase despite the early introduction of graduated weight bearing ambulation.

Figs 12.11A to E: (A) Radiograph of comminuted-fracture in the middle-third of the tibia and fibula. (B) Radiograph obtained through the functional brace. The original shortening was accepted as being inconsequential. (C) The fracture healed uneventfully without additional shortening or angulation. (D and E) The patient demonstrates the aesthetic appearance of his fractured extremity and his ability to kneel with full flexion of the knee.

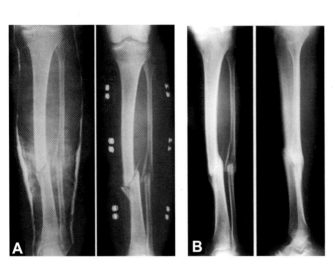

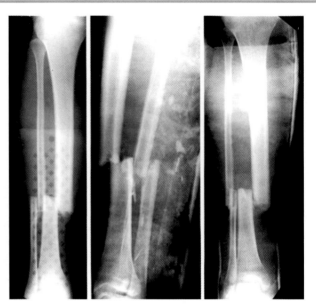

Figs 12.12A and B: (A) Composite radiographs of fractures of the tibia and fibula in their middle-third. (B) Antero-posterior and lateral radiographs of the healed fractures. Notice the maintenance of the original shortening.

Fig. 12.13: Composite photograph of a transverse, displaced fractures of the tibia and fibula. A manual reduction was carried out but the desirable mechanical stability was not achieved. The fragments displaced and the limb returned to the original shortening.

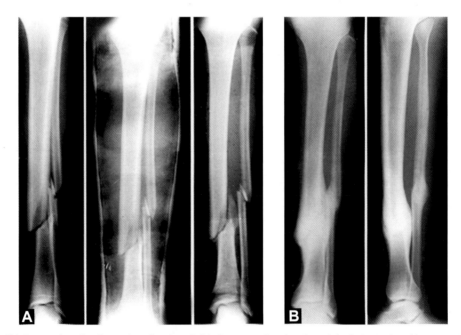

Figs 12.14A and B: (A) Composite of radiographs of a closed tibia fracture, showing the original shortening. No attempt was made to regain length. The other two radiographs show the tibia stabilized in the original above-the-knee cast; and later in the brace. (B) Radiograph of the healed tibia. The original shortening remained unchanged and the overall alignment was very acceptable.

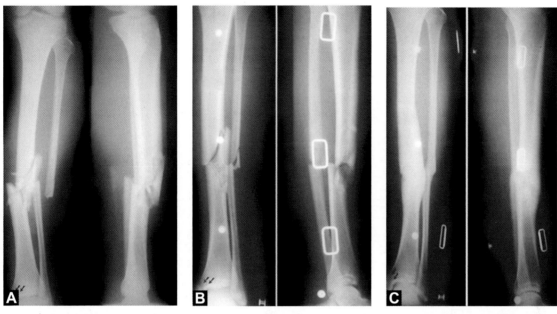

Figs 12.15A to C: (A) Radiograph of closed, comminuted fracture of the tibia and fibula in the middle-third of the diaphysis. Notice the original valgus deformity and the acceptable original shortening. (B) Radiographs in the functional brace. The angular deformity had been corrected at the time of application of the original cast. (C) Radiographs obtained after completion of healing. The fracture healed with a few degrees of varus.

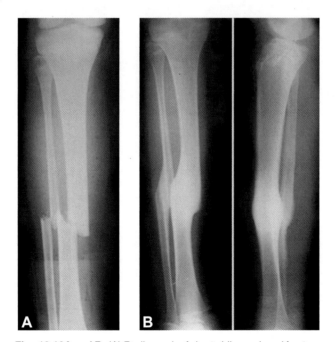

Figs 12.16A and B: (A) Radiograph of short oblique, closed fracture of the tibia and fibula. Notice the minimal original shortening. No attempt was made to regain length. (B) The fracture was treated with a functional brace and healed without additional shortening and good alignment.

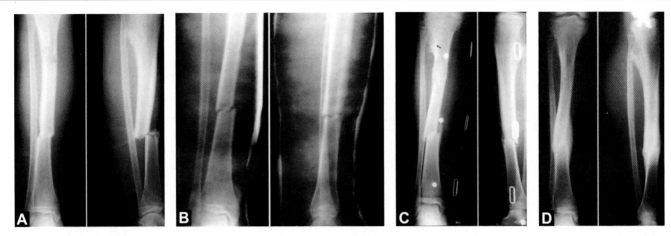

Figs 12.17A to D: (A) Radiograph of closed transverse fracture in the middle-third of the tibial diaphysis. Notice the initial varus attitude and the minimal shortening. (B) Radiographs taken through the above-the-knee cast after manual reduction of the fragments. (C) Radiographs showing the loss of reduction and the development of a mild varus deformity. (D) Radiographs showing the fracture solidly healed with an inconsequential varus deformity.

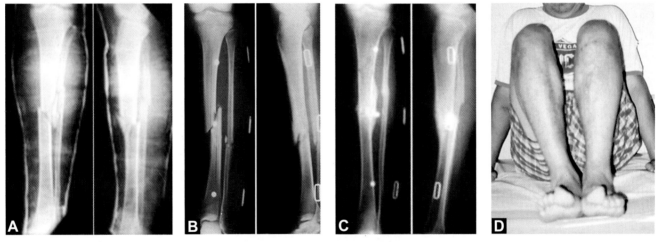

Figs 12.18A to D: (A) Radiograph of an oblique fracture in the middle-third of the tibial diaphysis, taken through the initial above-the-kne cast. (B) Radiograph obtained through the functional brace. (C) Radiographs showing the frature solidly healed with a mild recurvatum deformity. (D) Patient displays his lower extremities. Notice the residual, though temporary, atrophy of his left leg.

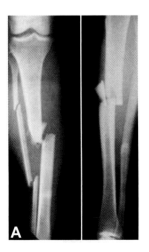
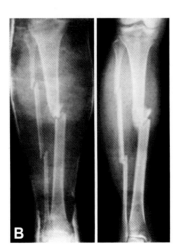
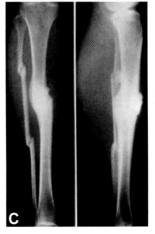

Figs 12.19A to C: (A) Radiographs of closed, comminuted fracture of the tibia and segmental fibula in the middle-third of their diaphyses. No attempt was made to regain length. The fragments were manually aligned. (B) Radiographs in the original cast and subsequent functional brace. (C) Radiographs showing the fractures healed without additional shortening and with very acceptable alignment.

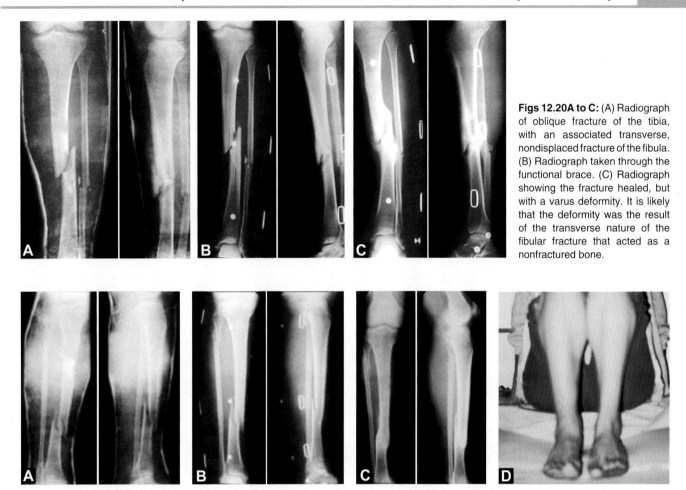

Figs 12.20A to C: (A) Radiograph of oblique fracture of the tibia, with an associated transverse, nondisplaced fracture of the fibula. (B) Radiograph taken through the functional brace. (C) Radiograph showing the fracture healed, but with a varus deformity. It is likely that the deformity was the result of the transverse nature of the fibular fracture that acted as a nonfractured bone.

Figs 12.21A to D: (A) Radiograph of oblique fracture of the tibia associated with an oblique fracture of the proxial fibula, taken through the initial above-the-knee cast. (B) Radiograph obtained through the functional brace. (C) Radiographs showing the fractures solidly healed, without additional shortening and with very acceptable alignment. (D) Patient exhibits his lower extremities.

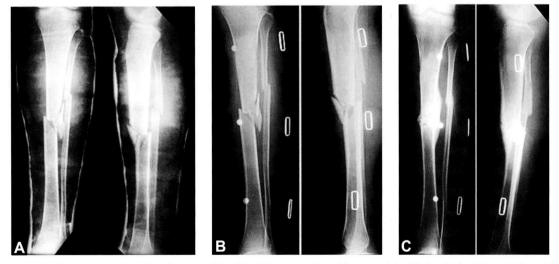

Figs 12.22A to C: (A) Radiographs of oblique fracture of the tibia with an associated fracture of the fibula, obtained through the original above-the-knee cast. No attempt had been made to regain length. (B) Radiographs in the functional brace. (C) Radiograph obtained after completion of healing. Additional shortening or angulaion did not occur.

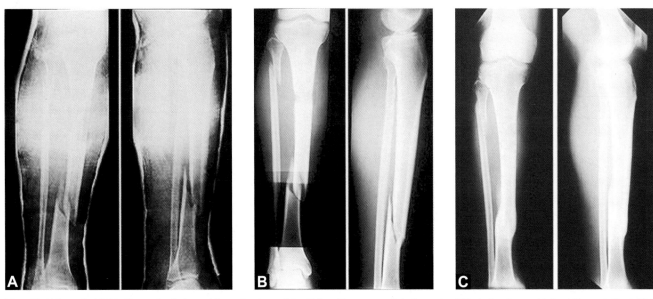

Figs 12.23A to C: (A) Radiograph of short oblique fracture of the tibia with an associated proximal fibula fracture, obtained through the initial above-the-knee cast. (B) Radiographs taken through the functional brace. (C) Radiographs showing the fracture solidly united without addtional shortening and in good alignment.

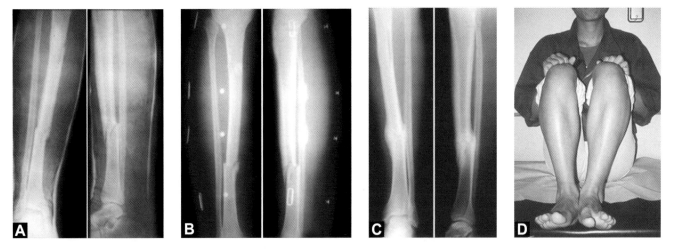

Figs 12.24A to D: (A) Radiograph of short oblique fracture of the tibial diaphysis and an associated fibular fracture. Notice the mild varus deformity. (B) Radiograph obtained through the functional brace. The deformity had been corrected during the application of the brace. (C) Radiographs showing the solidly united fracture. A partial recurrence of the varus deformity took place. (D) Patient displays his lower extremities.

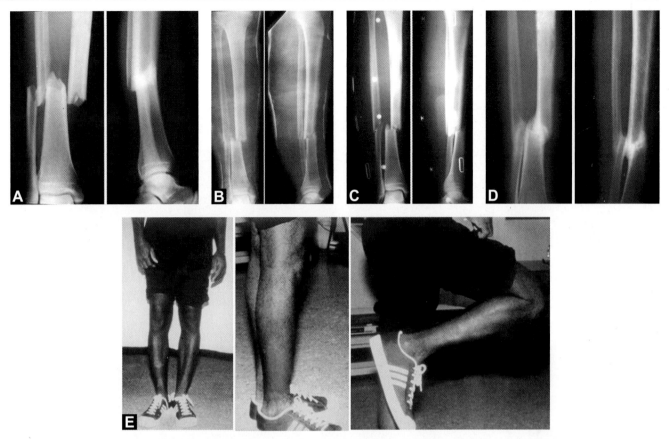

Figs 12.25A to E: (A) Radiograph of transverse fracture of the tibial diaphysis with an associated oblique fracture of the fibula at the same level. (B) The fracture was manually reduced and stabilized in an above-the-knee cast. (C) Two weeks later, the cast was replaced with a functional brace. (D) The fracture healed with a mild angular deformity. (E) Patient demonstrates the appearence of his legs and the flexion and extension of his knee.

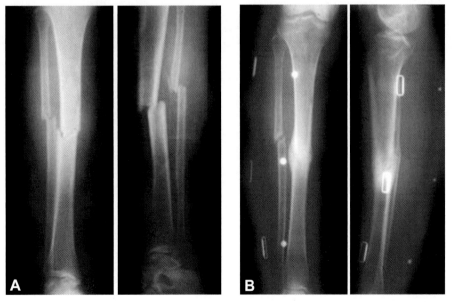

Figs 12.26A and B: (A) Radiograph of transverse fractures of the tibia and fibula at the same level. (B) The fracture was treated with a functional brace, and healed without shortening or angulation.

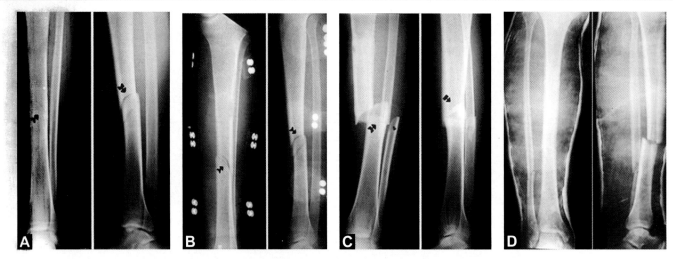

Figs 12.27A to D: (A) Radiograph of nondisplaced fracture of the tibial diaphysis treated with a functional brace. (B) Radiographs taken through the brace. (C) Patient discontinued the brace and sustained a refracture 7 months after the initial one. A trivial injury produced the fracture. Notice that no peripheral callus had developed following the initial fracture. (D) Seven months later, the fracture remained ununited. The patient has finally agreed to have surgery. No metabolic disorder has been identified to explain the absence of healing.

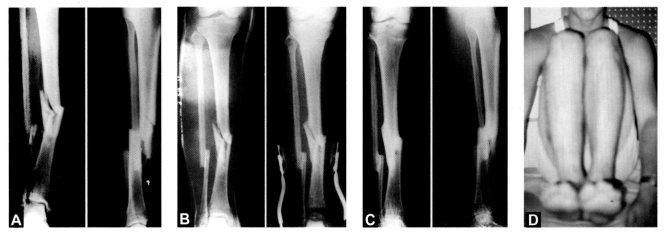

Figs 12.28A to D: (A) Radiograph of comminuted fracture of the tibial and fibular diaphyses. No attempt was made to overcome the shortening. (B) Radiographs obtained through the original above-the-knee cast and functional brace respectively. (C) Radiographs showing the fractures united without additional shortening or angulation. (D) Patient displays his lower extremities illustrating the inconsequential shortening of his fractured leg.

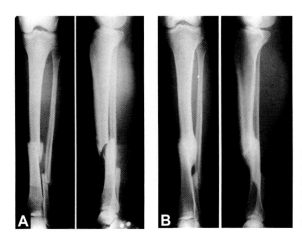

Figs 12.29A and B: (A) Radiograph of oblique fracture of tibia and fibula in the middle-third of the diaphysis. (B) The fracture was treated with a functional brace, and healed without additional shortening and with no angulation.

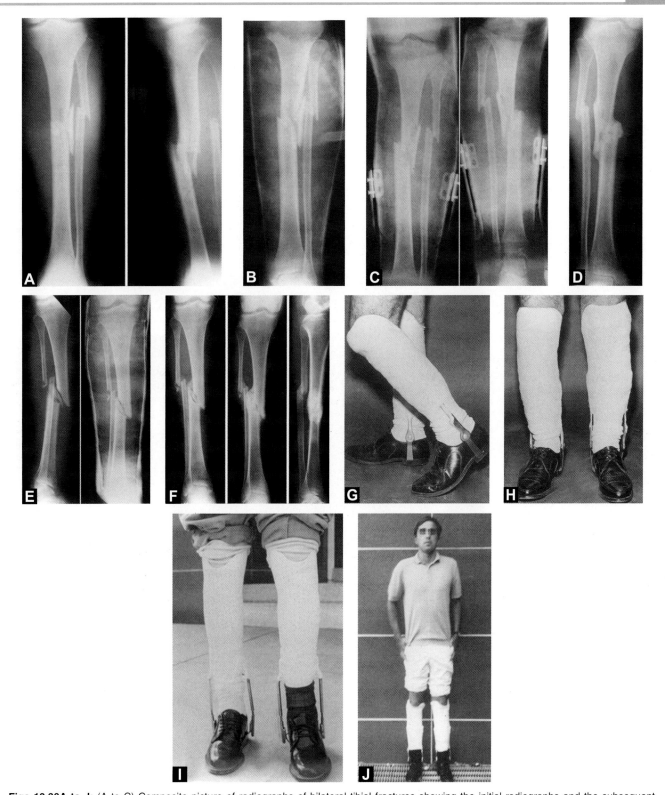

Figs 12.30A to J: (A to C) Composite picture of radiographs of bilateral tibial fractures showing the initial radiographs and the subsequent progress from above-the-knee casts to healing. The first set of radiographs belong to the right leg. Similar composite of radiographs pertaining to the left leg, Notice the maintenance of the original shortening in both lower extremities. (D and E) Illustration of the bilateral functional plaster of Paris braces. (F) The fractures united uneventfully. (G to J) Photos of the patients with original Plaster of Paris braces which were subsequently replaced with Orthoplast custom-made braces.

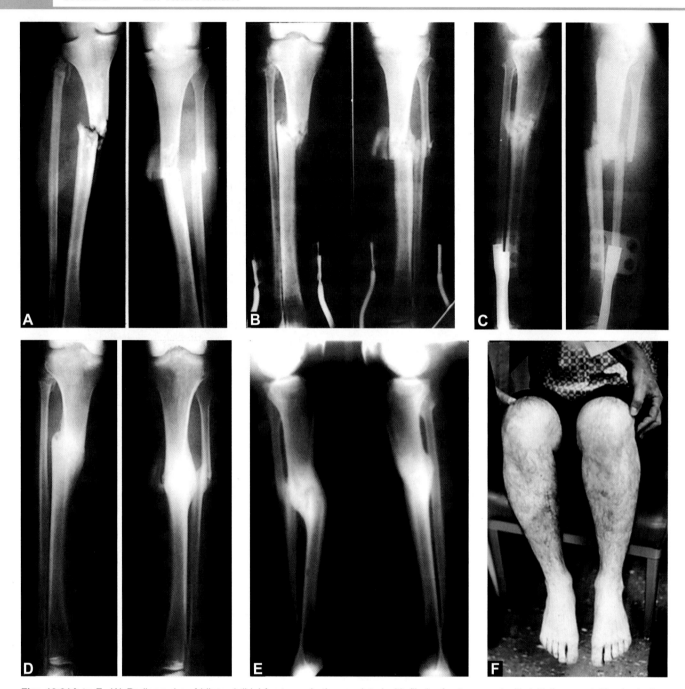

Figs 12.31A to F: (A) Radiographs of bilateral tibial fractures, both associated with fibular fractures and with initially acceptable shortening. (B and C) Because of a delay in the transfer of the patient to our facility, on account of other injuries, the functional bracing did not begin 4 weeks after the initial injury; these radiographs were taken 5 weeks later. (D and E) Radiographs obtained after completion of healing. (F) Patient shows his legs after removal of the braces.

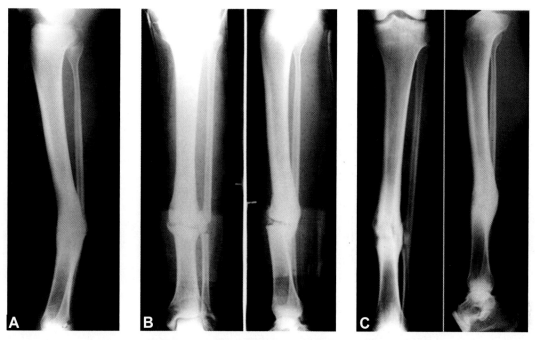

Figs 12.32A to C: (A) Radiograph of an old fracture of the tibia, allegedly treated with debridement and application of an above-the-knee cast. The fracture healed with a severe recurvatum deformity. (B) The deformity was corrected with an osteotomy of the tibia and an ostectomy of the fibula. (C) The tibia and fibula healed, but a stretch palsy of the peroneal nerve was recognized immediately after surgery. Apparently, the correction was carried out too rapidly. It did recover approximately 5 months later.

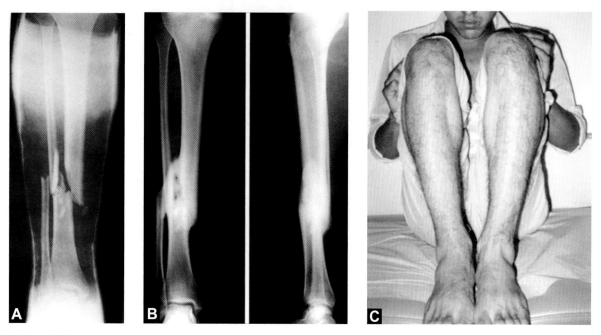

Figs 12.33A to C: (A) Radiograph of comminuted fracture of the tibial diaphysis. Notice the acceptable shortening of the extremity. No attempt was made to regain length. (B) The fracture was treated with a functional brace, and the fracture healed uneventfully. (C) The patient exhibits his lower extremities. Notice the mild, inconsequential shortening.

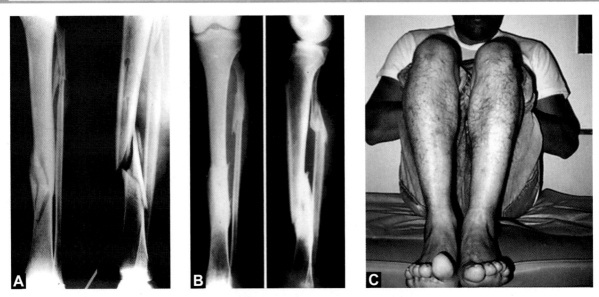

Figs 12.34A to C: (A) Radiographs of comminuted fracture of the tibial diaphysis with associated fracture of the proximal fibula. (B) The fracture was treated in a functional below-the-knee brace and healed uneventfully without angular deformity. (C) The patient exhibits his lower extremities.

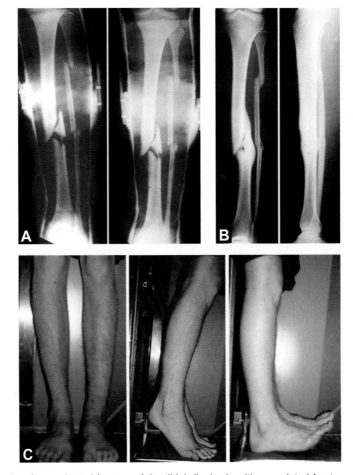

Figs 12.35A to C: (A) Radiographs of comminuted fracture of the tibial diaphysis with associated fracture of the proximal fibula. Notice the initial shortening. (B) The fracture was treated with a functional brace and heal uneventfully, without additional shortening and without angular deformity. (C) Patient demonstrates the overall alignment of the fractured extremity and the range of motion of his ankles following removal of the functional brace.

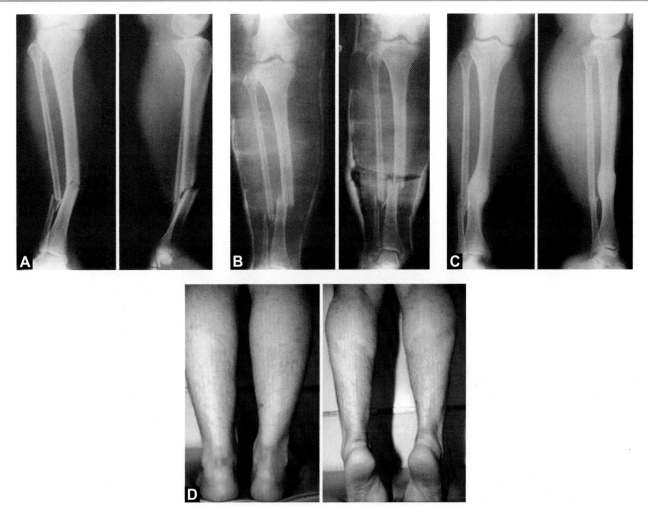

Figs 12.36A to D: (A) Radiograph of transverse, angulated fracture of the tibia and fibula at the same level. (B) Radiographs showing the tibia stabilized in an above-the-knee cast. The alignment of the fracture was unacceptable and needed correction. This was accomplished with wedging of the cast. (C) Radiographs showing the fracture solidly healed without shortening or angulation. (D) Patient demonstrates the appearence of his legs and his ability to stand on his toes.

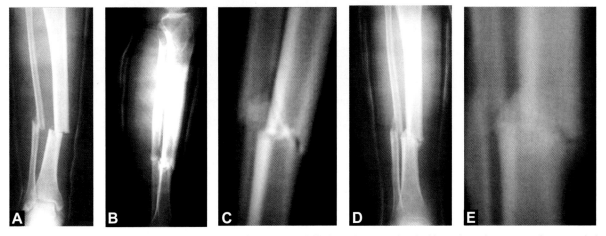

Figs 12.37A to E: (A) Radiograph of transverse fracture of the tibia and fibula at the same level with moderately severe valgus angulation but without displacement. (B and C) Radiographs showing the good alignment of the fragments and early callus formation. The fracture was treated in a below-the-kneee functional cast. (D and E) Radiographs obtained 3 months after the initial injury. The cast was discontinued and unassisted ambulation introduced.

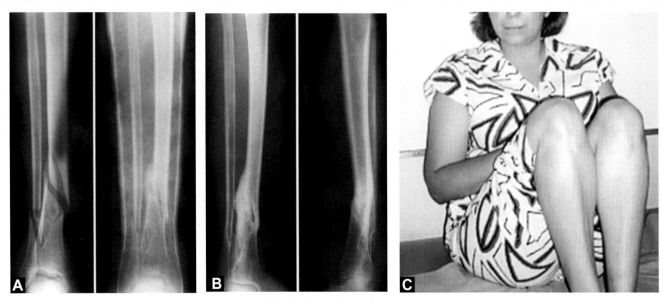

Figs 12.38A to C: (A) Radiograph of comminuted fracture of the distal tibia and fibula. The valgus deformity was corrected at the time of application of the stabilizing above-the-knee cast. (B) The cast was later replaced with a functional cast. The fracture healed with minimal shortening and good alignment. (C) Patient shows the appearance of her lower extremities.

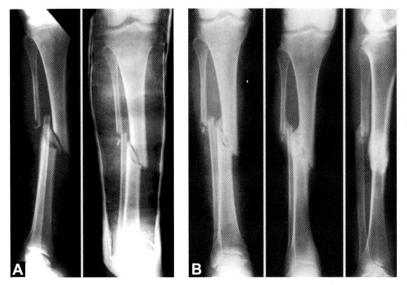

Figs 12.39A and B: (A) Radiograph of oblique fractures of the tibia and fibula in the middle-third of the diaphysis obtained originally and after application of the above-the-knee cast. Correction of the deformity at that time was incomplete. (B) Composite photograph of fracture until completion of healing. The malalignment was corrected at the time of application of the functional brace. The fractures healed uneventfully without increase of shortening or angulation.

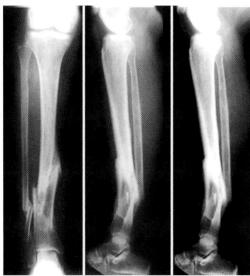

Fig. 12.40: Composite of radiographs showing the ill-effects of originally accepting recurvatum at the fracture site. Under weight bearing, the angular deformity increased.

REFERENCES

1. Sarmiento A, Latta LL. Closed fractures of the middle third of the tibia treated with a functional Brace. Clin Orthop. 2008 Dec; 466:3108-15.

2. Lovasz, Llinas A, Benya P, Bodey B, McKellop H, Luck Jr, and Sarmiento A. Effects of Valgus Tibial Angulation on Cartilage Degeneration in the Rabbit Knee. J Ortho Res. 1995; 13:846-53.

3. Sarmiento A, Latta LL. 450 Closed Fractures of the distal third of the tibia treated with a functional brace. Clin Orthop. 2004; 428: 261-71.

13

Fractures in the Distal-Third, Clinical Results and Representative Examples

In one of our studies, we reported on 450 (45%) fractures treated with a functional brace that were located in the distal third and analyzed them critically. The following is an abbreviated version of that article.[1]

One hundred and twenty six (28%) patients were female, and 324 (72%) were male. Their ages ranged from 16 to 82 years, average 33.5 ± 12.0 years. One hundred-eighty five (41%) fractures occurred in the left leg, and 265 (58.9%) occurred in the right leg. Eighty-eight (19.6%) fractures were comminuted; 104 (23%) fractures were oblique; 187 (41.6%) fractures were spiral; 61 (13.6%) fractures were transverse; and 11 (2.5%) fractures were segmental.

Fractures were considered low-energy produced if they were the result of direct blows, falls to the ground, falls from a bicycle or a kick on the leg. Fractures were considered high-energy produced if they occurred from an accident involving a bicycle and an automobile, a motorcycle accident, a motor vehicle accident or a pedestrian being hit by a motor vehicle. Three hundred eight (68.2%) were considered low-energy produced fractures, and 142 (31.6%) were considered high-energy produced fractures. The functional brace was applied at an average of 25.6 ± 27.5 days after the injury.

INITIAL CARE

Due to previous experience that had shown a higher incidence of varus deformity in fractures of the tibia with an intact fibula, special care was given to these fractures. If the fracture was oblique or comminuted, brace treatment was usually not recommended. If the fracture was transverse and there was no or minimal angulation on the initial radiograph, bracing was instituted. In this case, an effort was made to discourage patients from progressing too rapidly to full weight bearing ambulation. It is not known whether these patients followed instructions.

At the first follow-up 1 week later, the brace was removed and the leg was inspected. If discomfort and swelling were minimal, the patient was instructed on the appropriate way of donning and doffing the brace for hygienic purposes. This temporary loosening of the brace for hygienic reasons was to be done infrequently to avoid undesirable changes in the alignment of a fracture that still was intrinsically unstable. As the fracture experienced progressive healing, the frequency of brace removal was increased.

CLINICAL RESULTS

Healing Time

The average healing time was 16.6 ± 5.6 weeks, with a median of 15.9 weeks, and a mode of 13.4 weeks. Patients' age did not effect healing time. Patients younger than 35 years achieved healing on an average time of 16.3 ± 5.4 weeks, with a median of 15.6 weeks, and a mode at 15.4 weeks. Patients older than 35 years achieved healing at an average of 17.2 ± 6.0 weeks, with a median of 16.5 weeks and at a mode of 13.4 weeks. The earlier mode in the group of 158 patients older than 35 years may be a result of the slightly lower incidence of high-energy injuries (23.4% versus 34.6%) in the group of 292 patients younger than 35 years. This, however, was not reflected in the initial and final displacement and shortening values which were higher for those older than 35 years; (initial displacement 34.8% ± 24.6%, versus 29.3% ± 24.7%, $P < 0.02$; final displacement 32.2% ± 22.5% versus 25.6% ± 21.3%, $P < 0.02$. Initial shortening, 6 ± 4.9 versus 4.3 ± 4.6 mm, $P < 0.005$; and final shortening, 6.4 ± 5.0 mm versus 4.4 ± 4.6 mm, $P < 0.003$).

There was a difference in time to achieve healing for the 384 patients who had a brace applied in less than 6 weeks (16.0 ± 5.0 weeks), versus the 66 patients who had a brace applied after 6 weeks (19.7 ± 6.9 weeks; $P < 0.0001$).

Healing time was inversely proportional to the initial shortening (correlation coefficient (CC), 0.107; $P < 0.024$). Healing time did not correlate with any other parameter

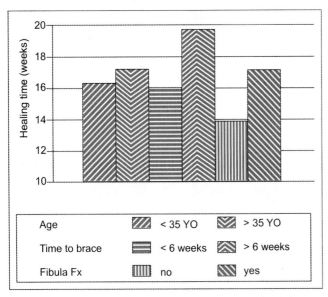

Fig. 13.1: A graph shows the degree of shortening in relation to time to bracing.

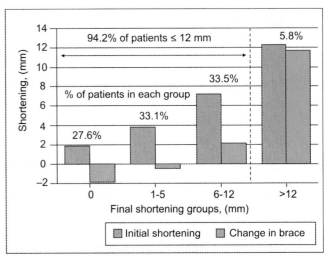

Fig. 13.3: Graph shows the final sagittal angular deformity that occurred during functional treatment. 1.3% of fractures experienced > 12° angulation. The patients who achieved healing with > 12 mm shortening had greater initial shortening (12.3 ± 8.2 mm versus 4.4 ± 4.5 mm for patients who achieved healing with ≤ 12 mm shortening, P < 0.03). The amount of shortening change during treatment was greater in the small group of patients who achieved healing with > 12 mm shortening (11.7 ± 9.4 mm, versus 0.5 ± 4.2 mm P < 0.03). This change in leg length was accompanied by a change in displacement during treatment (30.0% ± 24.5 %, versus 3.5% ± 20.3%, P < 0.02).

measured. In the 77 tibial fractures in which the fibula was intact (17%), the healing time was less if the fibula was fractured (13.8 ± 4.0 weeks versus 17.1 ± 5.8 weeks; P < 0.0001).

Shortening

The average shortening was 5.1 ± 4.8 mm; range, 0 to 25 mm; 4 mm median, and 0 mm strong mode. Final shortening was highly correlated with final displacement (CC, 0.560; P < 0.0001). The 424 (94.2%) patients who achieved healing with ≤ 12 mm shortening had a higher %age of high-energy injuries 31.8%), than the 26 patients who achieved healing with > 12 mm shortening (11.5%).

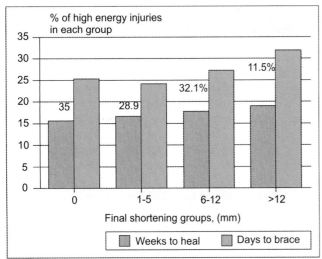

Fig. 13.2: A graph shows shortening that occurred after application of the functional brace. Fractures that healed with 12 mm or greater represented 5.8% patients in the study.

There were two patients that ended up with 25 mm of shortening. Both were young males, 25 years old and 38 years old. Both were injured in a fall, both had a distal spiral oblique tibial fracture with an associated distal fracture of the fibula, both had a significant change in shortening and displacement during treatment. Final angulation was ≤ 4° in all planes for each. They were braced later, 5 weeks, and healed more slowly, 23 weeks, than the average patient (Figure 13.1).

Between these groups, the cause of the change in displacement and shortening during treatment was not clear because there were no statistical correlations with age, time to bracing, time to achieve healing, initial displacement, final displacement, or angulation in any plane with the group of patients with shortening > 12 mm. Only the change in displacement (CC, 0.519; P < 0.007) and the change in shortening (CC, 0.553; P < 0.003) were observed as shown in Figures 13.2 and 13.3. The 11.5% of the patients with final shortening > 12 mm had changes in fracture position that occurred during the treatment.

The group with ≤ 12 mm final shortening (94.2% of the patients) showed significant correlation between shortening and age (CC, 0.232; P < 0.001), time to achieve healing (CC, 0.123; P < 0.011), initial displacement (CC, 0.409; P < 0.0001), final displacement (CC, 0.571; P < 0.0001), change in displacement (CC, 0.105; P < 0.03), initial shortening (CC, 0.492; P < 0.0001), and change in shortening (CC, 0.396; P < 0.0001). No significant correlation was found with either group for initial, final, or change in angle with angulation in either plane.

Comparing tibial fractures in which the fibula was intact with fractures with an associated fibular fracture, the initial shortening, 1.4 ± 2.5 mm versus 5.6 ± 4.8 mm and the final shortening, 1.0 ±1.9 mm versus vs. 6.0 ± 4.9 mm were significantly less, P < 0.0001, for the isolated tibial fractures.

ANGULATION

Four hundred and five fractures (90.0%) healed with < 8° angulation in any plane. The initial angulation of these 405 fractures (0.9° ± 4.4°) was not different than that of the 45 fractures that healed with > 8° in either plane (1.5° ± 4.4°). It was the change in angulation that occurred during treatment that made the difference (1.3° ± 4.9° versus 4.4° ± 6.2°, P < 0.0001).

There was no correlation between initial or final shortening and angulation in any plane. In the medial-lateral plane, 414 fractures (92%) healed with ≤ 8° angulation. Six fractures (1.3%) had greater than 12° varus angulation and 30 fractures had 9° to 12° varus. No patients had more than 8° valgus angulation. High-energy injuries accounted for 38.9% of all the fractures with > 8° varus, whereas the other 414 had 27.1% high-energy injuries. The initial angulation in the 6 fractures that healed with > 12° varus was 2.8° ± 3.6°; for the fractures with 9° to 12° angulation, only 3.2° ± 4.2 ° compared with those fractures that healed in the 5° to 8° range of varus; the 1° to 4° range of varus, no angulation, 1° to 4° valgus and 5° to 8° valgus which were: 2.4° ± 4.0°, 1.4° ± 4.3°, 0.2° ± 3.8°, 1.3° ± 4.6° and 2.9° ± 5.3°, respectively. There was no significant difference in the initial angulation in any of these groups, or a significant difference in the change in angulation during treatment. For the six fractures that healed with > 12° varus, the change was 12.2° ± 3.9°, and for the fractures that healed with 9° to 12° angulation, the change was 5.8° ± 4.4° compared with fractures that healed in the 5° to 8°

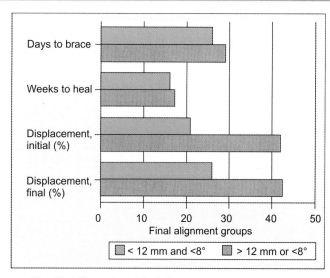

Fig. 13.5: Illustration of final alignment observed in fractures according to the initial displacement .

range of varus, the 1° to 4° range of varus, no angulation, 1° to 4° valgus and 5° to 8° valgus which were: 3.2° ± 4.0°, 1.6° ± 4.5°, 0.2° ± 3.8°, 1.7° ± 4.6° and 2.9° ± 5.2°, respectively,

If the fibula was intact, initial angulation of the tibia (in varus) was significantly greater, 1.8° ± 3.8°, than if the fibula was fractured, 0.8° ± 4.5°. The final angulation in the two groups however, was not significantly different; 2.7° ± 4.0° versus 2.2° ± 3.9°. If the fracture of the fibula was in the proximal-third (almost always associated with a spiral fracture of the distal-third of the tibia from a low-energy twisting injury), the tibial fracture behaved similarly to those with an intact fibula. The initial angulation was in varus, 1.7° ± 3.6° compared with 1.8° ± 3.7° for the intact fibula, and the final angulation was varus, 2.8° ± 3.2° versus 2.7° ± 4.0°, respectively (Figures 13.4 and 13.7).

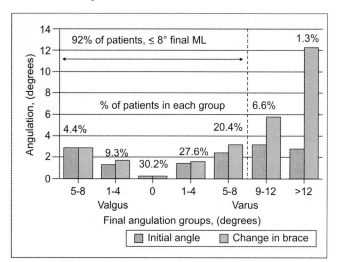

Fig. 13.4: Angulation in the medial-lateral plane compares final angulation with initial angulation and changes in the brace.

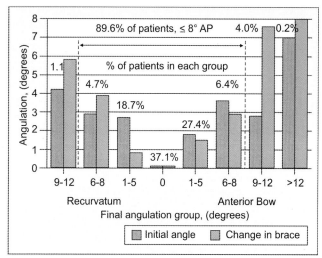

Fig. 13.6: A graph shows coronal angular deformity that developed during functional treatment.

The antero-posterior angulation for both groups also was similar. The only significant difference in position of the tibial fragments was in shortening which was 6.2 ± 4.2 mm for patients with a proximal fibular fracture, compared with 1.4 ± 4.5 mm for patients with an intact fibula.

In the antero-posterior plane, there were 424 fractures (94.2%) with ≤ 8° recurvatum or anterior bowing. There was a trend for greater initial angulation and change in angulation in the antero-posterior plane for fractures that healed with > 8° recurvatum or anterior bowing. The condition of the fibula had no measurable effect on the degree of initial or final angulation of the tibia in the AP plane (Figures 13.5 and 13.6).

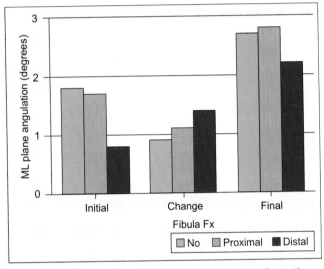

Fig. 13.7: A graph shows the angular changes according to the condition of the fibula.

Anatomic Alignment

The desirable final anatomical alignment of the tibia is angulation ≤ 8° in any plane and shortening ≤ 12 mm.

Using this criteria, patients were divided into two groups: Group I in the desirable final anatomic position and Group II outside the desirable final anatomic position. Besides there was no clear association between angular alignment in one plane versus the other or angulation in either plane with shortening, one might get the impression that to isolate patients who had angulation in any plane > 8° or shortening > 12 mm, one simply would add the number of patients with > 12 mm final shortening, 26 (5.8%), to the 36 (8.0%) patients who had 8° final medial-lateral plane angulation, to the 26 patients (5.8%) who had 8° antero-posterior angulation, obtaining 71 patients (15.8%) for Group II. But when the patients who had angulation > 8° in either plane were isolated, there were only 45 (10%), not 62 (13.8%) outside the range. When the patients in Group II were isolated, there were only 59 (13.1%). The mechanism of injury did not have a major impact regarding final alignment as 28.8% of the patients in Group II had fractures resulting from high-energy injuries, and

30.9% of the patients in Group I had high-energy injuries. The parameters that were significantly different between Group I and II were: time to bracing (3.3 ± 2.2 weeks versus 4.7 ± 3.3 weeks; < 0.002), initial displacement (29.9% ± 24.8% versus 23.7% ± 23%; P < 0.05), and final displacement (26.4% ± 21.4% versus 37.9% ± 23.2%; P < 0.002).

As expected, initial shortening had a significant influence, (4.4 ± 4.4 mm versus 8.0 ± 5.9 mm; P < 0.0001) along with the change in shortening during treatment 0.04 ± 4.0 mm versus 2.15 ± 6.3 mm; P < 0.01 (Figures 13.8 and 13.9). The initial angulation in either plane was not significantly different between Groups I and II. The change in angulation during treatment was significantly different for medial-lateral plane angulation (1.1° ± 4.7° versus 2.8° ± 6.0°, P < 0.03), and antero-posterior plane angulation (0.3° ± 4.6° versus 2.3° ± 7.2°, P < 0.03).

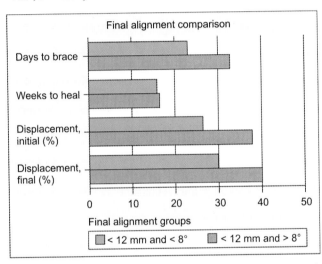

Fig. 13.8: A graph shows the final alignment in relation to days in brace, weeks to healing, initial displacement and final displacement.

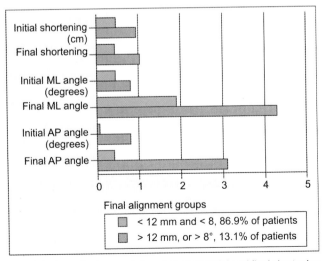

Fig. 13.9: A graph shows relations between initial and final shortening, initial shortening, initial and final medial lateral angulation, and initial and final angulation.

Joint Motion

No attempt was made to record ROM of the knee and ankle. We observed that the short time these joints are immobilized in the cast was not sufficient to create permanent limitation of motion. Furthermore, early ambulation in the long-leg cast and doing isometric exercises of all the surrounding musculature is likely to prevent joint stiffness.

DISCUSSION

Although no standard criteria exists regarding the most appropriate way to determine the precise date of healing of a fracture, it seems that the speed of healing in the current patients compares favorably with healing by patients in other studies of intramedullary nailing. For this study, we chose to quote data dealing exclusively with intramedullary nailing and ignored other methods of treatment, based on the fact that closed intramedullary nailing is the most commonly used treatment at this time. In this study, fractures healed at an average of 16.6 weeks, with a median of 15.9 weeks, a mode of 13.4 weeks, and a range from 1 to 40 weeks. Wiss and Stetson reported an average healing time of 28 weeks with a range of 12 to 104 weeks. In addition, they stated that 88% fractures healed within 6 months, 11% were considered delayed unions.[2] Court-Brown et al reported an average healing time of 16.7 weeks,[3] Gregory and Sanders reported 8% nonunion and 5% delayed union in 38 closed fractures.[4]

In the study of 1000 closed tibial fractures from which the current report is derived, the nonunion rate was 1.1%.[5,6] In the current study of 450 fractures located in the distal-third of the tibia, the nonunion rate was 0.9%. Wiss and Stetson reported a nonunion rate of 2%. The average time to healing was 28 weeks with a range of 12 to 104 weeks. Total 88% healed within 6 months, and there was a delayed union rate of 11% (healing time longer than 6 months).[2] Court-Brown et al reported a nonunion rate of 1.6% with intramedullary nailing.[3] Muscle compartment syndrome is a complication that usually occurs within the first few hours after the initial injury regardless of the method of treatment used. However, the distal traction necessary to regain length and reduce the fracture increases the pressure to the muscles surrounding the fracture site. In addition, the extravasation of blood and bone marrow into the compartments of the leg during closed intramedullary nailing is likely to further increase muscle compartment pressures not yet dangerously elevated. Mawhinney et al reported an incidence of 12% compartment syndromes in tibial fractures treated with intramedullary nails.[7] Cortical necrosis is another complication from nailing, although it is rarely reported. Infection after nailing of closed fractures is low; however,[8-11] Bone and Johnson[12] reported a 4% incidence of infection in a group of 68 patients.[13] Court-Brown et al reported 1.6% infections.[14] Alho et al reported 2.1% infection in a group

of 93 closed tibial fractures.[15] Wiss and Stetson reported an infection rate of 5% in a group of 100 closed fractures treated with reamed intramedullary nails.[2]

Axially unstable fractures, such as oblique, spiral and comminuted fractures, and particularly those that show a lack of contact between major fragments, are prone to failure of the interlocking screws, as they become major weightbearing structures. Fracture of the interlocking screws usually results in production of shortening and angular deformity. The incidence of breakage of the intramedullary nail or locking screws or both is reported to range between 14% and 20%.[16]

Shortening after intramedullary nailing was reported by Bone and Johnson to be 10 mm in 5% of 100 patients[13] and 3.4% in 21 patients by Hooper, et al.[17] In our study, the mean shortening was 5.1 mm. Most closed tibial fractures initially experience less than 0.5 cm of shortening. The minimal shortening in our patients largely is attributable to the fact that only axially unstable fractures with initial shortening less than 15 mm were treated with a functional brace. At our institution, intramedullary nailing or plating were the preferred methods of treatment for axially unstable fractures with initial shortening greater than 15 mm. The shortening is not likely to have produced a limp. Patients with closed fractures located on the distal-third of the tibia rarely experience shortening greater than 2 cm because the soft tissue envelope at that level is very thin. Greater displacement of the fragments is likely to create an open wound. Open fractures usually are not suitable for functional bracing.

The angular deformities measured in patients in this study were in most instances acceptable from the cosmetic point of view, as 405 (90.0%) patients had less than 8° of angular deformity. These figures are comparable to those reported in the literature dealing with intramedullary nailing. Deformities in this range are not likely to produce osteoarthritis later. Merchant and Dietz, based on a review of 37 patients who had tibial fractures with a follow-up of nearly 30 years, concluded that angulation of healed fractures of the distal tibia was not related to functional deficit. They additionally stated that the clinical and radiographic results were unaffected by the amount of anterior or posterior and varus or valgus angulation and the level of the fracture. Other investigators have studied the effect of angular deformities on the adjacent joints, and have found that minor deformities do not alter pressure distribution on the articular cartilage in the adjacent joints in a significant way.

We did not discuss rotary deformities in this study, which in retrospect was a mistake. We concluded earlier that such deformities were extremely rare with functional bracing, and their development usually was iatrogenic because of failure to expose the normal extremity during the initial casting to duplicate the alignment and shape of the normal extremity into the fractured limb.

The most common undesirable sequela of intramedullary nailing is knee pain. Court-Brown et al reported an incidence of knee pain in 48% of patients, and 24.4% patients required removal of the nail. They stated that removal of the nail often did not resolve the pain.[18] Keating et al reported the need for removal of the nail because of knee pain in 80% of 61 patients and after 16 months, the pain had not resolved in 22 of these patients (36%).[19] Toivanen et al reported knee pain in 86% of patients who had a transtendinous approach, and 81% in patients who had a paratendinous approach. They additionally stated that 69% of their patients had anterior knee pain at an average of 1.5 years after nail removal.[20,21]

Although not a panacea, functional bracing does not require surgical intervention, and therefore infection, cortical necrosis, and knee pain are not possible complications.

There are fractures of the distal tibia which preclude bracing techniques, and which are best treated with plate fixation, nailing, or external fixation. It seems that the majority of closed fractures at this level of the diaphysis can be treated successfully with a functional brace, provided their initial shortening is < 15 mm and the angular deformity after closed manipulation does not exceed 5°. The minimal shortening and angular deformities thought to be acceptable with our current protocol are not complications, but simply inconsequential deviations from the normal.

REPRESENTATIVE EXAMPLES

Some of the representative examples illustrating the fractures in distal-third of tibia are shown in Figures 13.10 to 13.47.

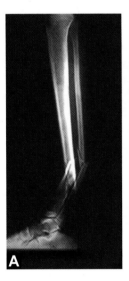
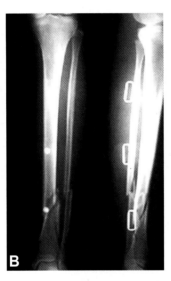
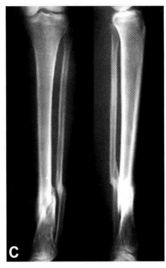

Figs 13.10A to C: (A) Radiograph of oblique fracture of the tibia and fibula in the distal-third of the diaphysis. A severe recurvatum deformity was present and corrected manually at the time of application of the initial above-the-knee cast. (B) Fourteen days later, the cast was replaced with a functional brace. (C) The fracture healed with good alignment and with shortening identical to that seen at the time of the injury.

Figs 13.11A to C: (A) Radiograph of long spiral fracture in the distal-third of the diaphysis, with an associated fracture in the proximal fibula. (B) After 10 days of stabilization in an above-the-knee cast, a functional brace was applied. (C) The fracture healed with excellent alignment and with minimal shortening.

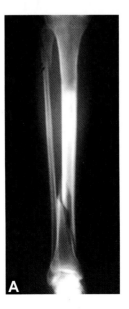
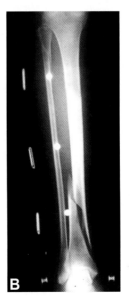
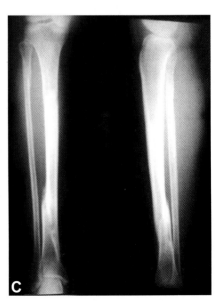

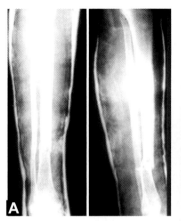
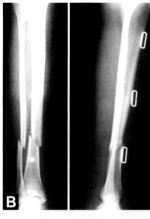
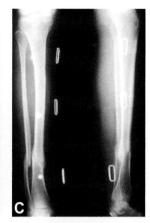

Figs 13.12A to C: (A) Radiograph of short oblique fracture of the distal tibia and fibula that was reduced and stabilized in an above-the-knee cast. Notice the recurvatum angulation. (B) Radiograph after the application of the functional brace 12 days after the initial injury. Notice the corrected recurvatum. (C) Radiograph obtained 6 months later showed the fracture solidly united with good alignment and minimal shortening.

Figs 13.13A to C: (A) Radiograph of oblique fracture of the distal tibia and proximal fibula. No attempt was made to regain length. (B) Radiograph showing the fractured tibia stabilized in a functional brace. The molding of the extremity gives the mistaken impression that an attempt to regain length was made. (C) The fracture healed with the same shortening it had experienced initially.

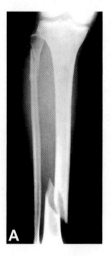
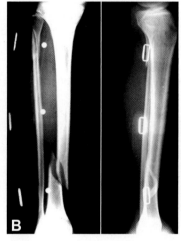
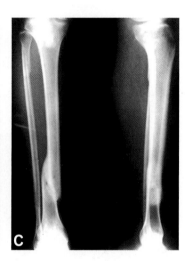

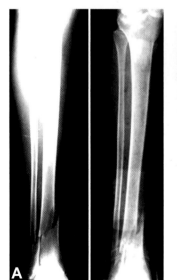
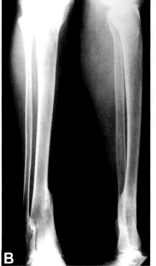

Figs 13.14A and B: (A) Initial radiograph and the one taken through the functional brace. (B) Radiographs obtained after solid union had taken place. There is a minimal and inconsequential varus angulation.

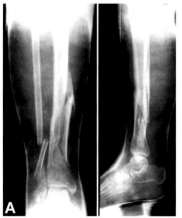
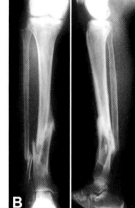

Figs 13.15A and B: (A) Radiograph of comminuted fracture of the distal tibia and fibula. Notice the improper stabilization of the ankle in equinus. This attitude predispose to the increase in the deformity. (B) Radiographs showing the fractures healed, but the tibia healed with a moderate degree of recurvatum. It is very likely that this degree of deformity did not produce a limp or lead to later arthritic changes.

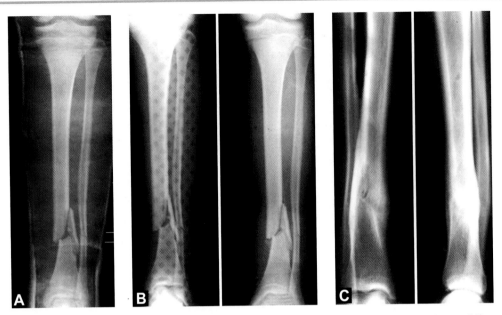

Figs 13.16A to C: (A) Radiograph of comminuted fracture of the distal tibia with an intact fibula sustained by a 14-year-old boy, stabilized initially in an above-the-knee cast. (B) Two subsequent radiographs showing the progressive healing of the fracture. (C) The fracture healed with a mild varus angulation.

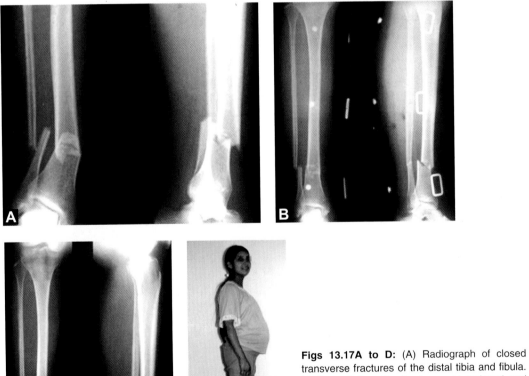

Figs 13.17A to D: (A) Radiograph of closed transverse fractures of the distal tibia and fibula. Under sedation, the fracture was reduced and stabilized in an above-the-knee cast. (B) The cast was replaced with a functional brace 2 weeks later. (C) The fracture healed uneventfully with no shortening and an inconsequential mild anterior angulation (D) The patient, pregnant at the time, later had a normal delivery.

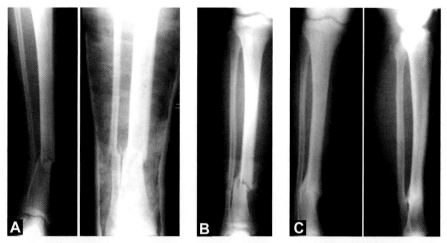

Figs 13.18A to C: (A) Radiograph of transverse, angulated fracture of the distal-third of the tibia and fibula, initially stabilized in an above-the knee cast. (B) Radiograph obtained through the functional brace that was applied 2 weeks after the initial insult. (C) Radiograph showing the fracture solidly healed.

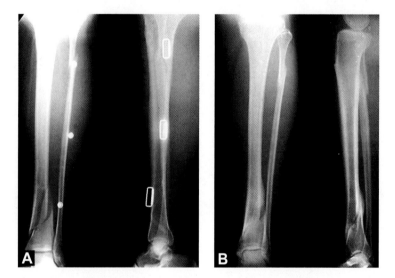

Figs 13.19A and B: (A) Radiograph of long oblique fracture of the distal-third of the tibia with an associated fracture of the proximal fibula. (B) The fracture was treated with a functional brace and healed uneventfully.

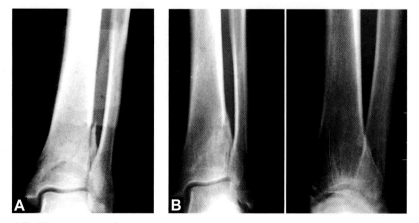

Figs 13.20A and B: (A) Metaphyseal fracture of the distal tibia treated with a functional brace. (B) The fracture healed without change in the position of the fragments.

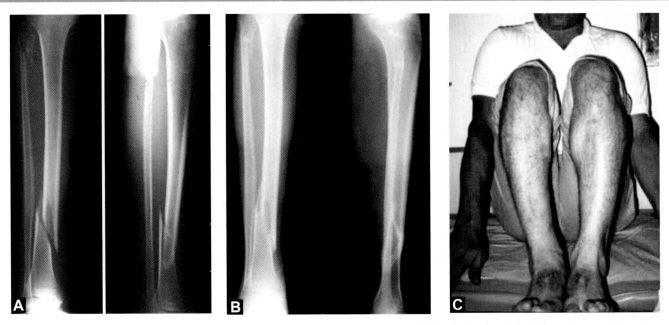

Figs 13.21A to C: (A) Radiograph of long oblique fracture of the distal tibia and proximal fibula. Notice the minimal shortening experienced at the time of the injury. (B and C) The fracture was treated in a functional brace and healed without additional shortening or angulation.

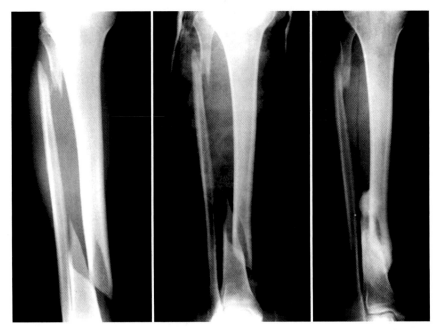

Fig. 13.22: Composite of radiographs showing the unchanged shortening of an oblique fracture of the distal tibia and proximal fibula.

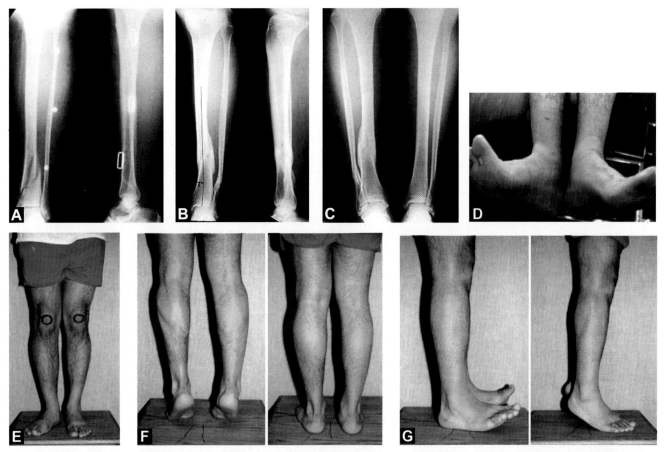

Figs 13.23A to G: (A) Radiograph of oblique fracture of the distal and proximal fibula. The fracture was treated with a functional brace. (B) However, the external rotary deformity that developed at the time of the injury was not corrected. The fracture healed uneventfully. (C) Radiograph suggesting the rotary deformity by the different relationship between the tibia and fibula in the two legs. (D to G) Patient demonstrates the rotary deformity and overall appearance of his lower extremities.

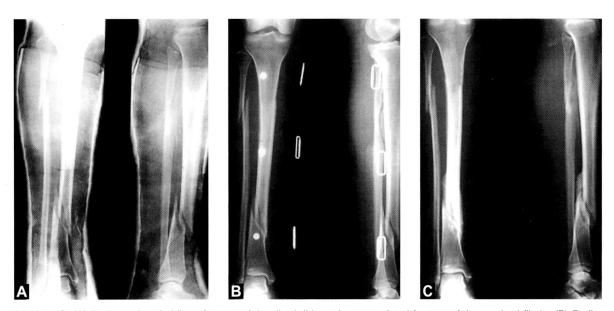

Figs 13.24A to C: (A) Radiographs of oblique fracture of the distal tibia and an associated fracture of the proximal fibula. (B) Radiographs obtained through the brace, suggesting that at the time of application of the brace, the fragments were better realigned. (C) The fractures healed uneventfully without additional shortening or angulation.

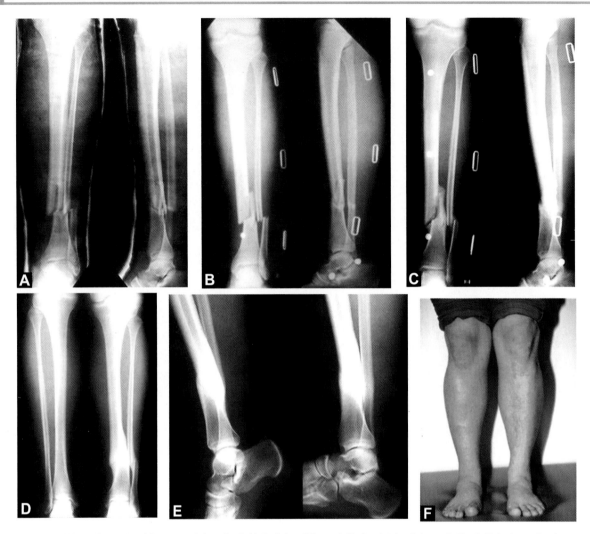

Figs 13.25A to F: (A) Radiograph of fracture of the distal-third of the tibia and fibula obtained through the initial above-the-knee cast. (B) Radiograph taken 2 weeks later through the functional brace. (C) Radiographs taken 4 weeks later showing early callus formation and maintenance of adequate alignment. (D and E) Radiographs of both tibias showing the mild and inconsequential angular deviation. (F) The appearance of the lower extremities after completion of healing.

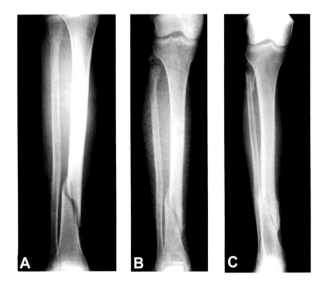

Figs 13.26A to C: (A) Radiograph of oblique fracture of the distal tibia and proximal fibula. The displayed minimal shortening is the one found in the vast majority of closed tibial fracture. (B) Radiograph taken through the brace. (C) Final radiograph demonstrating that despite the early introduction of weight bearing, dictated by symptoms, the initial shortening did not change.

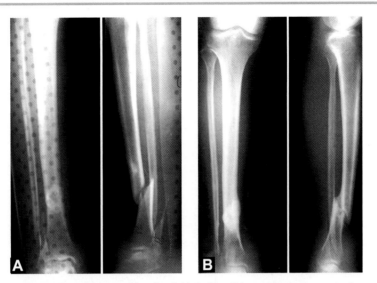

Figs 13.27A and B: (A) Radiograph of oblique fracture of the distal-third of the tibia and fibula demonstrating a mild recurvatum deformity at the fracture site. (B) The fracture healed with very acceptable length and alignment.

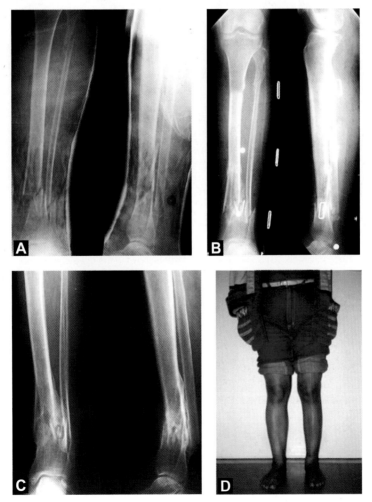

Figs 13.28A to D: (A) Radiograph of comminuted fracture of the distal-third of the tibia and fibula shown through the initial above-the-knee cast. Notice the translatory deformity. (B) The alignment of the fragments was improved during the application of the functional brace. (C) The fracture healed uneventfully with inconsequential mild recurvatum. (D) Appearance of the patient's lower extremities.

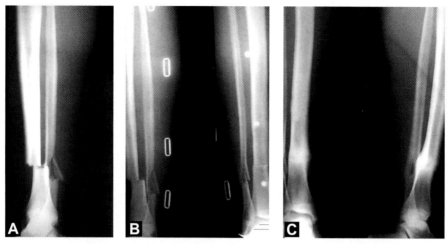

Figs 13.29A to C: (A) Radiograph of transverse fracture of the distal-third of the tibia with an associated comminuted fracture of the fibula at the same level. (B) Radiograph obtained through the functional brace. (C) Radiograph illustrating the healed fractures without shortening or malalignment.

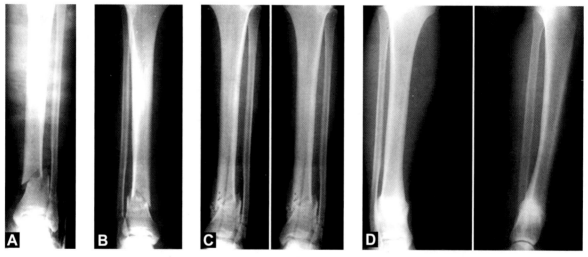

Figs 13.30A to D: (A) Radiograph of transverse fracture of the distal-third of the tibia and fibula taken through the initial above-the-knee cast. (B) Radiograph obtained through the functional brace. (C) Subsequent radiograph showing the development of mild varus deformity at the fracture site. (D) The fracture healed with a moderate varus angulation.

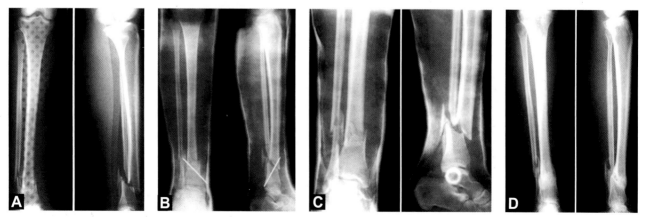

Figs 13.31A to D: (A) Initial radiograph of fracture in the distal-third of the tibia and fibula. (B) The treating resident felt that a transfixion pin would ensure maintenance of stability. (C) The pin was removed 3 weeks after the initial injury and a brace was applied. (D) The fracture healed uneventfully.

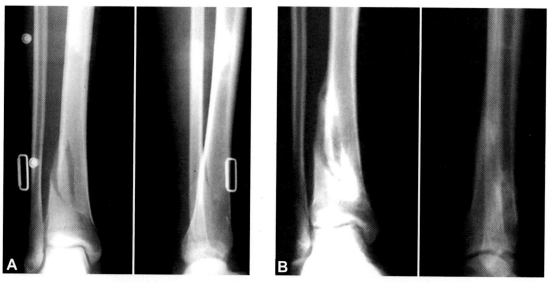

Figs 13.32A and B: Sequential radiographs of an oblique fracture of the distal tibia that healed without additional angulation or shortening.

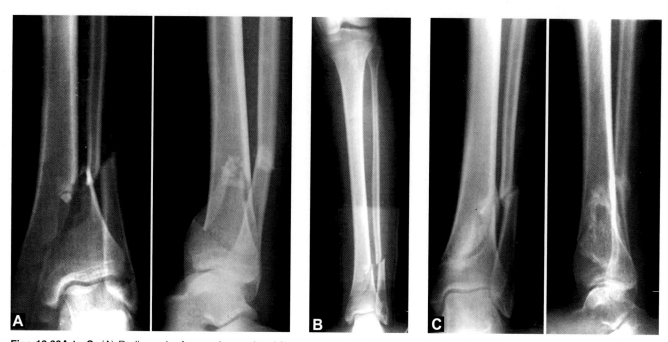

Figs 13.33A to C: (A) Radiograph of severely angulated fracture in the distal tibial metaphysis with an associated fibular fracture. (B) After reduction and stabilization of the fracture in an above-the-knee cast, a functional brace was applied. Distal swelling prevented the application of the brace for 15 days. (C) The fracture healed uneventfully.

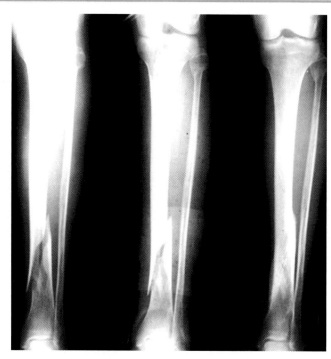

Fig. 13.34: Composite of radiographs demonstrating that the original shortening does not increase above and beyond that observed at the time of the injury, despite the early introduction of weight bearing activities.

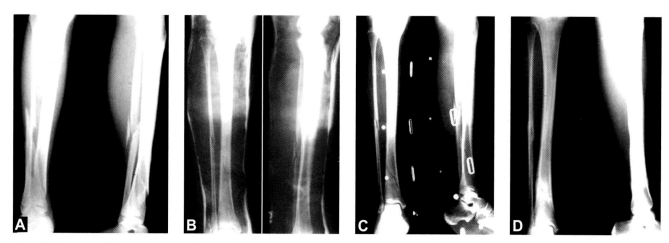

Figs 13.35A to D: (A) Radiograph of oblique fracture of the tibial diaphysis with an associated oblique fracture of the fibula. (B) Radiographs obtained through the initial above-the-knee cast showing anatomical alignment of the fragments. (C) Radiographs taken 2 weeks later illustrating the maintenance of alignment and shortening in the functional brace. (D) Radiographs showing solid healing of the fracture without change in the position of the fragments.

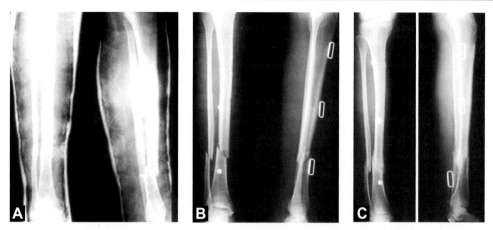

Figs 13.36A to C: (A) Radiograph of short oblique fracture of the tibia and fibula taken through the initial above-the-knee cast. A mild varus deformity is present. (B) Radiographs showing the fractured tibia in the functional brace. Notice that the mild varus deformity was corrected at the time of application of the brace. (C) The fracture healed without change in the length or alignment of the fragments.

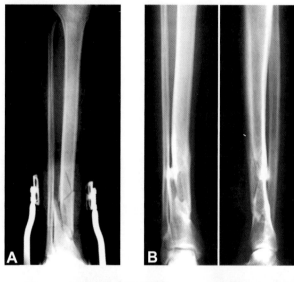

Figs 13.37A and B: (A) Radiograph of an oblique fracture of the distal tibia and fibula obtained through a functional brace. (B) Radiographs showing the healed fracture, without obvious deformity and without additional shortening.

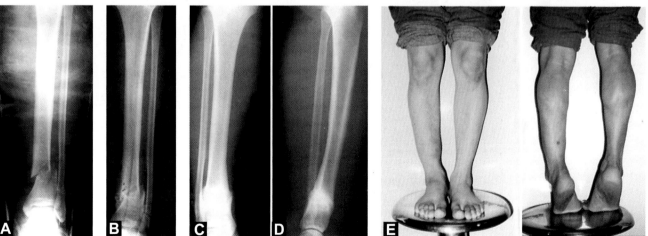

Figs 13.38A to E: (A) Radiograph of a very short oblique fracture of the tibia and fibula, taken through the initial above-the-knee cast. (B) Radiograph showing a mild varus deformity that appeared after the application of a functional brace. (C and D) Radiographs showing the solidly healed fracture with an inconsequential varus angulation. (E) Appearance of the extremities. The varus angular deformity can be readily recognized.

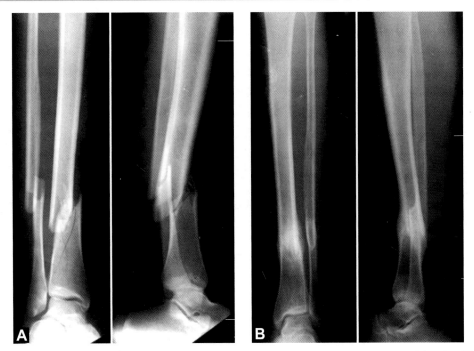

Figs 13.39A and B: (A) Radiographs of a short oblique fracture of the tibia and fibula. Notice the recurvatum deformity. (B) The fracture was treated with a functional brace, and healed with a minimal recurvatum angulation.

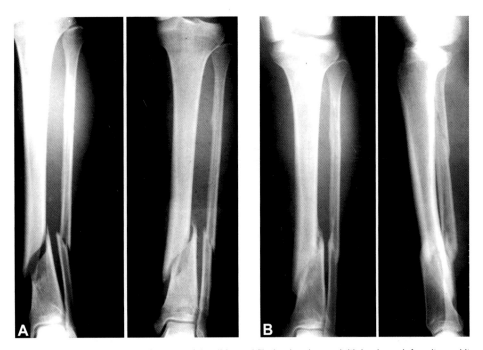

Figs 13.40A and B: (A) Radiographs of oblique fracture of the tibia and fibula showing an initial valgus deformity and its correction in the functional brace. (B) The fracture healed without additional shortening and no angulation.

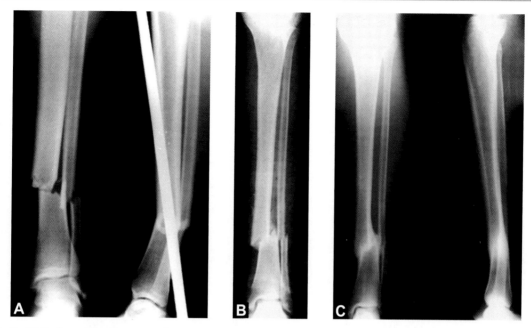

Figs 13.41A to C: (A) Radiographs of transverse fracture of the tibia and fibula. Notice the valgus deformity at the fracture site. (B) Radiograph in the functional brace. The angular deformity was corrected at the time of application of the initial above-the-knee cast. (C) The fractures healed uneventfully with a very mild recurvatum angulation.

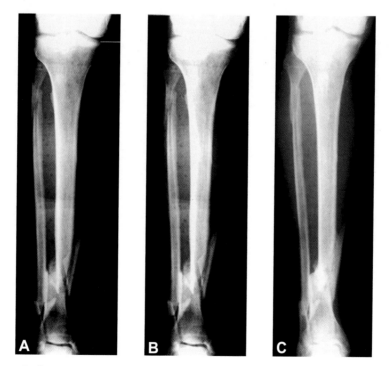

Figs 13.42A to C: (A) Radiograph of comminuted fracture of the tibia and fibula at the same level, taken in the functional brace, which was applied 12 days after the initial injury. (B) Radiograph taken 4 weeks later. (C) The fracture healed uneventfully without additional shortening or angulation.

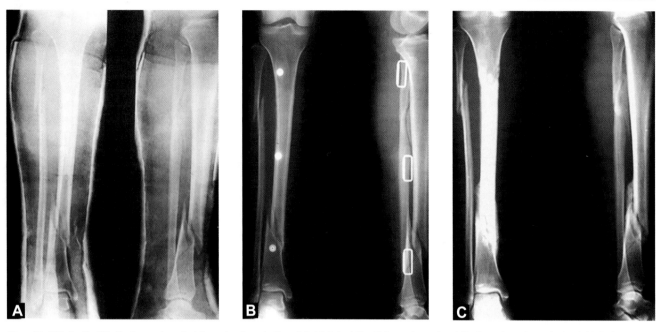

Figs 13.43A to C: (A) Radiographs of oblique fracture in the distal-third of the tibia and proximal fibula, taken through the initial above-the-knee cast. (B) Radiographs in the functional brace showing correction of the mild varus deformity seen in the cast. (C) The fractures healed uneventfully without additional shortening or angulation.

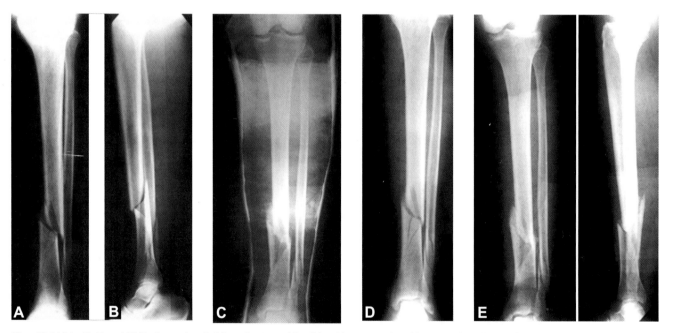

Figs 13.44A to E: (A and B) Radiographs of oblique fracture of the tibia with an associated fracture of the fibula. (C) Radiograph obtained through the above-the-knee cast. (D) Radiograph taken in the functional brace. (E) Radiograph illustrating the healed fractures with good alignment.

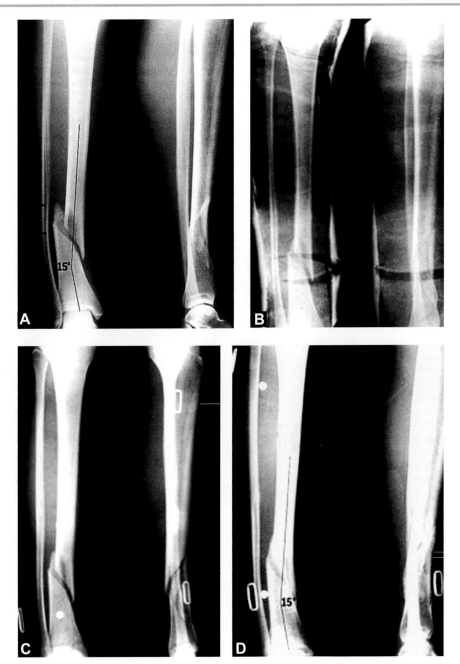

Figs 13.45A to D: (A) Composite of radiographs of a patient with an oblique fractures of the distal-third of the tibia without an associated fibular fracture. (B) A resident tried to correct the severe varus deformity by wedging the cast. Needless to say, the effort was unrewarding, since correction of a varus deformity cannot be accomplished as long as the fibula is intact. (C) Mistakenly, a functional brace was applied. (D) The fracture healed with the initial severe angular deformity. It did not get worse, probably due to the ultimate abutment of the distal fragment against the musculature in the area, which prevented additional displacement. Fracture of this type should not be treated with functional braces, unless the deformity is corrected through an osteotomy of the fibula at a short distance from the tibial fracture.

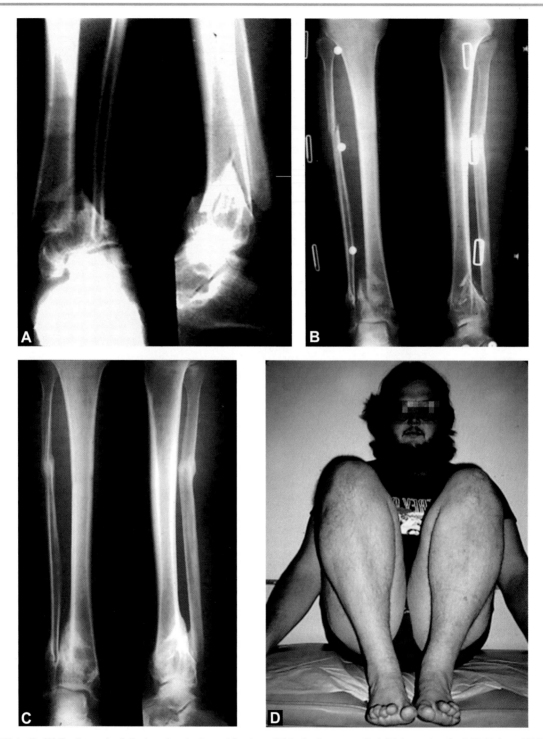

Figs 13.46A to D: (A) Radiograph of displaced metaphyseal fracture. (B) In the brace applied 17 days after the initial injury. (C) Radiograph taken after healing of the fracture. (D) The obese patient demonstrates the cosmetic appearance of the injured extremity.

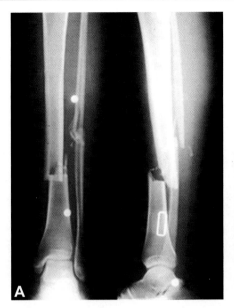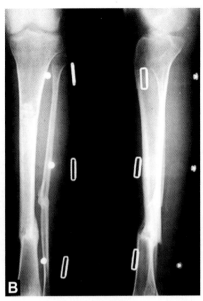

Figs 13.47A and B: (A) Radiographs of closed tibial and fibular fractures with mild overriding of the fragments. (B) Radiographs taken after the removal of the brace showing solid healing of the fractures and acceptable alignment.

REFERENCES

1. Sarmiento A, Latta LL. 450 Closed Fractures of the distal-third of the tibia treated with a functional brace. Clin Orthop. 2004; 428: 261-71.
2. Wiss DA, Stetson WB. Unstable fractures of the tibia treated with reamed intramedullary nails. Clin Orthop Relat Res. 1995; 315:56-63.
3. Court-Brown CM, Will E, Christie J, McQueen M. Reamed or unreamed nailing for closed tibial fractures. J Bone and Joint Surg. July 1996; 78B:580-3.
4. Gregory P, Sanders R. The treatment of closed, unstable tibial shaft fractures with unreamed interlocking nails. Clin Orthop Relat Res. 1995; 315:48-55.
5. Sarmiento A, Sharpe MD, Ebramzadeh E, Normand P, Shankwiler J. Factors influencing the Outcome of Closed Tibial Fractures Treated with Functional Bracing. Clin Ortho Relat Res. 1995 Jun; (315):8-24.
6. Sarmiento A. On the behavior of closed tibial fractures: clinical and radiological correlations. J Orthop Trauma, 2000; 14(3):199-205.
7. McKellop HA, Llinas A, Sarmiento A. Effects of Tibial Malalignment on the Knee and Ankle. Ortho. Clin. N. Amer. 1994 Jul; 25:3.
8. Hooper GJ, Keddell RG, Penny ID. Conservative management or closed nailing for tibial shaft fractures. A randomized prospective trial. J. Bone and Joint Surg. 1991 Jan; 73B:83-5.
9. Koval KJ, Clapper MF, Elison PS, Poka A, Bathon GH, Burgess AR. Complications of reamed intramedullary nailing of the tibia. J Ortop Trauma. 1991; 5:184-9.
10. Ricciardi-Pollini PT, Falez F. The Treatment of Diaphyseal Fractures by Functional Bracing. Results in 36 Cases. Et al J Orthop Traumatol. 1985 Jun; 11(2):199-205.
11. Williams J, Gibbons M, Trundle H, Murray D, Worlock P. Complications of nailing in closed tibial fractures. J Orthop Trauma. 1995; 9(6):476-81.
12. Alho A, Ekelan A, Stromsoe K et al. Nonunion of Tibial Shaft Fractures treated with locked intramedullary nailing without bone grafting. J. Trauma. 1993; 34(1):62.
13. Bone LB, Johnson K.D. Treatment of tibial fractures by reaming and intramedullary nailing. J. Bone and Joint Surg. 1986; 68A(6):877-87.
14. Court-Brown CM, Keating JF, McQueen MM. Infection after intramedullary nailing of the tibia. Incidence and protocol for management. J Bone Joint Surg Br. 1992; 74-B (5):770-16
15. Alho A, Eckeland A, Stromsoe K, Folleras G, Thorensen B. Locked intramedullary nailing of tibial fractures. J Bone Joint Surg. 1990; 72B:805-11.
16. Cole D, Latta LL. Fatigue failure of interlocking tibial nail implants. Orthop Trans Bone Joint Surg. 1992; 16-3A:663.
17. Hutson J. The Ilizarov System in Fracture care. Techniques in Orthopedics. 2002; 17:1-111.
18. Court-Brown CM, Gustilo T, Shaw AD. Knee pain after intramedullary nailing of proximal third tibia fractures. J Orthop Trauma. 1997; 11:103-5.
19. Kenwright J, Richardson JB, Goodship AE, Evans M, Kelly DJ, Spriggins AJ, Newman JH, Burrough SJ, Harris JD and Rowley DI. Effect of Controlled Axial Micromovement on Healing of Tibial Fractures. Lancet. 1986 Nov; 2(8517):1185-7.
20. Toivanen JA, Honkonen SE, Koivisto AM, Jarvinen MJ. Treatment of low-energy tibial shaft fractures. Plaster cast compared with intramedullary nailing. Int Orthop. 2001; 25(2):110-3.
21. Toivanen JA, Vaisto O, Kannus P, Latvala K, Honkonen SE, Jarvinen MJ. Anterior knee pain after intramedullary nailing of fractures of the tibial shaft. A prospective, randomized study comparing two different nail-insertion techniques. J Bone Joint Surg Am. 2002; 84-A(4):580-5.

14

The Segmental Fracture, Results and Representative Examples

It is customarily accepted that segmental fractures are a greater problem than non-segmental fractures frequently present. It is assumed, without empirical evidence to support the view, that the second or third fracture unfavorably influence the healing process. The fact is that the number of fractures, or the type of fracture have little to do with the manner in which fractures heal, since the healing process is determined by the response of the surrounding soft tissues, not by the bone pathology itself. More important than the type of tibial fracture is the condition of the fibula, which dictates the influences of alignment of the bone.

Segmental fractures are not necessarily produced by injuries of higher energy, when compared to those resulting from lower energy produced fractures. The initial energy that produces segmental fractures may be as great or as low as, that resulted in non-segmental fractures, therefore, the initial shortening observed in segmental fractures may even be of an inconsequential degree. Since the degree of initial shortening is the single most important feature in determining whether the closed functional treatment is appropriate, segmental fractures that show acceptable initial shortening are amenable to nonsurgical functional care. However, if acceptable alignment of the extremity cannot be easily attained simply by manual pressure, then a more radical surgical intervention is required. Oftentimes mild angular deformity of the middle fragment is acceptable providing the knee and ankle joints are parallel.

We reviewed our experiences with closed segmental tibial fractures that were managed with functional cast or braces. The following is an abbreviated version of the original publication.[1]

Thirty-one fractures were identified. The mean age was 35 years (age group 16 to 86). The mechanism of injury as shown in Table 14.1, where as the location of associated fracture of fibula is shown in Table 14.2.

Table 14.1: Mechanism of injury		
	Fracture	%
Motorcycle accidents	3	0.27
Pedestrian vs. auto	28	49.1
Falls.	16	28
Motor-veh accident	9	15.7
Unknown mechanism	1	1.75

Four patients had associated musculoskeletal injuries.

Table 14.2: Location of associated fracture of fibula		
	Fracture location	%
Proximal-third	15	26.3
Middle-third	18	31.5
Distal-third	18	31.5
Segmental	6	10.5

The initial versus the final shortening was: 4.34 mm – 4.1 mm. The initial medio-lateral angulation versus the final angulation was: 4.49° – 5.07°: The initial antero-posterior angulation versus the final angulation was: 5.53° – 3.81°. The initial displacement versus the distal displacement was: 22.94% versus 24.75%.

We have documented the fact that closed segmental fractures that experience initially acceptable shortening and the angular deformity can be brought to acceptable degrees, and can be successfully managed by closed functional care using a functional cast or brace.

REPRESENTATIVE EXAMPLES

Some of the Representative examples illustrating segmental fractures are shown in Figures 14.1 to 14.18.

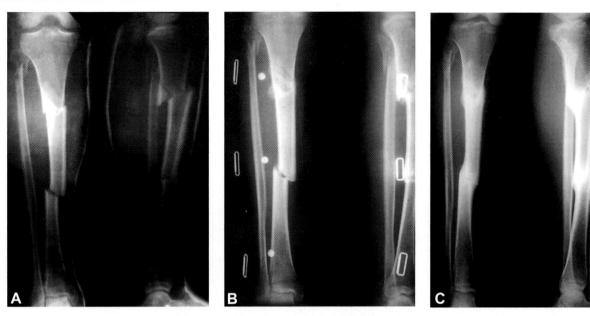

Figs 14.1A to C: (A) Segmental fracture of the tibia with an associated fibula fracture. Notice the acceptable shortening. (B) The limb was stabilized in a functional brace. (C) The fracture healed uneventfully with excellent alignment.

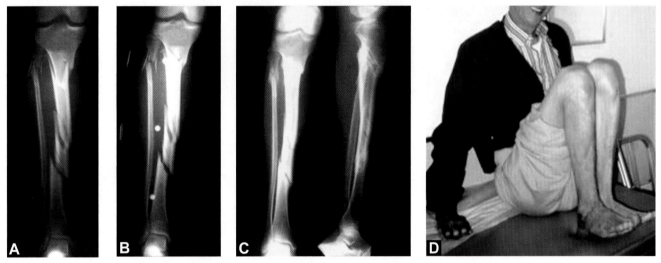

Figs 14.2A to D: (A and B) Radiographs of double segmental fracture of the tibia. Notice the minimal shortening of the extremity. The fracture was eventually stabilized in a below-the-knee functional brace. (C and D) Radiograph of the fractured tibia demonstrating healing and excellent alignment without additional shortening. The photograph illustrates the range of flexion of the knee joint.

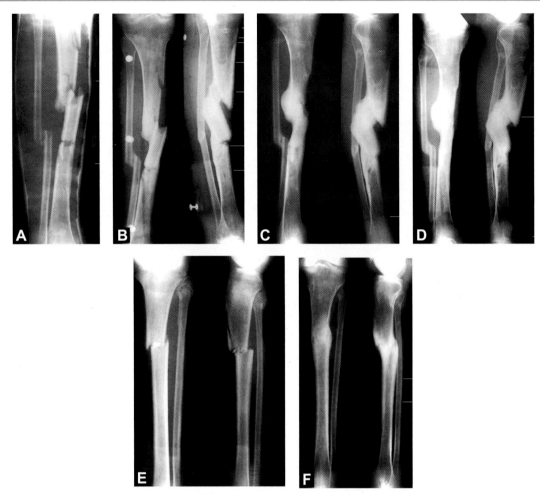

Figs 14.3A to F: (A to D) Sequential radiographs of an open fracture of the right tibia, sustained by a 49-year-old man struck by an automobile. The patient had also sustained a closed fracture of his opposite tibia. (E and F) The fractures united uneventfully.

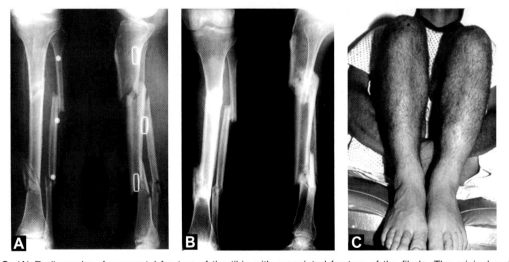

Figs 14.4A to C: (A) Radiographs of segmental fracture of the tibia with associated fracture of the fibula. The original malalignment was manually corrected. The limb was stabilized in a below-the-knee functional brace a few days later, when the acute symptoms and signs had subsided. (B) Radiograph obtained after completion of healing. The initial shortening remained essentially unchanged. (C) Appearance of the lower extremities. Notice the shortening of the left leg. A shoe insert had been given to the patient upon completion of healing, which a few months later eliminated as he felt that the shortening was not producing a limp.

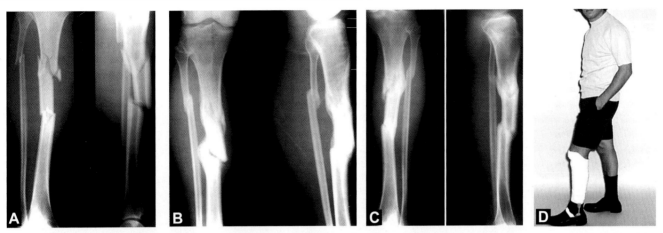

Figs 14.5A to D: (A) Radiographs of segmental fracture of the tibia with an associated fracture of the fibula. Notice the minimal shortening of the extremity. (B) The second radiograph shows the appearance of the tibia stabilized in a below-the-knee functional brace. (C) Radiograph taken after completion of healing and cosmetic appearance of the fractured limb. (D) The patient wearing the functional brace.

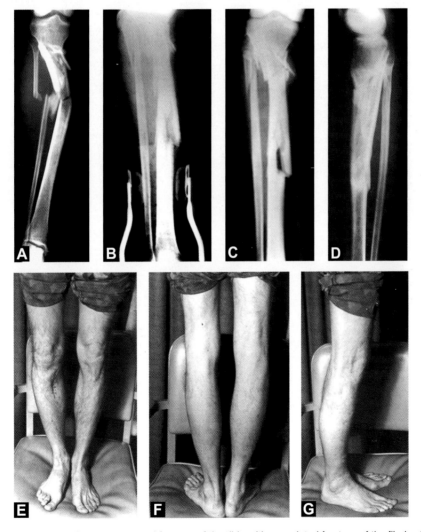

Figs 14.6A to G: (A to C) Radiographs of open-segmental fracture of the tibia with associated fracture of the fibula. After the acute symptoms and signs subsided, a below-the-knee functional brace was applied. (D) The fracture healed uneventfully and the original shortening did not increase. (E to G) Photographs of the patient's legs demonstrating the acceptable cosmetic appearance of the injured extremity.

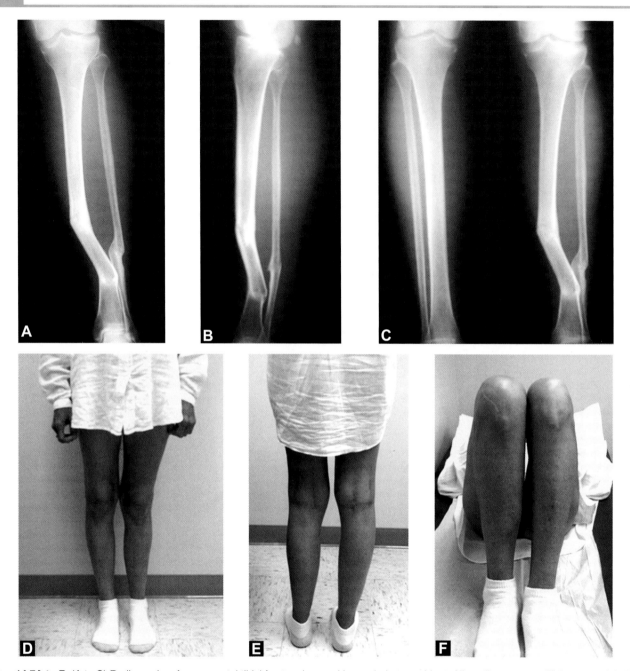

Figs 14.7A to F: (A to C) Radiographs of a segmental tibial fracture incurred in an airplane accident. Allegedly severe multiple-system injuries took place, which probably justified the acceptance of a severe deformity. She was first seen by us 35 years later with osteoarthritis of the opposite hip. A total hip arthroplasty was performed. (D to F) Standing films illustrating the angular deformity but relatively parallel relationship between the knee and ankle joints. Patient states that she had a meniscectomy performed prior to the airplane accident. The knee was asymptomatic.

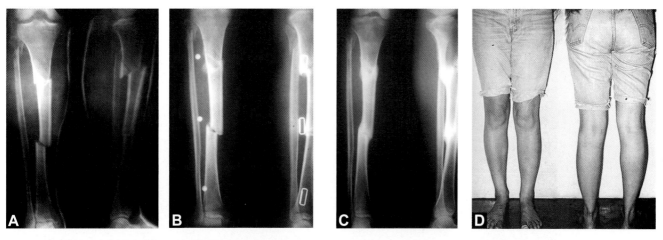

Figs 14.8A to D: (A) Radiograph of segmental fracture showing minimal initial shortening and acceptable angulation. (B) Radiographs taken in the functional brace. (C) Radiographs showing the healed fracture without additional shortening and very acceptable angulation. (D) Patient exhibits the cosmetic appearance of her lower extremities,

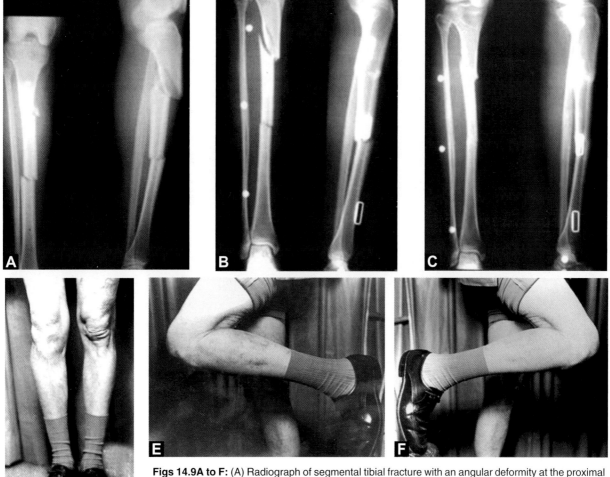

Figs 14.9A to F: (A) Radiograph of segmental tibial fracture with an angular deformity at the proximal level. (B) Radiographs in the functional brace. Notice that the angular deformity has been corrected. (C) The last radiograph before patient was lost to follow-up. It appears the fracture was healed at that time. (D) Appearance of the lower extremities when the patient was last seen. (E and F) Degree of motion of the knees.

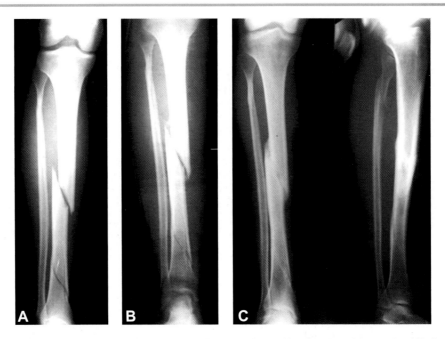

Figs 14.10A to C: (A) Radiograph of segmental fracture of the tibia associated with a fracture of the proximal fibula. The initial shortening was acceptable. Notice the non-displaced, stable nature of the distal fracture. (B) Radiograph in the functional brace. No attempt to gain length was made. (C) Radiographs obtained following healing of the fracture. No additional shortening took place. The absence of callus on the distal fracture shows the seminal role played by motion in the production of peripheral callus.

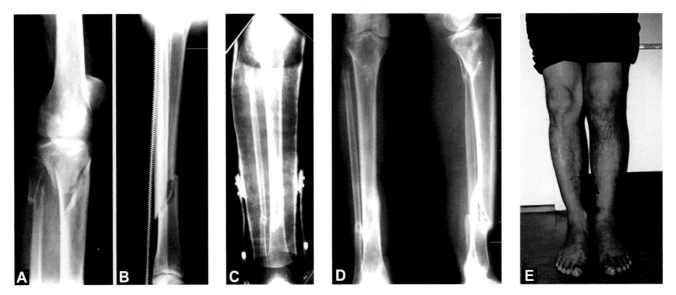

Figs 14.11A to E: (A and B) Radiograph of segmental tibial fracture with acceptable initial shortening. (C) Radiograph taken in the Plaster of Paris functional brace. (D) Radiographs taken after completion of healing. There is a residual but inconsequential mild angular deformity at the proximal level. (E) Appearance of the extremities a few weeks after the application of the cast-brace.

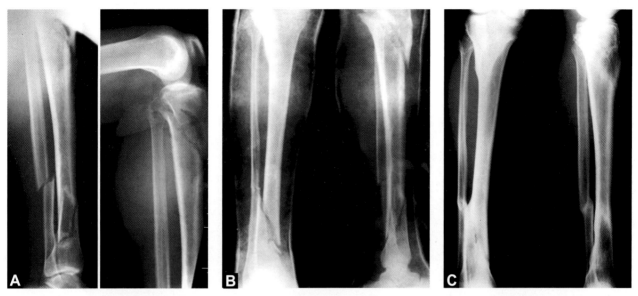

Figs 14.12A to C: (A) Radiograph of segmental tibial fracture with acceptable initial shortening. (B) Radiographs in the initial above-the-knee cast showing a varus deformity at the distal level. (C) The fracture healed uneventfully with a mild angular deformity.

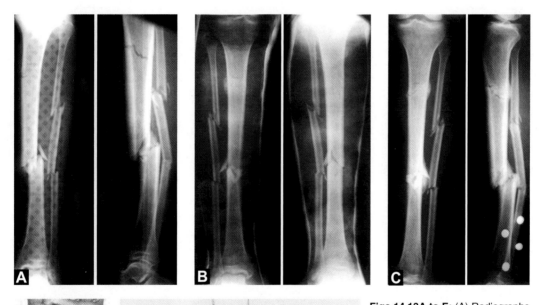

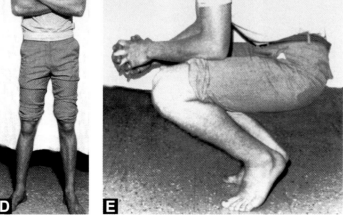

Figs 14.13A to E: (A) Radiographs of segmental fractures of the tibia and fibula. The proximal fracture was a nondisplaced and stable one. (B) Radiographs in the initial above-the-knee cast and in the below-the-knee functional cast. (C) The fractures healed without additional shortening and with a mild, inconsequential recurvatum at the distal level. (D and E) Patient demonstrates the cosmetic appearance of his lower extremities and the range of motion of his knees shortly after completion of healing.

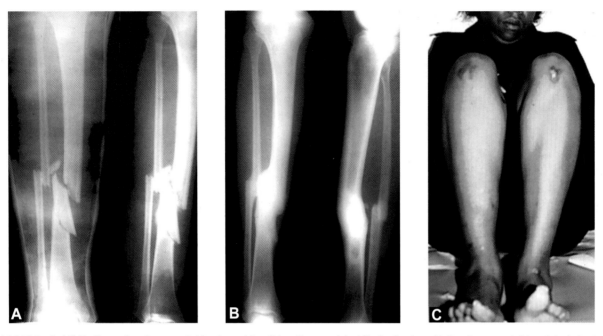

Figs 14.14A to C: (A) Radiographs of segmental fracture of the tibia with associated fibular fracture. Notice the acceptable original shortening. (B) No attempt was made to regain length. The fracture healed without additional shortening and very acceptable alignment. (C) Patient demonstrates the cosmetic appearance of her lower extremities and the inconsequential shortening of her fractured leg.

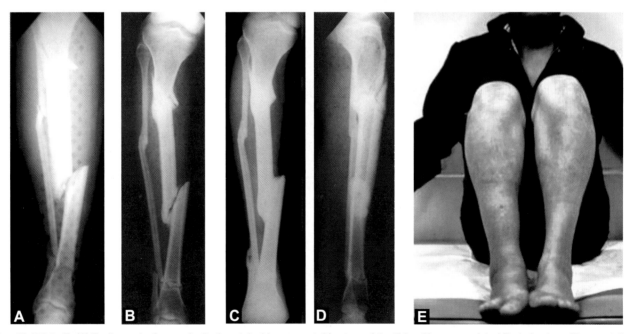

Figs 14.15A to E: (A) Radiograph of severely displaced double segmental fracture of the tibia with an associated fibula fracture. The most distal fracture was nondisplaced. The patient had associated multiple-organ injuries that delayed the appropriate early care of the fracture tibia. (B and C) Radiograph of the tibia showing the malalignment of the fragments and the initially accepted (unwisely) excessive shortening. (D) Radiograph illustrating the perhaps unacceptable shortening and angulation of the healed fractures. (E) Appearance of the patient's lower extremities. Notice the shortening, which was readily compensated with a heel- lift of half-centimeter.

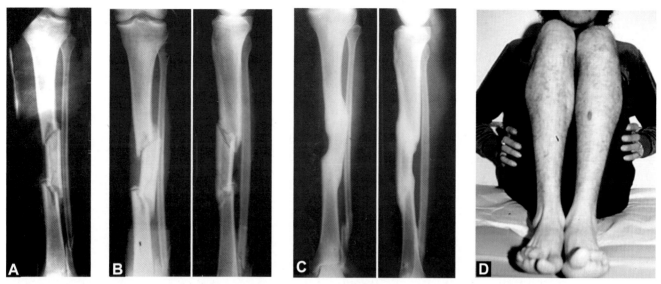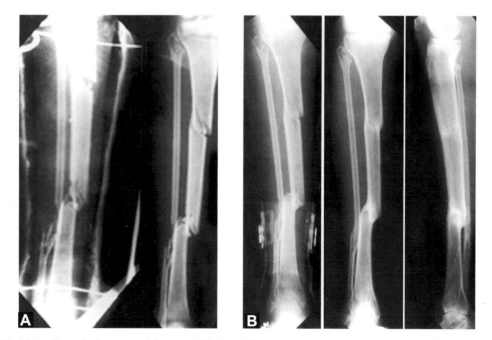

Figs 14.16A to D: (A) Radiograph of segmental fracture of the tibia associated with a distal fracture of the fibula. (B) Radiograph obtained 3 months after the initial injury. (C) The fracture healed uneventfully with additional shortening. (D) Patient shows the good alignment of his injured leg. Notice the residual temporary atrophy of his leg.

Figs 14.17A and B: (A) Radiograph of segmental fracture, initially stabilized with pins above and below the fractures. We have no information as to the amount of shortening the treating physician identified and corrected at the time of his initial encounter with the patient. We suspect the correction was of approximately 12 mm, based on the fact that the radiograph taken after removal of the pins showed that degree of shortening. In other words, the correction had been lost. (B) The limb was then stabilized in a brace. The fracture healed with acceptable degrees of shortening and angulation.

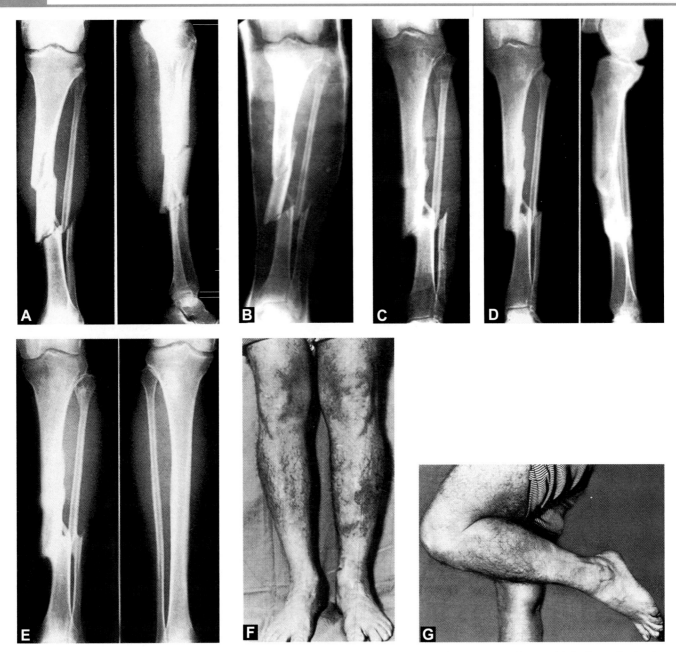

Figs 14.18A to G: (A) Segmental fracture of the tibia with associated fibula fracture. Notice the initial valgus deformity. (B) Radiograph after the application of the initial above-the-knee cast. The corrected valgus deformity reveals the true initial shortening of the limb, which was considered acceptable. (C) Radiograph obtained through the brace. Notice the maintenance of the original shortening. (D) Radiographs taken 3 and 6 months respectively following the initial injury. (E) Standing radiographs of both tibia illustrating the final shortening of the fractured tibia. (F and G) Clinical photographs of the lower extremities. It is virtually impossible to detect with accuracy which was the fractured limb.

REFERENCE

1. Sarmiento A, Latta LL. Functional treatment of Closed Segmental Fractures of the Tibia. Acta Chir Orthop Traumatol Cech. 2008; 75:325-31.

15

The Open Fracture

Despite great progress in the care of fractures, the open one remains a challenging one. Infections continue to occur even when the care is provided under the cleanest and most sophisticated environment. Once a fracture becomes infected, its elimination is either difficult or impossible to overcome. Powerful antibiotics to which many bacteria are sensitive are not effective if the drug does not reach the pathogenic organisms. If fracture fragments are avascular as a result of comminution and detachment from connecting blood vessels, no amount of antibiotics can be helpful. It is a frequently made mistake to believe that antibiotic administration alone is the best preventive measure of infection. Nothing can be further from the truth.

The obvious implication from this irrefutable fact is that the most important factor in the prevention of infection is a thorough early debridement of the wound after the initial injury and a prolonged "washing" of the area in order to remove, as much as possible, contaminated material. There are times when it is desirable to remove bony fragments that clearly demonstrate loss of all tissue attachment.

Open fractures heal more slowly than closed ones for reasons we do not clearly understand at this time.[1] The loss of the hematoma alone cannot possibly explain the phenomenon since the hematoma per se does not become bone. As we suggested earlier, if the hematoma were important in fracture healing, the injection of blood, taken from a distant vein, would accelerate healing. This is definitely not the case. By the same token, closed fracture associated with large hematomas, such as those that are result of higher energy levels, should heal faster, which once again is not the case.

Attempts to treat open fractures with plate fixation have clearly demonstrated an increase in the rate of infection. The trauma created by the surgical procedure adds to the damage produced by the injury itself. At this time, there is enthusiasm in some countries with the use of intramedullary nailing of open fractures, and some reports seem encouraging. However, the fact remains that in the absence of appropriate debridement of the wound, carried out under the best possible operating room environment, the results may be disastrous.

In general, it is best to treat open fracture with debridement and stabilization, either in a cast or with external fixation apparatus. Significant progress has been made recently with closed intramedullary nailing of the interlocking type. However, despite several reassuring reports, its final place has not yet been established.

The wound, in most cases, should be left open unless its damage is considered to have been minimal or moderate. If severe, it is best to leave it open and lightly packed with sterile dressings. It should be inspected and subjected to a second inspection approximately 24 hours later. Additional removal of damaged tissues that appears to have been inadvertently left behind should be removed. Prophylactic antibiotics should be continued until the clean granulation tissue is shown to cover the wound.

There is little to be gained from inspecting the wound on a frequent basis. Once the appearance of healthy healing tissues is seen after the debridements, it is best to leave the stabilizing cast in place and the wound undisturbed. Frequent inspections are likely to result in contamination with additional pathogenic organisms. Some investigators recommend early closure of the skin or skin grafting. This issue, however, must be placed in the proper perspective. Frequent inspection of the wound is not always necessary as Trueta so eloquently demonstrated some 60 years ago.

Early functional bracing in the management of open tibial fractures has only a minor place in the armamentarium of the orthopedic surgeon. Casting does not permit direct repeated care of the wound in the manner the external fixators or intramedullary nailing does.

The history of Trueta's contribution to the field of fracture care is fascinating and enlightening. Trueta was an orthopedic surgeon from Barcelona, Spain, during the Spanish Civil War of the 1930s. Allegedly, the casualties became overwhelming during the retreat of the Republican Army as Franco's troops advanced into Catalonia. It had become impossible to appropriately manage open fractures with then accepted method of repeated wound cleansing while the fractured limb was resting on a plaster splint.

The hospital where Trueta did his work could no longer accommodate the high number of wounded soldiers, so their transfer to another institution in a distant town became necessary. Rather than leaving the wound exposed to the air, a circular cast was applied directly over the wound. In that manner, the soldier was then sent to the distant hospital.

It was then discovered that upon inspection of the wounds a few days later, their appearance was found to be much better than what the orthopedists were accustomed to seeing in their own institutions. Based on those experiences, the management of open fractures was radically changed. The overall prognosis improved dramatically.

It must be recognized that at that time penicillin had not as yet been discovered. While Trueta was serendipitously covering open fractures with Plaster of Paris, Winett Orr, a surgeon from the Unites States was simultaneously treating osteomyelitis in the same manner and with equally encouraging results.

Trueta's lessons have been forgotten for the most part. Currently, open wounds are either closed primarily or secondarily using sophisticated skin grafting techniques. Indeed, a great deal of progress has been made in this area. However, to believe that the Trueta treatment has no place in today's armamentarium is a mistake. The patient recovery and rehabilitation is expedited exponentially. The addition of early ambulation further assists in the healing of the fractures. The tensile stresses on the soft tissues of the injured limb, injured brought about by the early active ambulation, encourages their more rapid healing. The belief that skin defects should be protected from ambulation is erroneous. The alignment of collagen fibers of the normal helix is expedited by repeated tensile stresses imposed upon them.

The following is an example of an open fracture of the tibia successfully managed with the Trueta method of debridement, followed by stabilization with pins above and below the fracture, and subsequently transferred to a below-the-knee functional cast (Figure 15.1A to G).

A reason as to why open tibial fractures are not frequent indications for functional casting and bracing is that in too many instances the initial shortening is unacceptable. In closed axially unstable fractures, as we have thoroughly discussed in a previous chapter, we do not experience additional shortening beyond the one observed immediately after the initial insult. This has led us to practice that if the initial shortening is acceptable in a closed fracture, the shortening can be accepted and ambulation permitted in anticipation of having the initial shortening unchanged. This is not always true with open fractures since determination of the initial shortening is difficult and often unreliable.

The following is a good representative example of the recurrence of shortening of axially unstable fracture that we have repeatedly illustrated in previous chapters. This recurrence easily occurs in open fractures, which as rule have a greater degree of initial shortening.

This is why we use functional casting, followed by functional bracing, only in open fractures that are the result of relatively minor trauma showing acceptable shortening, and an easily corrected angular deformity.

Open fractures produced by low-velocity bullet do not, as a rule, require debridement of the wound which is usually small. Cleansing of the wound, preceded and followed by a few days of prophylactic antibiotic therapy suffices. However, at the earliest sign of infection aggressive surgery should be performed.

With the healing of open fractures, particularly those in long bones, the surgeon confronts a number of questions of great importance. If a cast is being used, for example in the treatment of a tibial fracture, when should the patient be allowed to bear weight on the affected extremity? If an external fixator is used, when can it be safely removed? In regards to the first question, our answer is: if the fracture occurred as a result of a very high energy injury that produced extensive soft tissue damage and major distraction between the bony fragments as well as considerable shortening of the extremity that required traction to minimize that shortening, the early introduction of weight bearing would result in prompt recurrence of the initial shortening. Therefore, under this circumstance, non-weight bearing ambulation should be delayed until further soft tissue repair has taken place. If the initial shortening was not extreme, gradual increase in weight bearing can be introduced.

The appropriate time for removal of the metallic pins used with an external fixator is also a challenging question. If the fracture is axially unstable, i.e. comminuted or oblique, and required initial traction to overcome excessive shortening, removal of the pins prior to strong intrinsic stability of the soft tissues will likely result in a recurrence of shortening if treated in a cast (Figure 15.2). Another problem in this situation is the fact that in the fractured fibula heals faster than the tibia, in such a manner that when the "frame" is remove and weight bearing ambulation is introduced, a varus deformity readily develops.

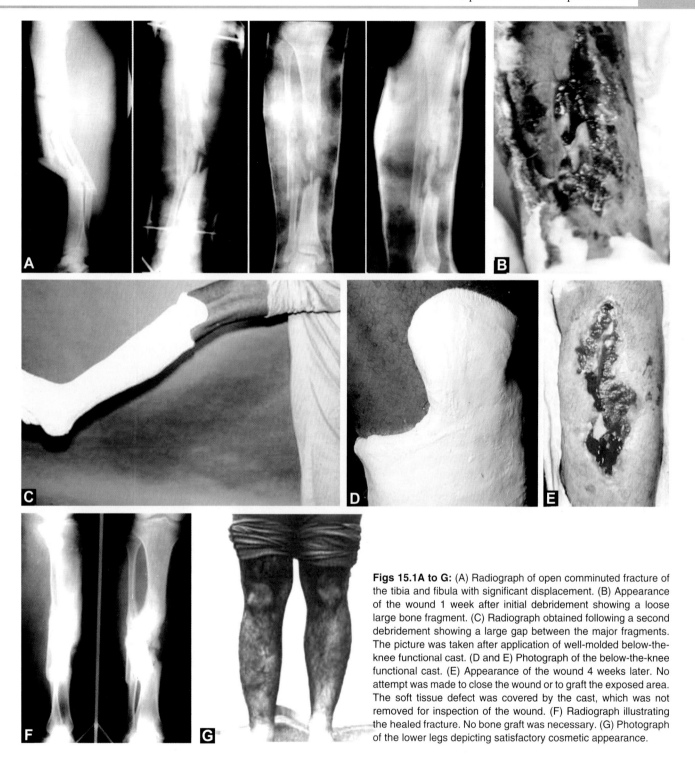

Figs 15.1A to G: (A) Radiograph of open comminuted fracture of the tibia and fibula with significant displacement. (B) Appearance of the wound 1 week after initial debridement showing a loose large bone fragment. (C) Radiograph obtained following a second debridement showing a large gap between the major fragments. The picture was taken after application of well-molded below-the-knee functional cast. (D and E) Photograph of the below-the-knee functional cast. (E) Appearance of the wound 4 weeks later. No attempt was made to close the wound or to graft the exposed area. The soft tissue defect was covered by the cast, which was not removed for inspection of the wound. (F) Radiograph illustrating the healed fracture. No bone graft was necessary. (G) Photograph of the lower legs depicting satisfactory cosmetic appearance.

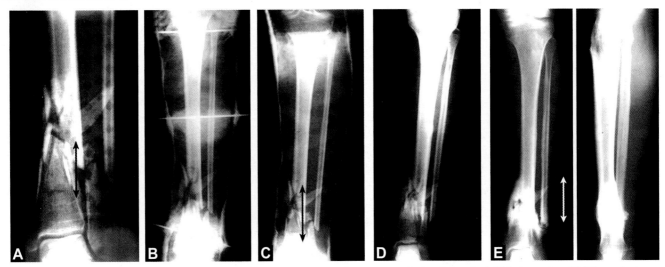

Figs 15.2A to E: (A) Radiograph of open comminuted fractures of the distal tibia and fibula. Notice the initial shortening. (B) The patient was initially treated at another community where the treating surgeon elected to carry out debridement of the wound and stabilization of the fracture with two pins. He, obviously, tried to regain length by traction prior to the placement of the pins. (C) Radiographs obtained after removal of the pins. Notice the recurrence of shortening to the initial degree. (D) Radiograph in the functional brace. showing progressing healing. (E) Final radiographs showing the healed fractures with good alignment and an acceptable degree of shortening.

Some of the representative examples illustrating open fractures are shown in Figures 15.3 to 15.19.

Amputation surgery is usually considered by the people at large and by the surgical profession as well, as a difficult decision. Its importance should not be minimized, however, it must be placed in its proper perspective. Sometimes, the need to amputate is not a sign of defeat, but a victory.

A trans-tibial amputation that can be followed by the proper fitting of a prosthesis carries a rather minor disability. The disability is in some instances of a lower degree than that produced from a partially anesthetic limb, particularly if accompanied with joint pain and ankylosis. A return to certain types of work is less likely to be precluded for the amputee than for the disabled counterpart.

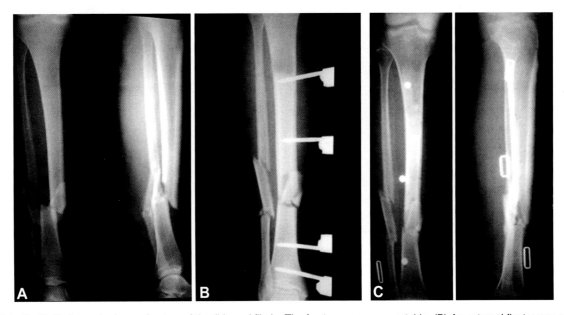

Figs 15.3A to C: (A) Radiograph of open fracture of the tibia and fibula. The fracture was very unstable. (B) An external fixator was used and the wound was left open. (C) The pins were removed 3 weeks after the initial insult and then stabilized, first in an above-the-knee cast and then in a below-the-knee functional cast. The fracture healed with good alignment and length. Since the period of joint immobilization was short, the range of motion of the ankle and knee was minimally impaired.

If appropriate prosthetic resources are available, the rehabilitation of the below-the knee amputee usually is rapid and effective. However, it is implied that the amputation procedure was properly carried out. We continue to make reference to below-the-knee amputees, rather than above-the-knee amputees, simply because the performance of the latter is significantly more compromised. Therefore, it behooves the surgeon to attempt, as much as possible, to save the knee joint when considering a lower extremity amputation. The same applies to the upper extremity where preservation of the elbow joint is of great importance.

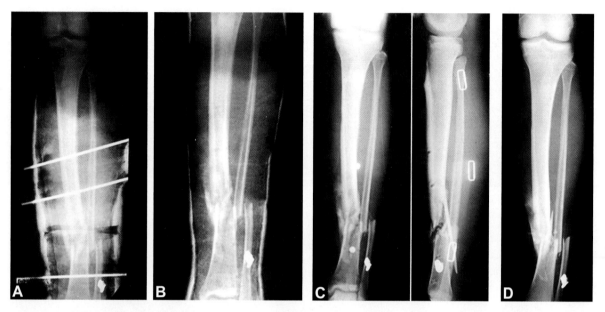

Figs 15.4A to D: (A) Radiograph of open fracture of the tibia stabilized with "pins-above-and-below." (B) After 2 months in the frame, a below-the-knee cast was applied. (C) Radiographs demonstrating the onset of a varus deformity shortly after a brace was applied. (D) One year later, the fracture was healed but with a severe and unacceptable deformity. It is very likely that the deformity occurred because the "frame" immobilized the tibia but left the fibula non-immobilized, and therefore subject to the healthy influence of motion at the fracture site. With the fibula healed at the time of application of the brace, the ubiquitous varus deformity developed.

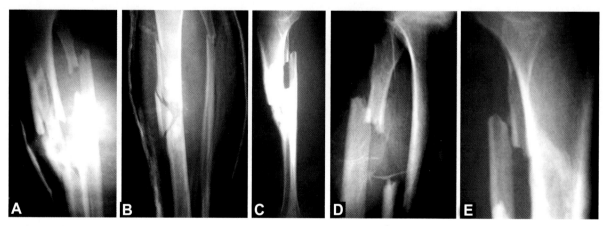

Figs 15.5A to E: (A) Radiograph of open fracture. Notice the degree of shortening, best illustrate by the fibula. (B) Radiograph obtained after attempts were made to regain length. Restoration of length in comminuted, axially unstable fractures does not prevent recurrence of shortening. (C) Radiograph obtained after completion of healing. Notice the recurrence of shortening. (D and E) Composite photograph illustrating the initial and final shortening, which for all practical purposes is identical.

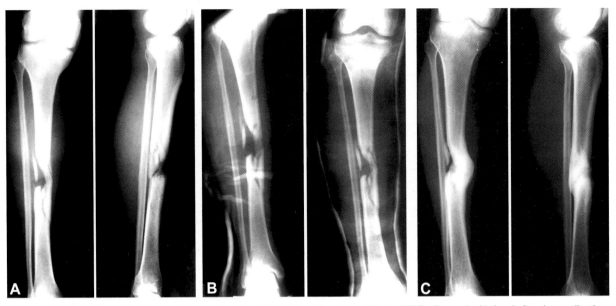

Figs 15.6A to C: (A) Radiograph of low-grade open fracture of the tibia with an intact fibula. (B) Radiograph obtained after the application of an above-the-knee cast, (C) which was held in place till the fracture showed evidence of union. This type of fracture has a tendency to angulate into varus under weight bearing conditions.

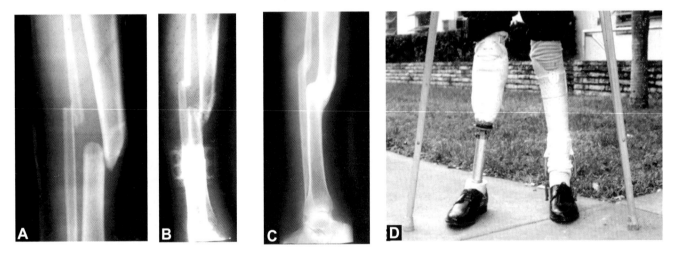

Figs 15.7A to D: (A) Radiograph of minimally open oblique, displaced fracture of the tibia with an associated fibula fracture. (B) The initial shortening was considered acceptable in light of the fact that the opposite extremity had been amputated at the time of the accident. It was anticipated that because of the low grade open nature of the fracture, no additional shortening would take place. (C) Radiograph taken through the brace showing no change in the length of the extremity. (D) Photograph of patient with the left lower extremity braced and the amputated right leg stabilized in a temporary plaster prosthesis.

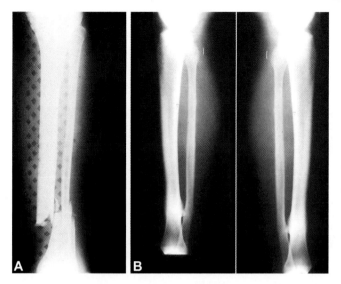

Figs 15.8A and B: (A) Radiograph of displaced closed fracture of the distal tibia. (B) After obtaining a stable reduction, the fracture was treated with a functional brace. The fracture healed uneventfully.

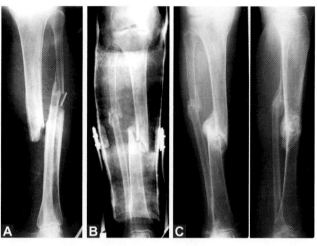

Figs 15.9A to C: (A) Radiograph of severe open fracture of the tibia and fibula with unacceptable shortening. (B) During the debridement of the wound, the fracture was reduced and found to be stable. An above-the-knee cast was applied, and 4 weeks later replaced with a functional Plaster of Paris functional cast. (C) The fracture progressed to healing with maintenance of the reduction and alignment.

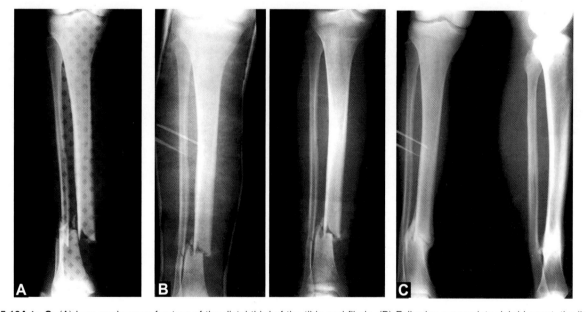

Figs 15.10A to C: (A) Low-grade open fracture of the distal-third of the tibia and fibula. (B) Following appropriate debridement, the limb was stabilized in an above-the-knee cast, which was replaced with a functional brace upon confirmation of uneventful soft tissue healing. (C) The fracture healed uneventfully.

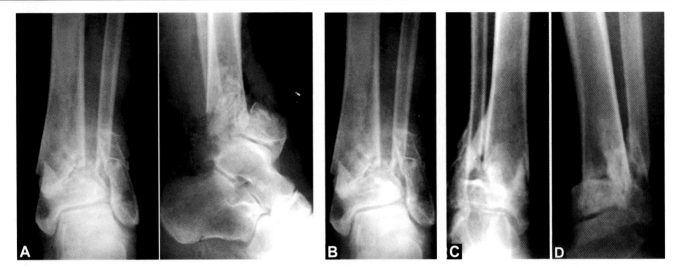

Figs 15.11A to C: (A) Radiographs of open (Type I) intraarticular comminuted fractures of distal tibia and fibula. (B) Through manipulation, the alignment of the fragments was improved. Through further manipulation, the deformity was improved. (C) The fracture healed with a deformity. It is likely that surgical treatment with metallic fixation would have rendered a better-appearing radiological appearance but a less functional ankle.

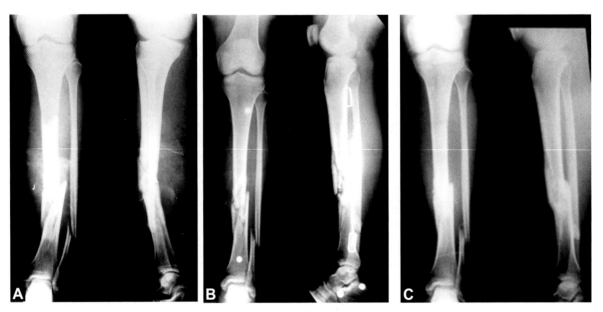

Figs 15.12A to C: (A) Radiograph of a low-grade open fracture of the tibia. Notice the varus angular deformity associated with minimal shortening. (B) Radiograph in the brace, which was applied 3 weeks after the initial injury. Notice the correction of the angular deformity. (C) Radiographs taken after completion of healing. No additional shortening took place.

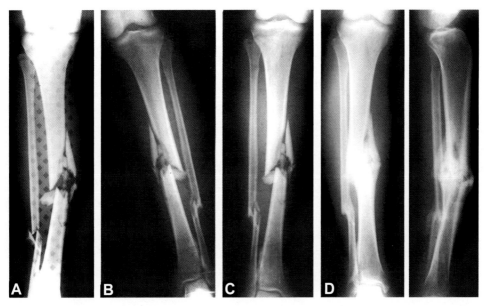

Figs 15.13A to D: (A) Radiograph of open fractures of the tibia and fibula produced by a low-velocity bullet (B) Radiograph obtained in the functional brace after stabilization of the fracture in an above-the-knee cast for 2 months. Notice the shortening that took place at the fracture site, indicative of the damage to the soft tissues. (C) Radiograph suggesting progressive healing with maintenance of length and alignment, but with a mild varus deformity. (D) The patient elected to discontinue the brace and developed deformities in the sagittal and coronal views.

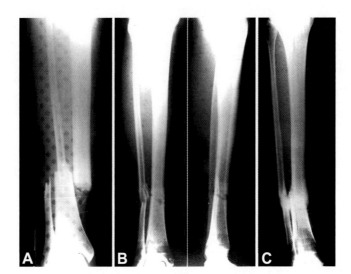

Figs 15.14A to C: (A) Radiograph of open transverse fracture of the tibia and fibula at the same level. (B) Radiographs of the tibia stabilized in a functional brace. The reduction obtained in surgery had been maintained. (C) The fracture healed but with mild angular deformity. Experiences such as this one, prompted us gradually to further limit the use of functional braces in open fractures.

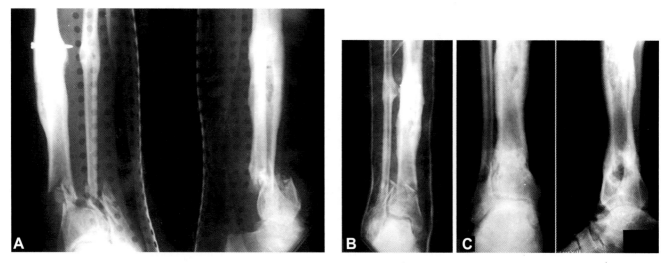

Figs 15.15A to C: (A) Radiograph of open metaphyseal fracture with severe displacement but relatively minor soft tissue defect. (B) Radiograph obtained after closed reduction by manipulation. (C) Radiograph demonstrating the healed fracture in good alignment.

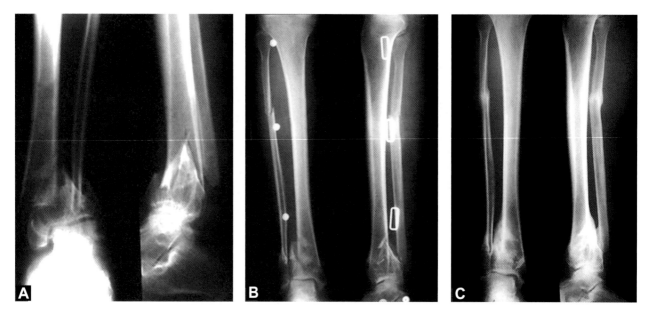

Figs 15.16A to C: (A) Radiograph of severely displaced closed fracture of the tibia and associated fibular fracture. (B) After the fracture was reduced manually and stabilized in an above-the-knee cast and later transferred to a functional brace, active motion of the ankle became possible. Weight bearing was gradually increased according to symptoms. (C) Radiograph of the fracture obtained after completion of healing.

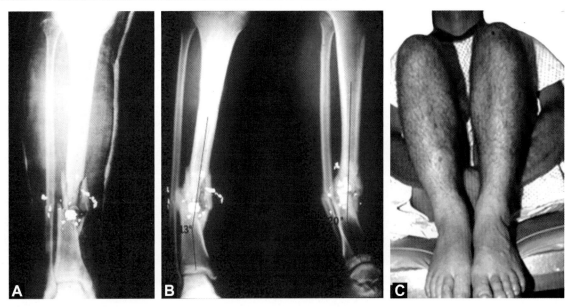

Figs 15.17A to C: (A) Radiograph of a comminuted fracture of the distal tibia produced by a low-velocity bullet. Notice that the fibula, though fracture is a transverse, is non-displaced one. (B) The non-displaced nature of the fibular fracture led to the development of a severe varus deformity. The fracture healed in that manner. (C) The appearance of the lower extremities illustrating the unacceptable varus deformity.

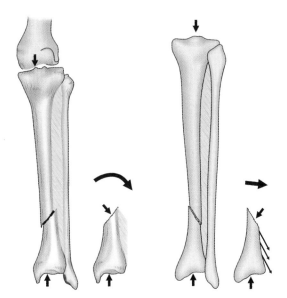

Figs 15.18: In the case of the fractured tibia with an intact fibula, the direction of the fracture determines whether or not a varus deformity is likely to occur. If an oblique fracture runs from proximal to distal and from lateral to medial, the tendency of the proximal fragment to drift into varus is partially or completely prevented by the abutment between the two fragments.[2-5]

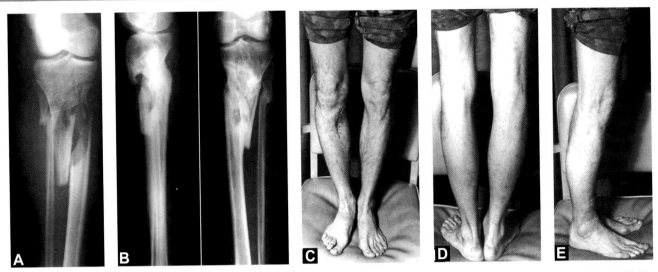

Figs 15.19A and B: (A) Radiograph of comminuted open fracture (Type II) of the proximal tibia with associated fracture of the fibula. (B) The fracture was treated initially with an above-the-knee cast and early ambulation. As soon as the acute symptoms subsided, a below-the-knee brace was applied. The fracture healed uneventfully. (C to E) Demonstrate the appearance of the extremity and the scar over the proximal aspect of the leg.

REFERENCES

1. Tscherne H, Oestern HJ. A new classification of soft tissue damage in open and closed fractures. Unfallheilkunde. 1982; 85(3):111-5.
2. Latta LL, Sarmiento A. Mechanical Behavior of Tibial Fractures. Symposium on Trauma to the Leg and Its Sequela. C.V. Mosby: St. Louis, MO 1981.
3. Latta LL, Sarmiento A. Fracture Casting and Bracing. ASOP Publishing Inc. 2008.
4. Rosa G, Savarese A, Chianca I, Coppola D. Treatment of Fractures of the Lower Limbs with Functional Braces. It al J Orthop Traumatol. 1982 Sep; 8(3):301-8.
5. Sarmiento A, Latta LL. Functional Bracing in Management of Tibial Fractures. The Intact Fibula. AAOS Symposium on Trauma of the Leg and Its Sequela. Moore TM (Ed). The C. V. Mosby Company. 1981; 278-98.

16

Pathological Fractures

The authors' experience with functional treatment of fractures through pathological bone is very limited. The few clinical cases (Figures 16.1 to 16.4), here presented are examples of such situations.

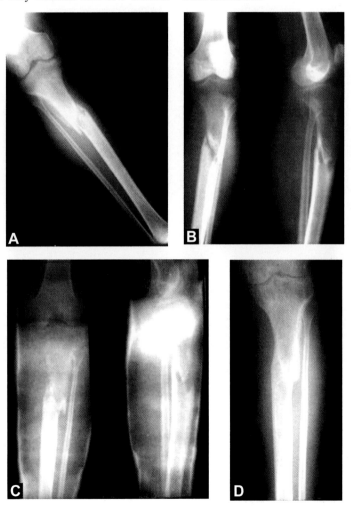

Figs 16.1A to D: (A) Radiograph of fracture of the proximal tibia treated with an above-the-knee cast. (B) Two months later, it was suspected that the high degree of mineralization could be secondary to a neoplastic condition. A biopsy revealed Paget's disease. (C) A below-the-knee functional cast was then applied, and weight bearing activities encouraged. (D) Two and one half months later, the fracture united.

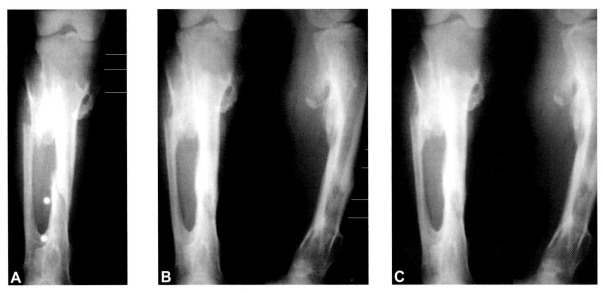

Figs 16.2A to C: (A) Radiograph of a fracture of the tibia sustained by a patient suffering from congenital multiple exostosis. (B) The fracture was stabilized in a prefabricated functional brace. (C) Radiograph showing the fracture solidly united 3 months after the initial injury.

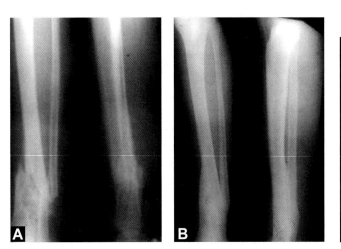

Figs 16.3A and B: (A) Radiograph of fracture of the tibia that occurred through an osteochondroma. (B) The fracture was treated with a functional brace. The initial malalignment was not corrected, and the fracture healed with a varus deformity.

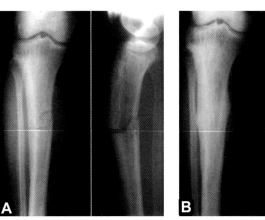

Figs 16.4A and B: (A) Radiograph of fracture of the proximal tibia that occurred through a bone affected with Paget's disease. (B) The fracture was treated with a functional brace and healed uneventfully.

17

Delayed Unions and Nonunions

Functional bracing of closed tibial fractures has revealed a high rate of success as depicted by the 1.5% nonunion rate and angular deformities where 90% patients healed their fractures with less than 6° of deformity.[1,2] However, the method, as we have repeatedly emphasized, is not a panacea, and close adherence to a simple protocol is essential.

Nonunions continue to plague the treatment of tibial fractures, particularly open fractures. Despite significant progress in this area, this complication threatens success.

The lessons we learnt from the functional treatment of acute closed fractures with a functional bracing method taught us that functional bracing has a relatively few applications in the management of open fractures. This is why, for all practical purposes, we have limited the functional treatment to closed fractures and to a relatively small number of low-grade open fractures that meet the criteria prescribed for closed fractures, such as acceptable original shortening and correctable angular deformity.

Encouraged by the success in the care of closed fractures we applied the functional method to nonunions that had been referred to us, following the treatment of fractures by other various methods, e.g. plating, closed treatment, external fixation, and intramedullary nailing. Others have reported instances of spontaneous union of delayed unions and nonunions following the application of weight bearing casts.

CLINICAL EXPERIENCES

We treated 73 fractures of the tibial diaphysis that failed to demonstrate healing within the usually anticipated time of 4 to 6 months. This material was previously published.[6] The following is an abbreviated version of the original article.

The patients were treated in one of three different ways: (1) Ambulation in a below-the-knee functional cast or brace. (2) Fibular ostectomy, followed by early ambulation in a below-the-knee functional cast or brace. (3) Fibular ostectomy followed by bone grafting and early ambulation in a below-the-knee functional cast or brace. The use of a functional cast or brace and weight bearing ambulation were the common denominators in the three sub-groups. These functional treatment modalities were based on the authors' clinical and laboratory experiences that indicated that rigid immobilization is not necessary for spontaneous repair of acute fractures, and that activity and physiologically controlled motion at the fracture site is conducive to osteogenesis.[1-26] We extrapolated that similar premises could be made applicable to the treatment of delayed unions and nonunions of the tibial diaphysis.

Material and Methods

The common denominator was early weight bearing ambulation in below-the-knee casts or braces. In 11 (15%) patients, the cast or brace constituted the entire treatment protocol; in 52 (71.2%) patients the cast or brace was applied after an ostectomy of the fibula was performed; and in 10 (13.6%) patients, an autogenous bone graft was placed over the pathological defect following fibular ostectomy.

Six (8.2%) patients were lost to follow-up. Three of the patients lost to follow-up were from the Miami group (10.3%) and the remaining three (16.6%) were from the USC group.

This report is the product of a retrospective study. During the time the reported patients were treated by us, others within the department were treating similar conditions by conventional means of plating, nailing, bone grafting or external fixation. An effort was not made to compare the results obtained in the two groups.

From the group of 67 patients available to follow-up, 51 (76.1%) patients were male and 16 (23.6%) were female. The patients' age ranged from 16 to 67 years, with an average of 27 years, a median of 24 years and modes of 19, 23 and 30 years.

Fifty (75%) patients had open fractures; of these patients, 35 (70%) were male; and 15 (30%) were female. Seventeen (25%) patients had closed fractures; of these, 12 (70.5%) were male and 5 (29.4%) were female.

The original mechanism of injury was a motor vehicle injury in 39 (58.2%) patients; gunshot wounds in 20 (29.8%); a direct blow or a fall in seven (10.7%); and one (1.4%) a simple twisting in a patient with a metastatic lesion. Those patients with gunshot-related fractures had their initial injury at a mean and mode of 10 months. Those with motor vehicle related fractures had their injuries at a mean of 10 months and modes of 9 and 11 months.

The treatment received at the time of the initial injury was casting exclusively in 21 (31.3%) patients; plate osteosynthesis in 29 (43.3%) patients; intramedullary nailing is six (8.9%) patients; and external fixation in 11 (16.4%) patients. We have no accurate data regarding the number of surgical procedures the patients had prior to the institution of the functional treatment discussed in this paper since many of them were referred to our institutions from different sources, often without medical records. At the initiation of the functional treatment, none of the reported patients had internal devices in place.

The level of the fracture was the proximal-third of the tibia in 12 (17.9%) patients; of these, five (41.6%) were delayed unions and seven (58.3%) were nonunions. Twenty-two (32.8%) were in the middle-third of the tibia. Of these, three (13.6%) were delayed unions and 19 (86.3%) were nonunions. Thirty-one (46.2%) were in the distal-third of the tibia; of these, six (19.3%) were delayed unions and 25 (80.6%) were nonunions. Two (2.9%) were segmental. From this group, one was a delayed union and one was a nonunion.

Since there are no uniform criteria in the literature regarding a precise definition of delayed union union and nonunion, we arbitrarily chose to use the unscientific, though popular system, that calls a delayed union of a fracture that fails to unite within the 5th and 9th month following the initial injury and a nonunion, the fracture that fails to unite after 9 months. Two different radiographic views demonstrated the pathology. Fifteen (22.3%) conditions were delayed unions and 52 (77.6%) were nonunions. Of the 15 delayed unions, 12 (80%) were males and three (20%) were females. Of the 52 nonunions, 39 (75%) were males and 13 (25%) were females. Of these 52 nonunions, 44 (84.6%) nonunions were classified as hypertrophic and eight (15.3%) as atrophic. All eight patients with atrophic nonunions were males. In the group of 44 hypertrophic nonunions 31 (70.4%) were males and 13 (29.5%) were females.

Prior to the initiation of the functional treatment, patients with delayed union had been disabled from 5 to 9 months with a median of 7 months. Patients with nonunion had been disabled between 9 months and 8 years with a median of 11 months and a mode of 10 months. The six (8.9%) patients who failed to respond to the functional treatment, which will be discussed under RESULTS, had been disabled for periods of time ranging from 7 to 14 months, with an average of 11 months.

The below-the-knee functional cast was molded in the shape of a patellar tendon bearing prosthesis that allowed free range of motion of the knee. It was used in 36 (53.7%) patients. The below-the-knee functional brace permitted unencumbered motion of the knee and ankle joints and was used in 31 (46.2%) patients. Seven (22.5%) of these braces were pre-fabricated and 24 (77.4%) were custom-made. The custom-made braces were manufactured with **Orthoplast** (Johnson and Johnson).

The functional treatment instituted for the pathological conditions consisted exclusively of cast or brace in nine (13.4%) patients; fibular ostectomy followed by cast or brace in 48 (71.6%) patients; and ostectomy, followed by bone graft and cast or brace in 10 (14.9%) patients.

The authors assisted orthopedic residents in training in the reading of radiographs and in diagnosing the pathology. A rigid criterion was not used to determine what conditions should be treated simply with a functional cast or brace, a fibular ostectomy followed by bracing, or an ostectomy followed by bone grafting and subsequent bracing. In all instances, the functional method of treatment was applied to patients whose affected tibial diaphysis had only deformities that were esthetically acceptable. We felt that carrying out this treatment modality in patients with gross angular deformities would have resulted in an increase of angulation at the fracture site. The 11 patients whose treatment consisted only of casting or bracing, had pathological conditions that seemed to have minimal instability at the site of injury. We chose to add a graft to 10 (14.9%) nonunions simply because of a history of multiple previous unsuccessful surgical attempts to overcome the pathological condition and the presence of a large defect between the major fragments.

The choice between the different modalities was not based on scientific grounds. We were in the process of studying the possibility of using functional braces in the management of delayed unions and nonunions of the tibia, and had no grounds to suspect that one approach was better than the others. Pathological conditions where motion at the fracture site was minimal, received the cast or brace without osteotomy or bone graft. All others had a fibular ostectomy.

An ostectomy of the fibula was performed in the combined group of 58 (86.5%) patients (ostectomy alone and ostectomy plus bone graft). The ostectomy was performed opposite to the fracture in 35 (60.3%) patients, approximately 2 cm above or below the lesion in 23 (39.6%) patients. The amount of bone removed was 1 cm in most instances.

In the group of patients who did not have an ostectomy of the fibula, the functional cast or brace was applied on the day the pathological diagnosis was made. In the group of patients who had a fibular ostectomy, with or without a bone graft, the below-the-knee cast or brace was applied on an average of 7 days postoperatively and a maximum of 35 days. All patients were encouraged to bear weight on the extremity to a degree determined by the intensity of symptoms. Under no circumstances were patients encouraged to bear full weight in the presence of significant pain.

We did not record information concerning patients' smoking habits and degree of ingestion of alcoholic beverages. We were not able to obtain adequate data concerning the number of surgical procedures to which the patients had been subjected prior to the initiation of the functional treatment.

No measurement of shortening of the tibia was made before the institution of treatment. The treatment was considered to be a salvage one and we assumed that the existing shortening would be a small price to pay for the attainment of healing. Limbs with pronounced angular deformity, which was not thought to be correctable at the time of the fibular ostectomy, were not treated in a functional manner and were, therefore, not part of this report.

Results

From the original group of 73 patients, six (8.2%) were lost to follow-up. Five of these patients had open fractures and one had a closed fracture. In the remaining group of 67 patients available to follow-up, six (8.9%) failed to respond to the treatment protocol.

For the delayed unions, the period of stabilization in the below-the-knee cast or brace, the mean time was of 3 months with a range between 2 and 5 months. For the nonunions, the range was 2½ months and 13 months, with a median time of 4 months and modes of 4 and 5 months. According to the patients, gender, the 39 males with nonunion healed at a median time of 4 months with modes of 4 and 5 months. The 13 female patients with nonunion healed at a median time of four months. The 12 male patients with delayed union healed at a median time of 3 months. The three females with delayed unions healed on an average time of 2.6 months.

In the group of nine patients treated exclusively with a cast or brace, one (11.1%) failed to unite. In the group of 48 patients treated with ostectomy and bracing, three (6.2%) failed to unite. In the 10 patients treated with ostectomy, bone graft and bracing, two (20%) failed to achieve union. Five of the six patients who failed to heal their fractures had open fractures.

From the six failures, five (83.3%) were nonunions; and one (16.6%) was a delayed union. Three (60%) of the five nonunions were hypertrophic and two (40%) were atrophic. Five (83.3%) patients had open fractures; one (16.6) had a closed fracture.

From the group of 39 patients who had sustained the initial injury in a motor-vehicle accident, four (10.2%) failed to unite their nonunions, and two (10%) from the group of 20 patients who had gunshot produced injuries failed to unite their nonunions. There were no failures among those who originally had injuries produced from direct blows or falls.

From the group of 15 delayed unions, one (6.6%) failed to unite. From the group of 52 nonunions, five (9.6%) failed to unite. Of the five failed nonunions, three (60%) were hypertrophic, and two (40%) were atrophic.

The failure rate according to the level of the fracture was as follows: In the group of 12 fractures located in the proximal-third, one (8.3%) failed to unite. In the group of 22 lesions located in the middle-third of the tibia, two (9%) failed to unite. In the group of 31 lesions located in the distal third of the tibia, three (9.6%) failed to unite. No failures occurred in the two segmental fractures.

Shortening of the ostectomized fibula ranged from no measurable shortening to 10 mm, with a mean shortening of 3 mm in the delayed union group and 5 mm in the nonunion group. A nonunion at the fibular ostectomy site was recorded in 10 (14.9%) instances (Figures 17.1A to 17.2C). From these 10 patients, six (60%) had more than 10 millimeters of bone resection and four (40%) less than 10 millimeters. In all 10 patients with ununited ostectomies, the tibiae healed uneventfully.

Of the 58 patients who had an ostectomy of the fibula, two (3.4%) patients developed purulent drainage at the site of the ostectomy. One had had a bone grafting as part of the therapeutic approach. Both patients had open fractures. The infection promptly subsided in both instances under antibiotic administration and local care. The infection did not preclude the continuation of ambulation in the brace.

DISCUSSION

Currently, the most popular treatments for tibial nonunion are internal fixation with either plate osteosynthesis,[25,27-31] intramedullary nailing[32-34] and the distraction/stress system of Ilizarov.[33,36] The common rationale behind the surgical methods, i.e. plating and nailing, is the long-held belief by many that if immobilization is good for fracture healing, a greater degree of immobilization is necessary in the care of nonunion. There is strong evidence in the literature to conclude that motion at the fracture site is conducive to healing. We have conducted numerous clinical and laboratory studies dealing with acute injuries that indicate that motion at the fracture site, from weight bearing and the active use of the limb musculature and adjacent joints encourage osteogenesis.[11,15-18,24,25,37-43] Furthermore, the callus that eventually bridges the fracture possesses stronger mechanical properties than the one that forms in the presence of rigid immobilization.[5,10,11,16-18,42-44] Kenwright et al also demonstrated that micromotion at the fracture site expedited healing of fractures treated with external fixators.[7] Our investigation has documented that in acute axially unstable diaphyseal tibial fractures treated with functional below-the-knee braces, motion between the fragments at the end of the first post-injury week approached.[10,11,42] We also observed that the strength of the callus in fractures produced in experimental animals was also greater in those fractures that exhibit the greatest degree of motion.[10,16,17] The current preference for intramedullary nailing over plate osteosynthesis in the treatment of diaphyseal fractures seems to support the value of motion at the fractures site in fracture care. The nailing procedure, however, contrary to our reported method of treatment, was not designed for the primary purpose of increasing motion at the fractures. The performance of a fibular ostectomy, followed by the application of a below-the-knee cast or brace, indeed encourages additional motion at the nonunion site. Our reported findings suggest that activity and motion at the nonunion site favorably enhance osteogenesis.

In the recent past, the Ilizarov method of treatment of nonunions has further documented the value of motion at the fracture site, since this method calls for weight bearing during a rhythmic distraction/compression protocol.[36]

We wish we had carried out this study in a prospective, randomized manner. However, that was not the case. The project began simply with an idea, which we did not know might be valid. The senior author chose not to interfere with the preferences of other members of the department, who continued to treat similar conditions with other more conventional means. This, and the fact that in our study we included only patients with pathological limbs that were not infected and had minimal or no deformity, explains the small number of patients in our reported group. For example, Wiss' work was conducted at the same institution and during the same time period that 18 of our reported patients were treated by the functional bracing technique.[28,45]

In this retrospective analysis of 67 tibial delayed unions and nonunions, we observed a failure rate of 8.9%. Our failure rate is comparable to that reported by others in recent years using other treatment modalities. Wiss et al. reported a failure rate of 8% in a group of 49 patients treated by compression plating with an infection rate of 8% and fatigue fracture of the plate ogf 8%. Seventy-eight% of patients had an associated bone grafting procedures at the time of plating. In Wiss' report, 92% of patients healed their nonunions "in an average of 7 months without further intervention."[46] The period

of time before union in our series ranged from 2½ and 13 months. Carpenter and Jupiter reported a failure rate of 2.5% in a group of 16 patients with nonunion of distal metaphyseal fractures treated with plate osteosynthesis.[29]

Alho et al. obtained 100% union in a group of 25 patients treated with locked intramedullary nail without bone grafting. All patients had a fibular osteotomy. They identified infection as a complication in 3% patients.[32] Court-Brown et al. obtained 100% success in a group of 33 patients treated with exchanged intramedullary nailing.[7] Wiss and Stetson reported a failure to achieve union of 10.7% from a group of 47 patients treated with reamed intramedullary nailing. Infection developed in 13% of patients.[46]

De Bastiani et al had a failure rate of 7% in a group of 21 patients with hypertrophic aseptic nonunions treated with a unilateral fixator. In his report, he recorded a healing time of 150 days.[35] Simpson et al used posterolateral bone grafting in a series of 30 patients and found a failure rate of 3.4%.[31]

The above brief summary-review of the literature suggests that different treatment modalities are associated with a high degree of success. It appears to us that no clear advantages have been firmly documented to indicate that a given treatment is always superior to all others. It is likely that when appropriately performed, any of the above mentioned approaches render satisfactory clinical results. We believe that the use of functional braces, following ostectomy of the fibula, with or without additional bone grafting, is a viable method of treatment in aseptic delayed union and nonunion of the tibia, when a correctable angular deformity is present.

We did not report on the number of procedures our patients had prior to the initiation of the reported functional treatment using a cast or brace, since such information was not always available to us. Many patients have been referred to us from various sources without records or incomplete ones. It is doubtful that the addition of such information would have shed any further light into this complex issue.

We cannot offer a precise explanation as to why we experienced success in 91% of patients despite the fact that the method does not adhere to the traditional tenets that govern the current management of fractures and nonunions. We suspect that the ostectomy of the fibula and the introduction of weight bearing, constitute an episode similar to that of a new injury. This new "injury" provokes the biological responses that follow an acute fracture when graduated weight bearing and the resulting increased motion at the fracture site are introduced.[32,47]

REPRESENTATIVE EXAMPLES

Representative examples illustrating delayed unions and nonunion are shown in Figures 17.1 to 17.23

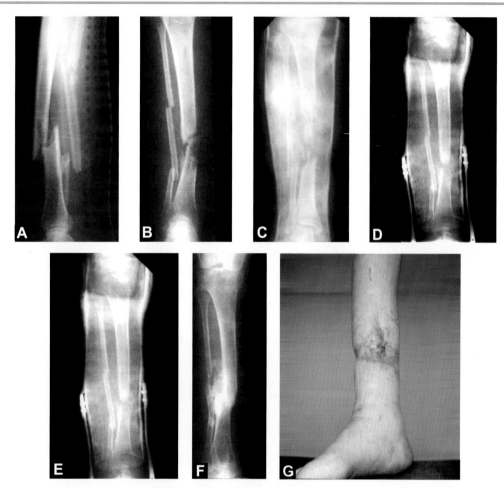

Figs 17.1A to G: (A) Radiograph of an open fracture of the tibia as a result of a motorcycle accident. (B) Eleven months later and after several surgical procedures, the fracture remained ununited, and draining purulent material. The patient requested an amputation. (C) A below-the-knee functional cast was applied, and the patient was encouraged to bear weight on her leg. The degree of draining increased significantly during the ensuing weeks, but began to decrease gradually. (D) The cast was then replaced with a below-the-knee functional brace made of Plaster of Paris. (E) Despite the fact that the wound was still draining, an autologous cancellous bone graft was placed over the nonunion site, using a posterior approach. (F) The fracture healed but the motion of her ankle was still limited a few months later. (G) Appearance of the extremity showing the healing of the skin.

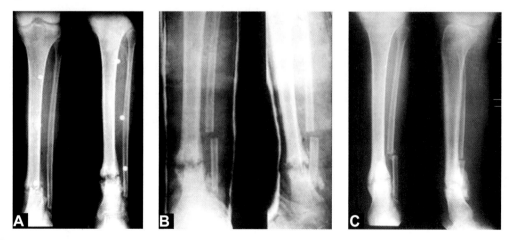

Figs 17.2A to C: (A) Radiograph of a well-established nonunion of a distal tibia following an open fracture treated with debridement and casting. (B) Radiograph taken after an ostectomy of the fibula was performed, and a below-the-knee functional cast was applied. (C) The nonunion healed within 5 months after the ostectomy.

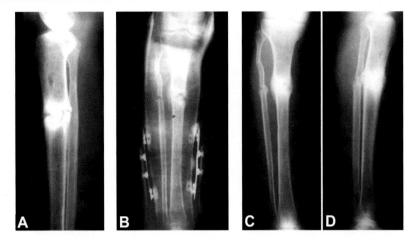

Figs 17.3A to D: (A and B) Thirteen-month-old nonunion of the tibia, initially treated with an external fixator. (C) The nonunion was treated with a below-the-knee functional brace after an ostectomy of the fibula was performed. The free fibular fragment was placed over the nonunion site. (D) The fracture healed uneventfully.

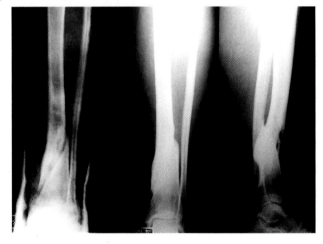

Figs 17.4: Composite radiographs of an open fracture of the distal tibia, showing no signs of union 6 months after the initial injury. The fracture had been treated with an above-the-knee cast. The cast was replaced with a functional brace and the fracture healed within the next 3 months.

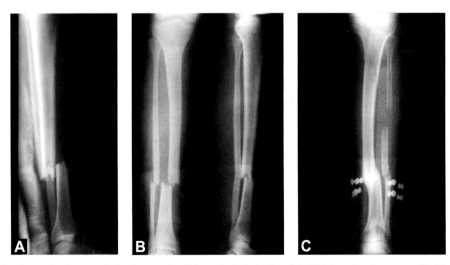

Figs 17.5A to C: (A) Radiograph of an acute fracture of the tibia and fibula in the distal-third of the diaphysis. (B) The fracture was treated with a functional brace, but failed to unite. (C) Four months after the fracture, an ostectomy of the fibula was performed and a functional brace reapplied. The fracture healed within the next 3 months.

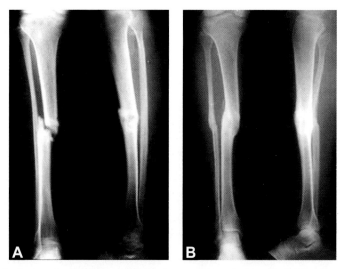

Figs 17.6A and B: (A) Radiograph of nonunited fracture of the tibia, not associated with a fibula fracture, obtained 10 months after the initial injury. The fracture had been treated with an above-the-knee cast. (B) An ostectomy of the fibula was performed and a functional brace applied. Union took place within the ensuing 3 months.

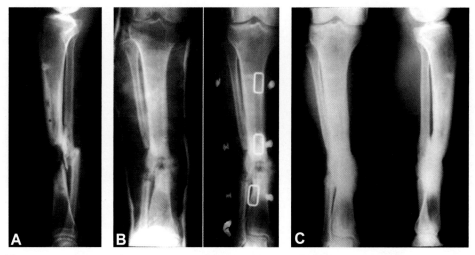

Figs 17.7A to C: (A) Radiograph of a 5-year old nonunion of a closed tibial fracture. The fracture was originally treated with a plate and screws. After failing to obtain union, an external fixator was used. The nonunion persisted. (B) A fragment of the fibula was resected and placed over the nonunion site. It was reinforced with pelvic bone. A functional cast-brace was then applied. (C) The fracture healed within the next 5 months.

Figs 17.8: Composite radiographs of an 8-year-old open fracture of the distal tibia that failed to unite despite external fixation, electrical stimulation and bone grafting. An above-the-knee cast had been in place all those years. A below-the-knee functional cast was applied and weight bearing encouraged. The fracture healed after an additional 5 months of active weight bearing ambulation.

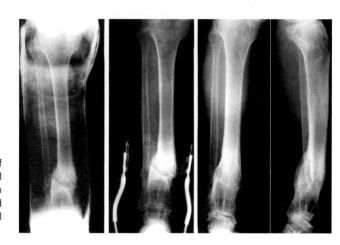

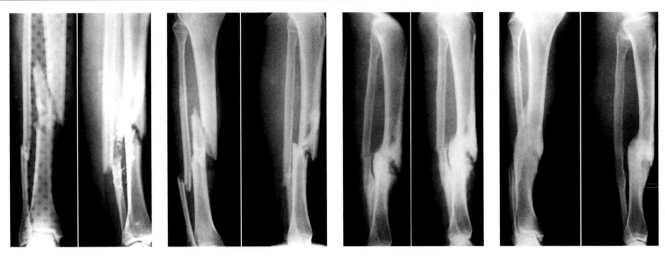

Figs 17.9: Composite radiographs of a nonunited fracture of the tibia 11 months after the initial insult. The fracture was being treated with a non-weight-bearing above-the-knee cast. An ostectomy of the fibula was performed slightly above the nonunion site, and a brace was applied. The fracture eventually healed.

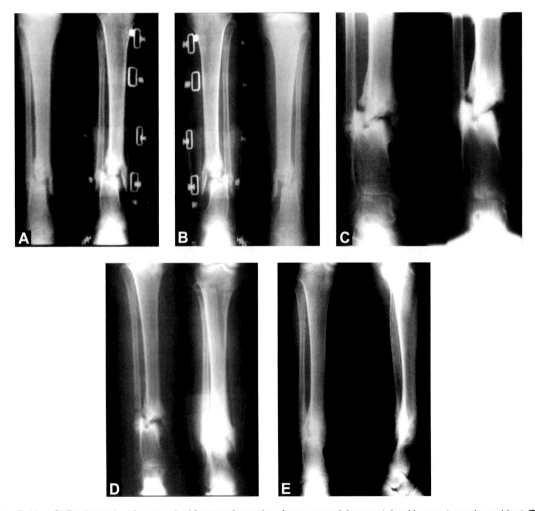

Figs 17.10A to E: (A to C) Radiographs of a nonunited fracture 9 months after an open injury sustained in a motorcycle accident. The nonunion was treated with an ostectomy of the fibula and the application of a functional brace. (D) Union progressed slowly. (E) The fracture united but the patient demonstrated significant stiffness of the ankle and subtalar joint, which was improving when the patient was last seen.

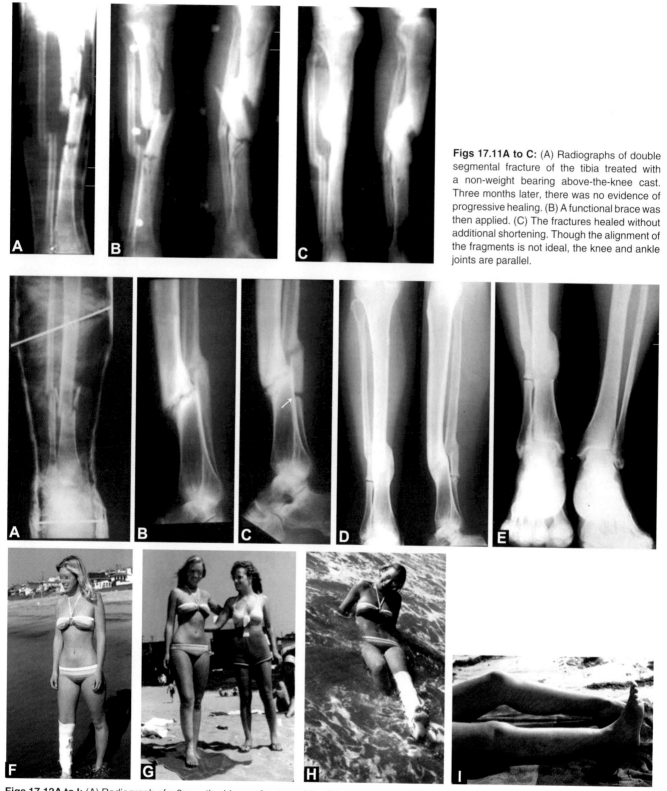

Figs 17.11A to C: (A) Radiographs of double segmental fracture of the tibia treated with a non-weight bearing above-the-knee cast. Three months later, there was no evidence of progressive healing. (B) A functional brace was then applied. (C) The fractures healed without additional shortening. Though the alignment of the fragments is not ideal, the knee and ankle joints are parallel.

Figs 17.12A to I: (A) Radiograph of a 8-month-old open fracture of the tibia apparently treated with an external fixator. There was no evidence of progressive healing. (B) Radiograph showing no evidence of union. (C) An ostectomy of the fibula was performed above the nonunion site, and a functional brace was applied. (D) The fracture healed but the fibular ostectomy remained ununited. (E) Radiograph comparing the two lower extremities. Though there is a difference in the length of the tibiae, it is inconsequential. (F to I) Photographs of the patient indulging in swimming activities. Notice the atrophy of the injured leg, which is assumed improved as return to normal activities became possible.

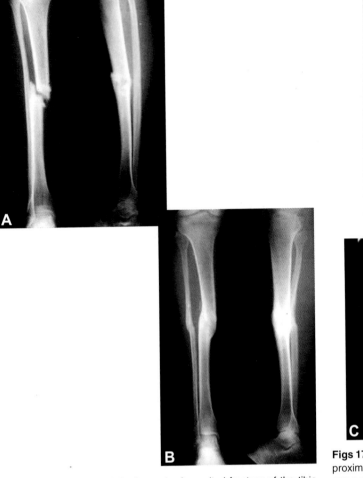

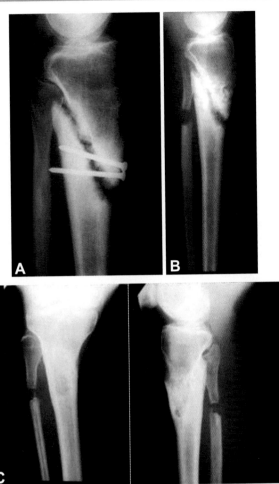

Figs 17.13A and B: (A) Radiograph of ununited fracture of the tibia without an associated fracture of the fibula. (B) Following an ostectomy of the fibula, the nonunion healed uneventfully.

Figs 17.14A to C: (A) Radiograph of a nonunited closed fracture of the proximal tibia treated originally with screw fixation. (B) The screws were removed and an ostectomy of the fibula was performed. A functional brace was then applied. (C) The fracture healed uneventfully and the ostectomized fibula remained ununited.

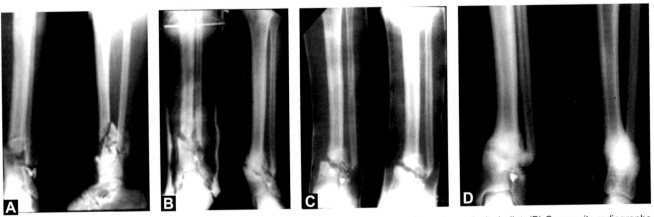

Figs 17.15A to D: (A) Radiograph of an open fracture of the distal tibia and fibula, produced by a low-velocity bullet. (B) Composite radiographs of the fracture, which had been initially treated with an external fixator. Notice the severe angular deformity that occurred after removal of the pins. (C) The fracture was surgically exposed and the deformity corrected. The fibrous union of the fibula was taken down. A below-the-knee functional cast was then applied. Three months later, there was minimal evidence of union. (D) Radiograph showing solid union of the fracture 5 months later.

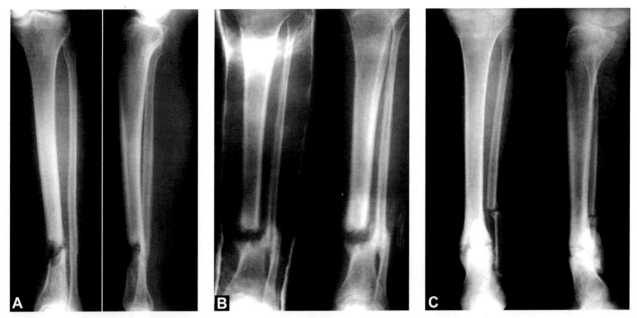

Figs 17.16A to C: (A) Radiograph of an open fracture of the distal tibia produced in a motorcycle accident. (B) Composite radiographs of the fracture showing a large gap between the fragments. Profuse drainage was present. (C) An ostectomy of the fibula was performed above the nonunion site and a functional brace was applied. The fracture united but the fibula remained ununited. Drainage persisted for a long time but eventually subsided spontaneously.

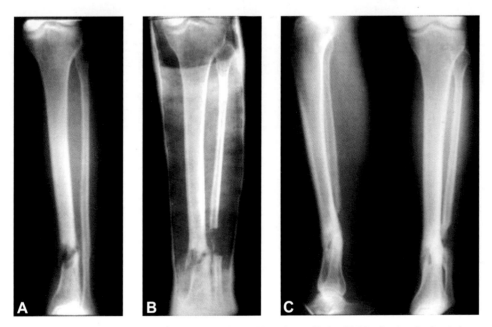

Figs 17.17A to C: (A) Radiograph of an open fracture of the distal tibia with an intact fibula. (B) The fracture had not shown signs of healing 6 months after the injury. A fibular ostectomy was then performed and a below-the-knee functional cast was applied. (C) The fracture united with a mild and inconsequential recurvatum deformity.

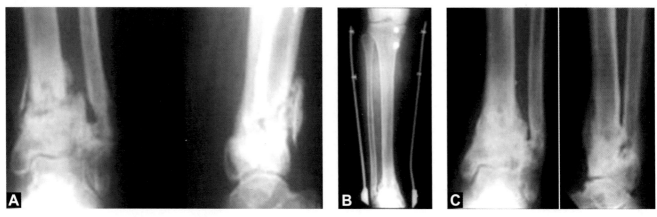

Figs 17.18A to C: (A) Radiograph of a delayed union of a fracture in the metaphyseal region of the distal tibia. Four months later, there was no evidence of bony union. (B) A functional brace was applied and activity encouraged. (C) The fracture united spontaneously.

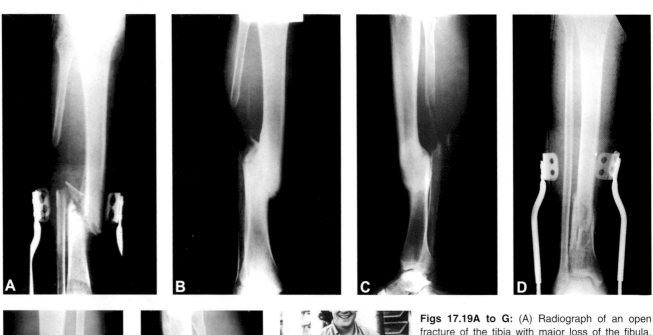

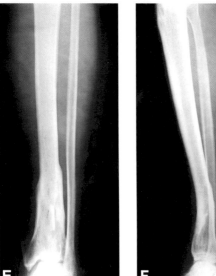

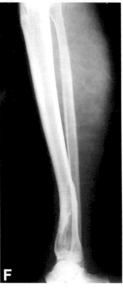

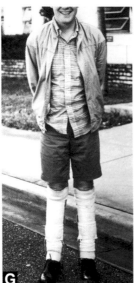

Figs 17.19A to G: (A) Radiograph of an open fracture of the tibia with major loss of the fibula. The fracture when first seen by us was 6 weeks old, and associated with minimal drainage. It was elected to accept the shortening in anticipation that if it became a problem to the patient, a lengthening procedure would be performed. A functional brace was applied. (B and C) The fracture healed uneventfully. (D to F) The patient had also sustained a closed fracture of the opposite tibia. (G) The patient wears a lift in the heel of the shoe and does not display a limp.

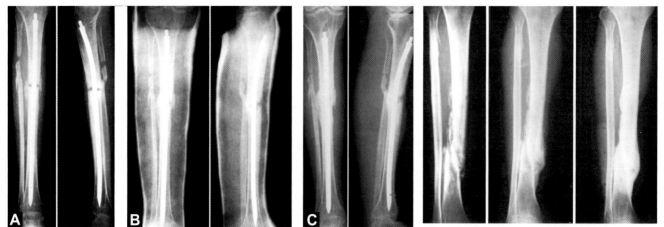

Figs 17.20A to C: (A) Composite of radiographs of united fracture of the tibia following closed intramedullary Lottes nailing. An ostectomy of the fibula was performed above the nonunion site. (B) A below-the-knee functional cast was applied. (C) The fracture united uneventfully.

Figs 17.22: Composite of radiographs showing a nonunited fracture of the tibia 6 months after the initial injury. Minimal drainage had persisted. A functional brace was applied and the patient encouraged to bear weight on his injured leg. The fracture united spontaneously and the drainage subsided.

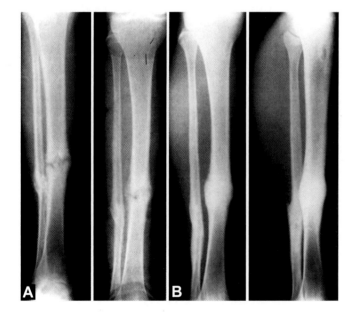

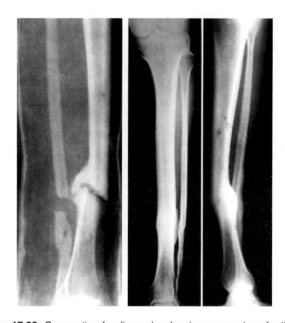

Figs 17.21A and B: (A) The composite of radiographs of a nonunited fracture of the tibia. The associated fibula fracture had healed uneventfully. (B) A functional brace was applied and the patient was encouraged to bear weight on his injured limb. The fracture united spontaneously.

Figs 17.23: Composite of radiographs showing a nonunion of a tibial fracture 7 months after the initial injury. An ostectomy of the fibula was carried out, and a functional brace applied. The fracture healed uneventfully.

REFERENCES

1. Sarmiento A, Sharpe MD, Ebramzadeh E, Normand P, Shankwiler J. Factors influencing the Outcome of Closed Tibial Fractures Treated with Functional Bracing. Clin Ortho Relat Res. 1995 Jun; (315):8-24.
2. Sarmiento A. On the behavior of closed tibial fractures: clinical and radiological correlations. J Orthop Trauma, 2000; 14(3):199-205.
3. Brown PW, Urban J.G. Early weight bearing treatment of open fractures of the tibia. An end-result study of sixty-three cases. J. Bone and Joint Surg. 1969; 51A(1):59-75.
4. Dehne E. Treatment of Fractures of the Tibial Shaft. Clin. Orthop. 1969; 66:159.
5. Sarmiento A, Burkhalter W, Latta LL. Functional Bracing in Delayed Union and Nonunion of the Tibia. Int Orthop. 2003; 27(1):26-9.

6. Bruggemann H, Kujat R, Tscherne, H. Funkionelle Frakturebehandlung nach Sarmiento an Unterschenkel, Unterarm und Oberarm. Orthopaede. 1983; 12:143.

7. Kenwright J, Richardson JB, Goodship AE, Evans M, Kelly DJ, Spriggins AJ, Newman JH, Burrough SJ, Harris JD and Rowley DI. Effect of Controlled Axial Micromovement on Healing of Tibial Fractures. Lancet. 1986 Nov; 2(8517):1185-7.

8. Kujat R, Tscherne H. Indications and Technic of Functional Fracture Treatment with the Sarmiento Brace. Zentralbl Chir. 1984; 109:1417.

9. Kujat R. Functional Treatment of Shaft Fractures of the Tibia with the Sarmiento Brace. Orthopade. Sept 1984; 13(4):262.

10. Latta LL, Sarmiento A. Mechanical Behavior of Tibial Fractures. Symposium on Trauma to the Leg and Its Sequela. C.V. Mosby: St. Louis, MO 1981.

11. Orfaly R, Keating JE, O'Brien PJ. Knee pain after tibial nailing: Does the entry point matter? J Bone Joint Surg Br. 1995; 77(6):976-7.

12. Resnick CT, Wagner KS, Sarmiento A. Changes in tibiotalar joint contact areas following experimentally induced tibial angular deformities. Clin Orthop. 1985 Oct; (199):72-80.

13. Roberts C, Ruktanonchai D, King D, Seligson D. Vascular compromise and amputation after intramedullary nailing of a tibial fracture. J Orthop Trauma; 1998 Feb; 12(2):136-8.

14. Sarmiento A, Latta LL. Functional treatment of Closed Segmental Fractures of the Tibia. Acta Chir Orthop Traumatol Cech. 2008; 75:325-31.

15. Sarmiento A, Latta LL. Closed Functional Treatment of Fractures. Springer-Verlag: Berlin 1981.

16. Sarmiento A, Schaeffer J, Beckerman L, Latta LL, Enis J. Fracture Healing in Rat Femora as Affected by Functional Weight Bearing. J. Bone Joint Surg Am, 1977; 59(3):369-75.

17. Sarmiento A, Mullis DL, Latta LL, Alvarez RR. A Quantitative, Comparative Analysis of Fracture Healing Under the Influence of Compression Plating vs. Closed Weight-Bearing Treatment. Clin Orthop. 1980; 149:232.

18. Sarmiento A, Latta LL. On the evolution of fracture bracing. J Bone Joint Surg Br. 2006; 88-8(2):141-8.

19. Sarmiento A, Latta LL. Functional Fracture Bracing. J. Amer Acad Orthop Surg. 1999; 7-1:66-75.

20. Suman RK. Orthoplast Brace for Treatment of Tibial Shaft Fractures. Injury. 1981; 13:133.

21. Suman RK. Functional Bracing in Lower Limb Fractures. Ital J Orthop Traumatol. 1983 Jun; 9(2):201.

22. Suman RK. The management of tibial shaft fractures by early weight in a patellar tendon bearing cast. A comparative study. J Trauma. 1977; 17(2):97-107.

23. Trueta J. The role of vessels in osteogenesis. J Bone Joint Surg Br. 1963; 45:402-6.

24. Trueta J. Blood supply and rate of healing of tibial fractures. Clin Orthop. 1974; 105:11.

25. Wolf JW et al. The Superiority of Cyclic Loading over Constant Compression in the Treatment of Long Bone Fractures. A Quantitative Biomechanical Study in Rabbits. Trans 26 Orthop Res Soc. 1980; 5:174.

26. Sarmiento A, Latta LL. Functional Fracture Bracing. A Manual. Lippincott, Williams and Wilkins: Philadelphia 2002; 82-147.

27. Bone LB, Johnson K.D. Treatment of tibial fractures by reaming and intramedullary nailing. J. Bone and Joint Surg. 1986; 68A(6):877-87.

28. Bonnevialle P, Bellumore Y, Foucras L, Hezard L, Mansat M. Tibial fractures with intact fibula treated by reamed nailing. Rev Chir Orthop Reparatrice Appar Mot. 2000; 86(1):29-37.

29. Carpenter CA, Jupiter J. Blade-plate reconstruction of metaphyseal nonunion of the tibia. Clinical Orthopedics Nov. 1996; (332):23:8.

30. Moore TM, Lester DK, Sarmiento A. The Stabilizing Effect of Soft Tissue Constraints in Artificial Galeazzi Fractures. Clin Orthop Relat Res. 1985 Apr; 194:189-94.

31. Simpson J, Ebrahim N, Jackson W. Posterolateral bone graft of the tibia. Clin Orthop. 1990; 251:200-6.

32. Alho A, Ekelan A, Stromsoe K et al. Nonunion of Tibial Shaft Fractures treated with locked intramedullary nailing without bone grafting. J. Trauma. 1993; 34(1):62.

33. Court-Brown C, Keating J, McQueen M. Exchange intramedullary nailing. Its use in aseptic tibial nonunion. J. Bone and Joint Surg. 1995; 77B (3):407-11.

34. Templeman D, Varecka T, Kyle R. Exchanged reamed intramedullary nailing for delayed union and nonunion of the tibia. Clin Orthop. 1995; (315):169-75.

35. De Bastiani G, Agostini S, Lesso P. Trattamento delle pseudoartrosi con fissatore esterno assiali. Anni della Societa Eliliana Romagnola di Ortopedia e Traumatología. 1990; XXXIII, fascicolo I:17.

36. Hutson J. The Ilizarov System in Fracture care. Techniques in Orthopedics. 2002; 17:1-111

37. McKellop HA, Sigholm G, Redfern FC, Doyle B, Sarmiento A, Luck J. The Effect of Simulated Fracture-Angulation of the Tibia on Cartilage Pressures in the Knee Joint. J Bone & Joint Surg. 1991; 73-A:1382-1390.

38. Sarmiento A. A Functional Below-Knee Cast for Tibial Fractures. J Bone and Joint Surg. 1967; 59:5.

39. Sarmiento A. A Functional Below-Knee Brace for Tibial Fractures. J. Bone and Joint Surg. 1970; 52(2):295-311.

40. Sarmiento A, Latta LL. Functional Fracture Bracing. The Tibia, Humerus and Ulna. Springer-Verlag 1992.

41. Sarmiento A. Functional Bracing of Tibial and Femoral Shaft Fractures. Clin Orthop Relat Res. 1972; 82:2-13.

42. Sarmiento A, Latta L, Zilioli A, Sinclair Wm F. The Role of Soft Tissues in the Stabilization of Tibial Fractures. Clin Orthop Relat Res. 1974; 105:116-29.

43. Sarmiento A. The functional bracing of fractures. J Bone Joint Am. Classics Techniques 2007; 89 Suppl 2 (Part 2):157-69.

44. Zych GA, Zagorski JB, Latta LL, McCollough NC. Modern Concepts in Functional Fracture Bracing - Lower Limb. In: AAOS Instructional Course Lectures.

45. Cole D, Latta LL. Fatigue failure of interlocking tibial nail implants. Orthop Trans Bone Joint Surg. 1992; 16-3A:663.

46. Wiss DA, Stetson WB. Unstable fractures of the tibia treated with reamed intramedullary nails. Clin Orthop Relat Res. 1995; 315:56-63.

47. De Smet K, Mostert AK, De Witte J, De Brauwer V, Verdonk R. Closed intramedullary tibial nailing using the Marchetti-Vicenzi nail. Injury. 2000; 31(8):597-603.

18

Tibial Condylar Fractures and Intra-articular Extensions

Refined instrumentation has made surgical stabilization of tibial condylar fractures a good treatment. It is, however, not a panacea. These fractures are often the result of major trauma in elderly patients; particularly those suffering from either atherosclerosis and or diabetes are very likely to develop complications such as infection and/or skin necrosis. These can be major complications that may even lead to amputation. Obviously, in the younger individual, the results are usually better.

All condylar fractures, in the absence of associated plateau depression, do not necessarily require surgery. The knee joint tolerates incongruity to degrees not generally known. Lansinger, from Sweden, Christensen,[1] from Denmark and Merchant,[2] from Iowa, among many others have reported on long-term follow-up of incongruous tibial condyles with most impressive clinical results. Lansinger, for example, states that he documented excellent results as long as 30 years after injury, in patients who had as much a 1 cm of step-off deformity at the fracture site. Though our experience is limited, we were able to obtain similar findings following the treatment of condylar fractures using articulated functional braces.[3]

We conducted laboratory studies using cadaver specimens that led to some very interesting observations. In human cadavers, we produced non-displaced osteotomies of the condyles that simulated the variety of fractures encountered in clinical practice: isolated fractures, of the lateral condyle, isolated fractures of the medial condyle and fractures of both condyles. With each of these fractures we studied the role of the fibula in the behavior of the tibial condylar fractures.

The laboratory specimens were subjected to vertical loading and the produced changes in the relationships of the fragments were monitored with cineradiography and photographs. We concluded that the changes seen in the laboratory corresponded very well with those observed in clinical situations: (1)

Medial condylar fractures readily collapsed into varus under vertical loading. (2) Lateral condylar fractures with intact fibulae did not collapse into valgus. It appears that the intact fibula, supporting the lateral condyle, prevents the collapse. (3) Fractures of the lateral condyle with an associated fibula fractures readily collapsed into valgus. (4) Fractures of both condyles with intact fibulae collapsed into varus. (5) Fractures of both condyles with associated fibula fractures were depressed evenly but without varus or valgus deformity (Figures 18.1 to 18.4). If the force applied had been increased, it is logical to assume that major depression would have been noticed that internal fixation of non-displaced or minimally displaced condylar fractures is not always necessary and that the treatment must also be based on the type of fracture and the condition of the fibula[3] (Figures 18.5A to E).

In our clinical study, we had assumed that ligamentous and meniscal injuries have been ruled out in our patients, before initiating the closed functional treatment. This work was done prior to the invention of the MRI, which I suspect would have revealed pathology that we could not identify through simple clinical examination. The lessons learnt from the project, however, should not be too quickly dismissed.

Years later, still suspecting that incongruity does not necessarily lead to late osteoarthritis, we conducted laboratory studies using adult rabbits to determine the effects of step-off deformities in the knee joint, with and without associated instability.[4,5] (See Chapter 1)

It is very likely that patients who become osteoarthritic, do so either because the incongruity was too severe; irreparable damage to the articular cartilage took place at the time of the original insult; or unrecognized associated ligamentous instability, or meniscal tears was present. We suspect also that when surgery is performed to reapproximate fractured fragments, particularly in comminuted fractures, major damage to the blood supply of the small fragments can be done.

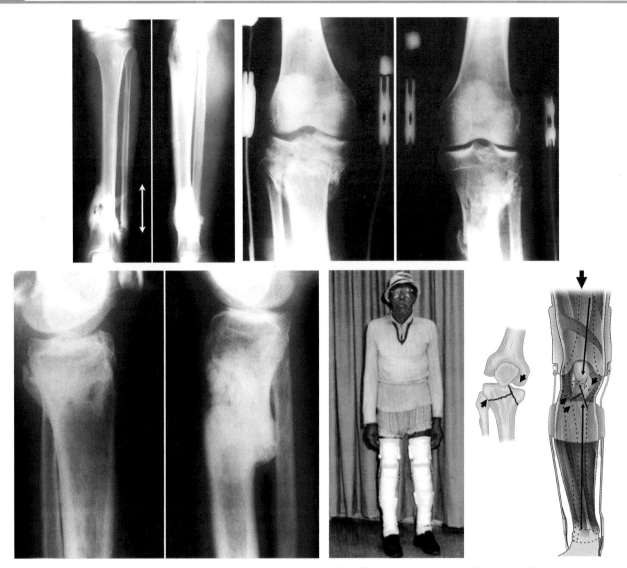

Figs 18.1: Fractures of the tibial condyles and proximal tibia. The transverse nature of the medial tibial condyle prevented a varus angular deformity.

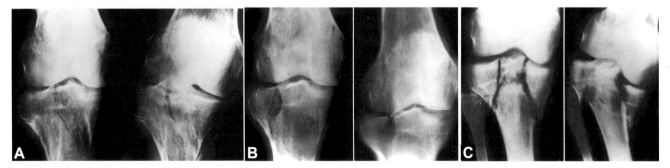

Figs 18.2: (A) Cadaver specimen of the proximal tibia with an artificially produced fracture of the medial condyle. Under vertical loading, the fracture collapsed into severe varus. (B) Artificially created fracture of the lateral condyle with an intact fibula. Under loading, the fracture did not collapse due to the support provided by the fibula. (C) Artificially produced bicondylar fracture with an intact fibula. Under vertical loading, the fracture collapsed into severe varus deformity.

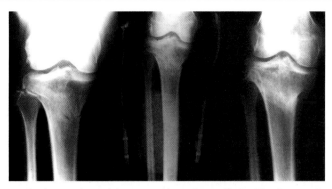

Fig. 18.3: Oblique fracture of the proximal metaphyseal fracture with an intact fibula. The fracture healed with mild varus deformity. The collapse was not severe because the fracture was rather transverse. Had it been more vertical, the varus deformity would have been severe.

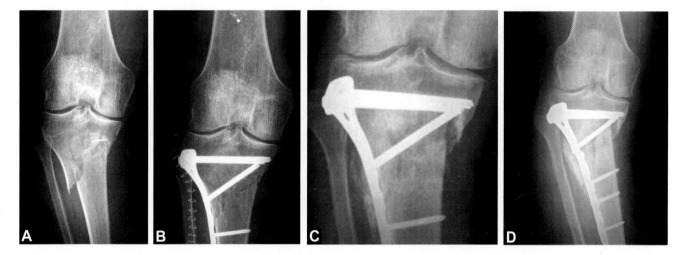

Figs 18.4A to D: (A) Oblique fracture of the proximal metaphysis of the tibia with an intact fibula. (B) A locked plate was placed on the lateral side after an anatomical reduction was obtained. (C) Within a few weeks, signs of collapse were taking place. The plate should have been located on the medial side since the intact fibula was providing good support to the fracture. (D) Severe collapse took place a few weeks later after the plate broke.

The next to clinical case vividly illustrates the important role that the fibula plays in the behavior of tibial fractures. In this instance, the bilateral condylar fracture was stabilized with a plate placed on the lateral side of the tibia, despite the fact the fibula was intact. In other words, it was ignored that the intact fibula was providing major support to the lateral condyle. The plate should have place on the medial side to enhance support to the more unstable unprotected side. The facture collapsed into varus "the unprotected condyler." Had the plate been located on the medial side, the chances are the collapse would have never occurred.

The following example is that of a patient, a homeless man, who sustained a fracture of both condyles of the tibia (Figure 18.6). It was felt his overall general condition precluded surgery. The fracture was gently manipulated under analgesia until satisfactory alignment of the fragments was achieved. An above-the-knee cast was applied and the patient was encouraged

to function as much as possible. Three weeks later, the cast was replaced with a brace that permitted free motion of the knee and ankle joints. Partial weight bearing was recommended. The fracture healed satisfactory, despite the absence of perfect anatomical reduction. The range of motion was good at the time of removal of the brace. A few weeks later, the knee extended fully and flexed normally. At this time, the knee is painless, however, the possibility of late arthritic changes is real.

INCONGRUITY

The thought that any post-traumatic incongruity in articular surfaces is unacceptable, has dominated the thinking of orthopedists for a very long time, and particularly since internal fixation of fractures became a reality. It is a logical feeling and a very difficult one to argue against. Who in his right mind would suggest that an incongruous joint is desirable?

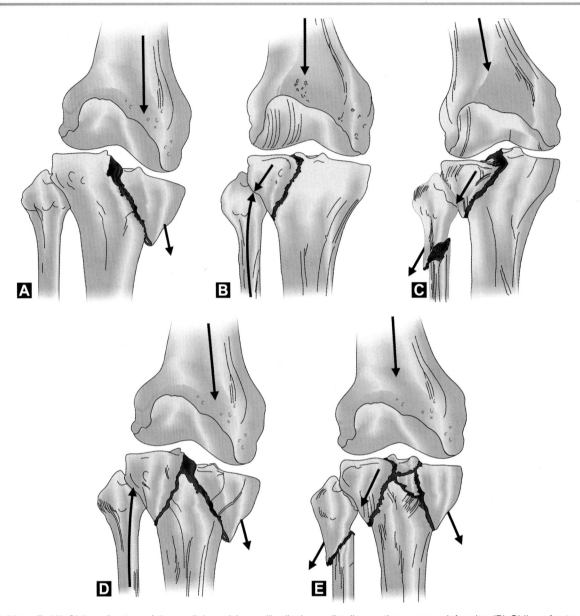

Figs 18.5A to E: (A) Oblique fracture of the medial condyle readily displaces distally creating a varus deformity. (B) Oblique fracture of the lateral condyle with an intact fibula does not displace further. (C) Oblique fracture of the lateral condyle with an associated fracture of the fibula displaces distally creating a valgus deformity. (D) Oblique fractures of both condyles with an intact fibula deform into a varus deformity. (E) Oblique fractures of both condyles, with associated fibular fracture depress evenly.

To some, the issue was settled long ago with a simple, primal answer: "Incongruity is evil and every possible effort must be made to correct it." However, is this an intelligent and scientific answer? It may not be. We often see incongruous surfaces that never developed osteoarthritic changes. Also, instances where anatomically restored congruity was followed by early degeneration of the joint.

A reasonable amount of clinical and experimental work has been conducted to elucidate those issues. The findings are interesting, but still inconclusive. The names of Lansinger from Sweden, and Kristensen from Denmark first come to mind. They conducted long-term follow-up reviews of patients whose intra-articular fractures of the knee and ankle had healed with a significant degree of incongruity. These investigators demonstrated absence of arthritic changes in many patients followed for as long as 30 years after the initial insult. Lansinger stated that as much as 1 cm step-off in the tibial condyles was compatible with good clinical results.

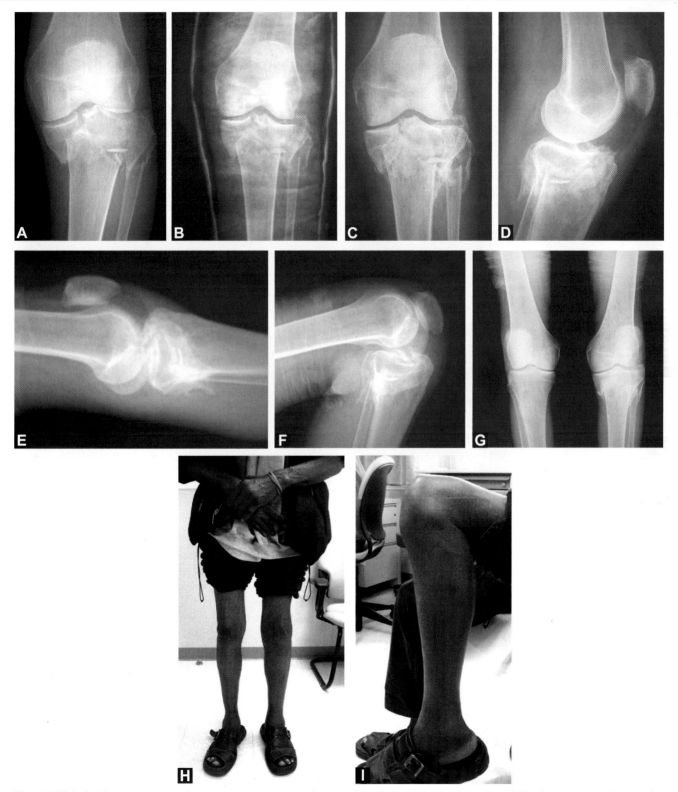

Figs 18.6A to I: (A) Bicondylar tibial fracture with an associated fracture of the fibula. Notice the deformity. (B) The fracture was reduced under analgesia. An acceptable realignment of the fragments us as obtained. An above-the-knee cast was applied. The patient was encouraged to walk bearing partial weight on the extremity. (C and D) Three weeks later, the cast was removed and an articulated brace was applied. (E and F) Radiographs of the knee showing the range of motion of the joint. (G) Standing films illustrating the residual valgus deformity of the injured leg. (H and I) Patient displays his lower extremities and the flexion of his knees. Six months later, he is still asymptomatic.

So where does the truth lie and how can we determine whether or not incongruity may be accepted? How much? in what joints? and under what circumstances?

As a result of my longstanding interest in the subject, we also studied the issue in our laboratories. Our work was done in experimental rabbits and the findings were most interesting (Figure 18.7). Doctor Adolfo Llinas from Colombia, a fellow in our laboratories, presided over the investigation. We created step-off deformities on the condyles of the femur. The depth of the step-off was arbitrarily designed to be comparable with the one most commonly seen in intraarticular tibial condylar fracture in the human (Figure 18.8).[4]

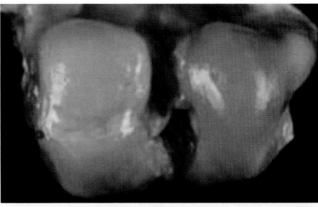

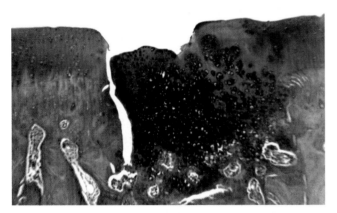

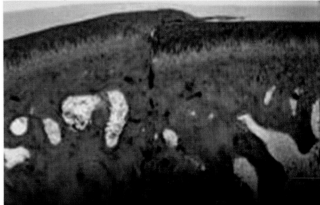

Figs 18.7: Specimen of the knee of the experimental rabbit with an artificially created incongruity followed by severance of the cruciate ligaments. Severe damage developed. In the previous study where incongruity was created but instability was not added, arthritic changes did not develop in the animals that were allowed to function normally.

Figs 18.8A and B: (A) Appearance of the articular surface of the femur after surgically created incongruity. (B) Microscopic example of the remodeling that occurs when the incongruous surface is not associated with joint instability.

The animals were divided into three groups: the first was immobilized in a long-leg cast; the second was not immobilized and allowed to run freely in the cage; and the third one was subjected to continuous passive motion of the operated joint.

The immobilized knees rapidly developed arthritic changes whereas the other two did not. There was no difference in the histological or anatomical results between the two groups of non-immobilized animals. In other words, continuous passive motion did not make matters any better. The important thing was weight bearing and motion.

Under the microscope, we demonstrated the presence of a tongue-like new cartilage extending from the high side of the step-off to the low side without arthritic changes developing.

Additional work was done by George Lovasz, from Hungary, also a research fellow in our laboratories. He added instability to the incongruous surface in the animal model by sectioning the cruciate ligaments of the knee. He concluded that incongruity, within the limits established in our original studies, was not important, but that added instability led to arthritic changes within a relatively short period of time.[5]

Their laboratory findings gave further credence to our anecdotal, undocumented perception that significant incongruity may be tolerated in many instances but associated instability encourages degeneration. We first made that observation during experimental clinical studies that we were conducting in patients with intra-articular knee fractures treated with functional braces.[6]

Many in the past have observed the absence of late arthritic changes in incongruous joints. The intra-articular fracture of the distal radius is a good example. Clinical arthritic changes are rarely seen, usually except in those instances where there is associated instability or when the fracture is the result of a severe impaction force. In this latter case, it is likely that initial irreparable pathological damage to the articular cartilage took place at the time of the traumatic event.

Fractures of the acetabulum have also illustrated the point that not all of them develop arthritic changes when

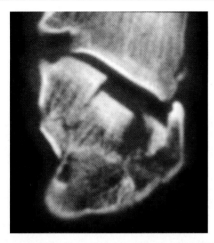

Figs 18.9: A comminuted intra-articular fracture of the tibio-talar joint. The impaction nature of the fracture may have damaged the cartilage to the point that surgical anatomical reapproximation of the fragments will not prevent later arthritic changes.

some incongruity was present and left unreduced. Several investigators recently studied the long-term follow-up of acetabular fractures and seem to have concluded that some degree of incongruity is compatible with good clinical results if the fracture was located in certain areas of the dome of the acetabulum. Those areas are the ones less likely to create instability. They however concluded that in general acetabular fractures that are anatomically reduced have a better prognosis.

It is our opinion that surgical repositioning of comminuted articular fragments can produce additional damage to an already damaged cartilage (Figure 18.9). We believe that the surgical dissection may further devascularize the subchondral bone. In addition, there is also strong experimental evidence that impact-fractures may produce severe and permanent damage to the cartilage. In other words, surgical reduction of intra-articular fractures produced through an impaction mechanism may not improve the final outcome. The reduction of devitalized fragments offers no benefits.

REFERENCES

1. Kristensen KD, Kiaer T, Blicher J. No arthrosis of the ankle 20 years after malaligned tibial-shaft fracture. Acta Orthop Scand. 1989:208-9.
2. Merchant TC, Dietz FR. Long-term follow-up after fractures of the tibial and fibular shafts. J Bone and Joint Surg. 1989 Apr; 71-A:599-606.
3. Sarmiento A, Kinman PB, Latta LL. Fractures of the Proximal Tibia and Tibial Condyles. A Clinical and Laboratory Comparative Study. Clin Orthop. 1979; 145:136.
4. Lippert FG, Hirsch C. The Three-Dimensional Measurement of Tibial Fracture Motion by Photogrammetry. Clin Orthop. 1974; 105:130.
5. Llinas A, McKellop H, Marshall J, Sharpe F, Lu B, Kirchen M and Sarmiento A. Healing and Remodeling of Articular Incongruities in a Rabbit Fracture Model. J Bone Joint Surg. 1993 Oct; 75(10):1508-23.
6. Delamarter R, Hohl M. The Cast Brace and Tibial Plateau Fractures. Clin Orthop. 1989; 242:26.

19

Notes on other Treatment Modalities

EXTERNAL FIXATORS

External fixation techniques are probably the first modern method of treatment for open tibial fractures. However, as it is true with all other methods of treatment, it may be associated with complications with pin-track infection being the most common. In addition, the rigid immobilization the system creates, oftentimes results in delayed union and nonunion. The enthusiasm generated by the success with current, more sophisticated techniques has sometimes led to heroic efforts to salvage some limbs, which for the ultimate benefit of the patient should have been ablated. Not infrequently, multiple surgical procedures are required over a period of many months, if not years, before the fracture is declared healed. By that time, the adjacent joints may be painful or partly ankylosed and some patients are unable to return to heavy labor. In addition, the psychological consequences of the injury and prolonged care should not be ignored, and the possibility of addiction to narcotics seriously considered.

The technique of bone lengthening and correction. of angular bony abnormalities described by Ilizarov in the Soviet Union has been enormously helpful. It is now possible to correct shortening of extremities to degrees that previously were considered unattainable and dangerous to attempt. He also extended the use of his technique to the care of open and difficult fractures.

One of us (A.S.) had the opportunity to hear Ilizarov present his experiences in the late 1970s in Lecco, Italy, allegedly on his first trip outside his country. Dean McEwen from Delaware and I were invited by the State Department to hear his presentations first hand.

I must admit that the experience was unforgettable. Ilizarov, using slides, showed in impressive examples of his results in a packed auditorium. He illustrated correction of nonunions associated with deformities that ordinarily we would have treated by primary amputation of the limb. He had lengthened extremities with congenital or post-traumatic conditions of grotesque degrees. He successfully managed to obtain union of congenital pseudoarthrosis of the tibia that no one had ever succeeded in curing. All this occurred in the remote Siberian city of Kurgan using bicycle spokes to fabricate a frame.

The concept fascinated me so much that I purchased the entire Ilizarov instrumentation that day. I brought it to the United States and did my best to encourage my associates, responsible for the trauma service, to use it. My efforts were futile. Now the procedure is being performed by many orthopedists around the world with success.

Ever since the moment I heard Ilizarov present his results, I was intrigued by the rationale he gave for the effectiveness of his distraction osteogenesis theory. Others had achieved various degrees of success in lengthening shortened extremities with a variety of gadgets. They had observed new bone filling the gap, but had also realized that the amount of shortening to be overcome was limited and that the quality of the new bone remained inferior for a very long time.

What Ilizarov demonstrated was the possibility of gaining greater degrees of length and the more rapid maturation of the bone at the distraction level. I readily noticed from his presentation, as well as from the number of patients shown to us by the Italian surgeons, that a great emphasis was placed on initiating weight bearing ambulation shortly after the performance of the surgical procedure. When performed in the upper extremity, active exercises and early use of the arm musculature was part of the postoperative protocol.

As a result of this observation, I was prompted to ask Ilizarov if he had thought about the possible value of motion at the fracture site, which was provoked by weight bearing and muscle activity. Since my conversation with him required a translator, I used the accordion as an example to describe the motions I suspected took place at the osteotomy and nonunion

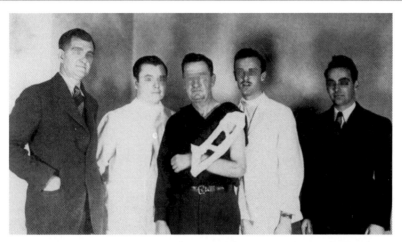

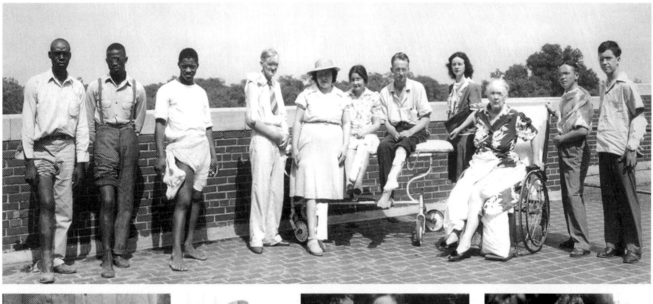

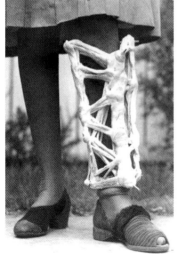

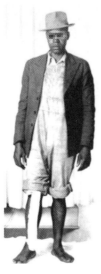

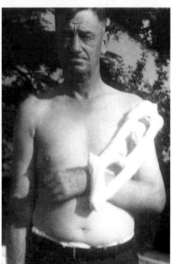

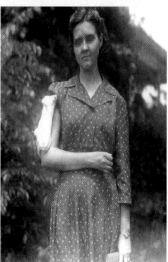

Fig. 19.1: Photographs of several patients treated by Austin T. Moore circa 1940. He eventually abandoned the method due to the frequent occurrence of pin-track infection. Doctor Moore, who appears on the top photograph, gave me these photos while serving as his residence between 1953-1956.

sites. The translator responded that the "professor" had not understood the question. It is possible I did not word the question correctly or that Ilizarov had not paid attention to my suggested mechanism. It is also possible that he had known that all along, but I failed to understand his philosophy.

Over the years, I have come to conclude that the accordion motion that definitely occurs with the Ilizarov system is the key to its success. Obviously, it is not immobilization. The distraction osteogenesis theory, in my opinion, loses a great deal of credence in the absence of intermittent compression and distraction. The fact that his results were obtained with the use of very thin bicycle spoke wires, gives further support to the view that stress and motion at the "fracture" site are essential for success.

The senior author had the opportunity and privilege to obtain my orthopedic residency education under Austin Moore, one of the great American pioneers in hip prosthetic replacement. The following photographs were given to me by Doctor Moore, which depict instances when he treated a variety of fractures with simple external fixation appliances (Figure 19.1). He did his work in the 1930s and 40s. His enthusiasm with the technique mellowed over the years, upon recognizing the frequency of pin-track infections and nonunions.

The following photos are only of historical interest, but serve as a lesson to illustrate the short life that virtually applies to all efforts to improve the human condition.

The fact that the fibula heals faster than the tibia, makes the recurrence of the tibial deformity a likely event. This reality increases the difficulties in determining when to remove the pins. If it is done before the fracture is intrinsically stable,

a recurrence of shortening is likely to rapidly take place. If postponed too long, the healed fibula fracture produces a varus angular deformity (Figures 19.2 to 19.4).

One of the most frequent complications from external fixation is infection around the pins. Frequent washing of the area lowers this problem, however, even in the presence of proper local care, infection can occur, which on occasion may degenerate into osteomyelitis that requires bone debridement (Figure 19.5).

Despite the above mentioned limitations of the method, external fixation remains the treatment of choice in the management of open tibial fractures. Neither plating, nor intramedullary nailing renders comparable results or fewer complications. Its place in closed fractures, likewise, is most appropriate in the management of axially unstable fractures that experience at the time of the injury an unacceptable shortening. It is difficult to justify its use in closed fractures that show acceptable initial shortening and correctable angular deformity.

This very useful and sound method of fracture stabilization has been greatly abused in recent years. In too many instances, this very expensive method is used in the treatment of closed, simple fractures that would have responded rapidly and more inexpensively to nonsurgical functional treatment without the risk of experiencing the common complication of pin-track infection and the delayed healing time that the rigid immobilization of the fracture creates by the unwise use of very stiff pins. We strongly believe that such rigid immobilization is detrimental. More flexible pins are more likely to render better results, as Ilizarov himself demonstrated.

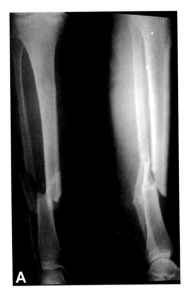 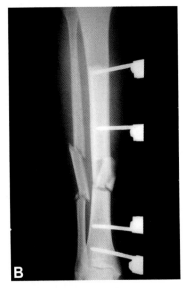 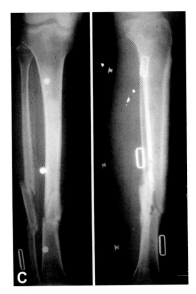

Figs 19.2A to C: (A) Radiograph of open fracture of the tibia and fibula. The fracture was very unstable. (B) An external fixator was used and the wound was left open. (C) The pins were removed 3 weeks after the initial insult and then stabilized, first in an above-the knee cast and then in a below-the knee functional cast. The fracture healed with good alignment and length. Since the period of joint immobilization was short, the range of motion of the ankle and knee was minimally impaired.

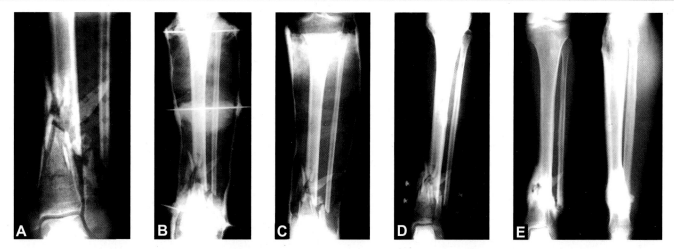

Figs 19.3A to E: (A) Radiograph of open comminuted fracture in the distal-third of the tibia, with an associated fracture of the fibula. Notice the degree of shortening. (B) The fracture was treated with debridement and, correction of shortening and stabilization in a cast that incorporate pins above and below the fracture. (C) Radiograph showing the early recurrence of shortening after removal of the pins. (D) Radiograph obtained through a plastic brace demonstrating further shortening of the limb. (E) Upon completion of union, the shortening of the limb had reached the initial shortening.

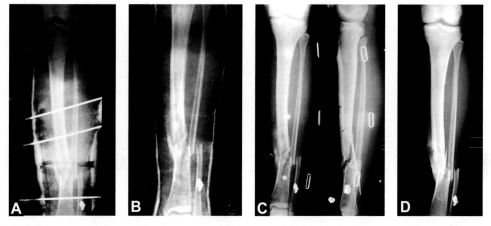

Figs 19.4A to D: (A) Radiograph of open fracture of the tibia treated with pins-in-plaster. A wedging procedure had been carried out to correct a deformity. (B) After transferring the limb to a cast, the limb began to experience shortening. (C) In the brace, the return to the initial shortening became obvious. (D) The last radiograph demonstrates the frequently seen recurrence of deformity due to the delayed healing of the fracture that rigid immobilization creates.

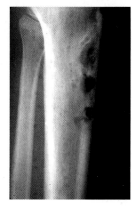

Fig. 19.5: Radiograph depicting osteomyelitis around loose pins in a fracture treated with an external fixator. Surgical debridement was necessary.

For the past several years, the senior author has had the privilege of observing with some frequency the work done by Doctor James Hutson at the University of Miami. He is a most skillful individual who has mastered and improved the Ilizarov method.[1] This experience has made me appreciate in a more scientific manner the true value of the system and its benefits. We anticipate that with time, the true place for the use of the method will be established and a more solid scientific foundation for the appropriate place and role for today's popular systems of fracture care will be determined.

REFERENCE

1. Hutson J. The Ilizarov System in Fracture care. Techniques in Orthopedics. 2002; 17:1-111.

20

Plate Fixation

Plating of tibial fractures was for nearly a century a popular method of treatment of tibial fractures. Militating against the method was the frequent complication of infection. The discovery of antibiotics partially resolved that problem. The initial plates and the technique recommended for their insertion were rather unsophisticated. It was not until Danis, a Flemish surgeon, proposed the technique of "compression" of the bony fragments that major progress in this area began to take place. However, his technique had remained imperfect, though the concept of rigid immobilization continue to gain acceptance in orthopedic circles.

Maurice Muller, an orthopedic giant in the second half of the 20th Century, learned about Danis' philosophy and converted the system into the one that dominated fracture care for the next 50 years. He and his group, the AO organization, working in concert with the manufacturing industry revolutionized fracture care. The technique, predicated in the concept of "rigid" immobilization and "interfragmentary compression" became a universally accepted method of treatment. The contribution to this school of thought made by people like Stephen Perren gave the project enormous credibility. The AO, success was greatly enhanced by the conduct of a parallel educational effort.[1]

Over time, the limitations of the method began to appear. The initial implication that following the plating procedure patients would be able to ambulate without a cast, proved to be wrong in most instances. Protection of the injured limb from full weight bearing became necessary.

Additional flaws in the system were recognized, despite the fact that plating had improved the care of fractures in a major way. The rigid immobilization of the fragments delayed healing, since peripheral callus in such an environment does not form. The "osteon-by-osteon" type of healing takes place very slowly, and means to accurately determine the progression of healing are unreliable, since the formation of mature crossing trabeculae cannot be seen until late in the process.[2-9]

The use of plating of diaphyseal fractures of the tibia has been eclipsed by the intramedullary nail. Plating remains however, one of the preferred methods of treatment for metaphyseal fractures and for fractures in the upper extremity.

Illsutration of fractures treated with plating are shown in Figures 20.1 to 20.3.

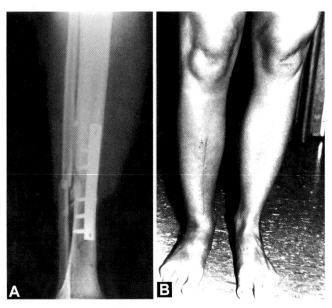

Figs 20.1A and B: (A) Radiograph of a plated tibial fracture showing restoration of length and anatomy to the injured limb. Though the film was obtained 2½ months after surgery, no obvious healing can be detected. As expected, peripheral callus had not formed. (B) The photograph demonstrates the readily visible surgical scar.

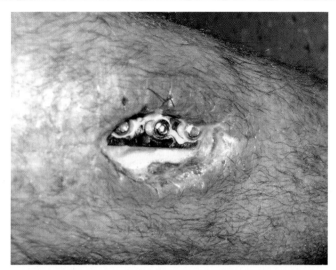

Fig. 20.2: Although the incidence of infection with plate osteosynthesis has decreased considerably over the years, it remains a likely complication, which in some instances defies early recovery. The removal of the plate is frequently mandatory in order to successfully obtain a cure.

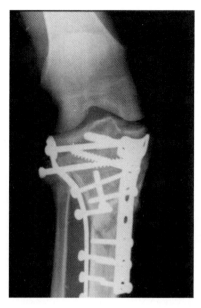

Fig. 20.3: Radiograph of a plated fracture of the proximal tibia. Despite the rigid fixation achieved, a varus deformity was perpetuated.

REFERENCES

1. Schlitch T. Surgery, Science and Industry. Palgrave-McMillan 2002.
2. Latta LL, Sarmiento A. Mechanical Behavior of Tibial Fractures. Symposium on Trauma to the Leg and Its Sequela. C.V. Mosby: St. Louis, MO 1981.
3. Latta LL, Sarmiento A. Fracture Casting and Bracing. ASOP Publishing Inc. 2008.
4. Park SH, O'Connor K, McKellop H, Sarmiento A. The Influence of active Shear or Compressive Motion on Fracture Healing. J Bone Joint Surg Am. 1998 Jun; 80(6):868-78.
5. Sarmiento A, Schaeffer J, Beckerman L, Latta LL, Enis J. Fracture Healing in Rat Femora as Affected by Functional Weight Bearing. J. Bone Joint Surg Am, 1977; 59(3):369-75.
6. Sarmiento A, Mullis DL, Latta LL, Alvarez RR. A Quantitative, Comparative Analysis of Fracture Healing Under the Influence of Compression Plating vs. Closed Weight-Bearing Treatment. Clin Orthop. 1980; 149:232.
7. Uhthoff HK. Prevention of bone atrophy through an early removal of internal fixation plates. An experimental study in the dog. Howmedica Trauma Workshop, New York. 1979.
8. Uhthoff HK, Dubuc FL. Bone structure changes in the dog under rigid internal fixation. Clin Orthop. 1970; 81:40-7.
9. Wolf JW et al. The Superiority of Cyclic Loading over Constant Compression in the Treatment of Long Bone Fractures. A Quantitative Biomechanical Study in Rabbits. Trans 26 Orthop Res Soc. 1980; 5:174.

21

Interlocking Intramedullary Nailing

The success of interlocking nailing of femoral fractures promptly resulted in exploring the possibility of using similar techniques in the management of tibial fractures. The success has been so great that today it has become the treatment of choice for many such fractures. In closed tibial fractures associated with significant soft tissue damage and initial major shortening and displacement, intramedullary nailing is the preferred treatment for many orthopedists. We question, however, the extension of the method at this time to the treatment of many low-energy fractures of the tibia for the following reasons:

The procedure is not free of complications. Infection is rare but it has been reported to range between 1 and 5%.[1-16] If the infection migrates down or up the shaft, management of the complication becomes a difficult and often unrewarding task.

In the process of applying traction to the extremity and then reaming the medullary canal we demonstrated, in cadaver specimens with mechanically produced fractures, that the muscle compartments of the leg experience significant elevation of pressure. We actually reproduced the mechanism of the classical compartment syndrome picture. This is easily explained in mechanical terms. When a fracture of the tibia occurs, bleeding takes place around the fracture. The leg shortens at the time of the injury to a degree determined by the severity of soft tissue damage. The girth of the extremity at that level increases to accommodate the bleeding. Fortunately, tamponade eventually stops the bleeding but, by that time, the compartmental pressures are elevated. In most instances, the increase in pressure is not high enough to produce a compartment syndrome. However, if under those circumstances traction is applied to the leg, its geometry changes and is forced to obtain the conical shape of the normal leg. This cannot take place without increasing the muscle compartment pressures. If, in addition, closed reaming of the medullary canal is done, the added bleeding and reamed material from the medullary canal produce further elevation of pressure. (See Chapter 1)

Since interlocking nails are usually inserted after applying traction to the fractured extremity, gaps between comminuted fragments are often increased. The interlocking screws perpetuate that separation until healing takes place. Weight bearing before healing is complete transfers weight bearing stresses to the screws at the screw-nail interface. This explains the high incidence of screw fracture, as high as 15 to 20% at this time. Removal of the broken screws can be an impossible task due to galling corrosion between the nail and the screws, a problem more likely to happen when the softer Titanium metal is used. Bending or breaking of the nail is not infrequent and when this complication occurs, the removal of the damaged nail becomes a major surgical undertaking. A broken nail is difficult to remove but a bent one can become an impossible task unless the fracture is surgically visually exposed and the two ends of the nail are separately removed (Figure 21.1).

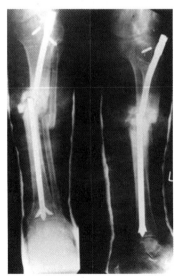

Fig. 21.1: A rare complication from an interlocking tibial nail. The nail broke after the patient attempted to ambulate without external support, shortly after surgery.

In previous studies, we have shown that the callus that forms in the presence of weight bearing and function is of a superior quality and that the initial shortening experienced in closed tibial fractures does not increase beyond that observed immediately after the initial insult. There are no standard criteria in the literature concerning determination of fracture healing. When rigid fixation methods are used, the difficulty in confirming union is increased because peripheral callus does not form in this environment. In our study the criteria used for healing were the radiological presence of bridging callus between the two major fragments and the patient's ability to walk without external support and without pain. Our fractures healed at an average of 16.6 weeks, with a median of 15.9 weeks, a mode of 14.4 weeks, and a range from 1 to 40 weeks. In this instance, we chose to compare our closed fractures with closed fractures treated by others with intramedullary nailing.

Court-Brown et al reported an average healing time of 16.7 weeks in nailed closed tibial fractures.[17,18] Wiss and Stetson reported an average healing time of 28 weeks with a range of 12 to 104 weeks.[16] Finkemeier et al stated that closed tibial fractures heal at approximately 16 weeks, with reamed fractures healing faster than those treated with unreamed nails (P = 0.040).[6] De Smet et al reported union at an average of 28.4 weeks using a flexible nail.[4] Bonnevialle et al reported a mean healing time of 25 weeks (range 8.5-68 weeks).[19]

In our study of 1000 closed tibial fractures from which this report is derived, the nonunion rate was 1.1%.[20] In the current study of 434 fractures located in the middle-third of the tibia, the nonunion rate was 0.9% indicating that, contrary to popular belief, the level of the fracture is not important regarding healing. Gregory and Sanders reported 8% nonunion in 38 closed fractures.[7] Wiss and Stetson reported a nonunion rate of 2%.[16] Court-Brown et al reported a nonunion rate of 1.6%.[17] Bonnevialle acknowledged 5.2% nonunions.[19]

Infection after nailing of closed fractures is low. Bone and Johnson reported a 4% incidence of infection in a group of 68 patients.[1] Court-Brown et al reported 1.6% infections[3] and Alho et al reported 2.1% infection in 93 closed tibial fractures.[21] Wiss and Stetson reported an infection rate of 5% in a group of 100 closed fractures treated with reamed intramedullary nails.[16] In our study, since surgery was not performed, no infections were encountered.

The use of interlocking screws has made possible the intramedullary nailing of many axially unstable fractures. However, under these circumstances weightbearing stresses are transferred to the screw, which under repeated loading may fracture or bend. Hutson et al review of the literature found out an incidence of breakage of intramedullary nails or locking screws or both, ranging between 14% and 20%.[22] Cole and Latta analyzed the mode and mechanism of failure of intramedullary nails and interlocking screws.[23]

Koval et al stated that 58% of patients who had intramedullary nailing of the tibia developed some complication attributable to the procedure. They acknowledged intraoperative complications in 10% of patients, with a propagation of a fracture during the insertion site of the nail in 6% of the procedures. They also identified peroneal palsy in 18% patients, usually transient.[10] Others have reported complications of various types such as vascular compromise, compartment syndromes and cortical necrosis.[1,6-9,11,12,15,24,25]

Shortening after intramedullary nailing was reported by Bone and Johnson[1] to be 10 mm in 5% patients and 3.4% in 21 patients by Hooper at al.[9] In our study, the mean shortening was 5.1 mm. At our institution, intramedullary nailing was the preferred method of treatment for axially unstable fractures with initial shortening greater than 15 mm. We do not have information as to the number of fractures treated surgically during the same period of time.

Intramedullary nailing does not consistently result in perfect alignment. Freeman et al using a criteria, where a fracture was considered malaligned if 5 or more degrees of angulation in any plane was measured, reported malalignment in 7% fractures located in the middle-third of the tibia; 58% in fractures located in its proximal-third; and 8% in its distal-third.[26]

The angular deformities measured in patients in this study were acceptable from the cosmetic point of view in most instances, as 405 (90.0%) patients had < 8° angular deformity. These figures are comparable with those reported in the literature dealing with intramedullary nailing.

There is strong suggestive evidence that angular deformities resulting from diaphyseal tibial fractures are rarely responsible for late degenerative arthritis in the adjacent joints. Merchant and Dietz, based on a review of 37 patients who had tibial fractures with a follow-up of nearly 29 years, concluded that 10-15° angular deformities were well tolerated and the deformity was not related to functional deficit. They stated that the clinical and radiographic results were unaffected by the amount of anterior or posterior and varus or valgus angulation at the level of the fracture.[27] Kristensen et al found no osteoarthritis of the ankle 20 years after malaligned tibial fractures and found out that ankle stiffness and associated pain is directly proportional to the length of immobilization.[28] It can be extrapolated that the early mobilization of all joints made possible by the functional brace minimizes temporary stiffness. We and other investigators have studied the effect of angular deformities on the adjacent joints, and have found that minor deformities do not alter pressure distribution on the articular cartilage in the adjacent joints in a significant way.[25-38]

We did not study rotary deformities in this article. We had long ago concluded that such deformity was extremely rare with functional bracing, and its presence is due to failure to correct it at the time of the initial reduction of the fracture. The use of intramedullary nailing does not guarantee the prevention of rotary deformity.

The most common undesirable consequence of intramedullary nailing is chronic knee pain. Court-Brown et al reported an incidence of knee pain in 56.2% of patients, most of them significantly younger. There was considerable functional impairment with 91.7% of patients experiencing pain on kneeling and 33.7% having pain even at rest. They stated that 24.4% patients required removal of the nail.[39] Keating et al reported the need for nail removal because of knee pain in 80% of 61 patients, and after 16 months, the pain had not resolved in 22 (36%) of these patients.[40] Bonneivialle reported that 50% of his patients complained of knee pain. However, 20% "felt cured" 5 months postoperatively.[6] Orfany et al stated that the incidence of knee pain can be reduced by using paratendinous incisions.[41] Quraishi et al reported 93.7% patients had anterior knee sensory disturbance, 96.8% had pain on kneeling. Twenty-six percent of his patients had their nail removed. Of these 53.5% had persistent anterior knee; 89.5% had anterior sensory knee disturbance; 71.4% had pain on kneeling. Metal removal did not facilitate the desired reduction of symptoms.[42] Toivanen et al reported knee pain in 86% of patients who had a transtendinous approach, and 81% in patients who had a paratendinous approach. They stated that 69% of their patients had anterior knee pain at an average of 1.5 years after nail removal.[43]

The residual shortening and mild angular deformities identified in most patients in the study should not be called complications since they are esthetically acceptable, and do not produce a limp or lead to late degenerative joint disease (Figure 21.2). They simply are inconsequential deviations from the normal. A glance at the ethos of Orthopedics during the last few decades readily demonstrates a growing obsession with the need to restore anatomical reduction of all fractures, as if such a premise was synonymous with better clinical results. Though anatomical reduction is very important in many instances, it does not mean that this is the case in all cases. A shortening of the tibia of 1 cm or less, does not produce a limp, creates a limp or leads to late undesirable changes in the adjacent joints. The same applies to angular deformities where angulation of 5° is not recognizable with the naked eyes in most instances and the deformity does not lead to arthritic changes. The exaggerated influence and control of education of the orthopedist by the implant manufacturing companies has been highly responsible for this harmful trend having led to a loss of objectivity that is converting the orthopedic surgeon into a cosmetic surgeon of the skeleton from the surgeon/scientist required to meet the exigencies of the time.[44-58]

Although functional bracing appears to render good results in the care of closed axially unstable fractures that experience initially < 12 mm of shortening and a corrected angular deformity < 8°, and in reduced, made stable closed transverse fractures, the role of bracing should not, at this time, be extended to fractures that experience initially > 12 mm of shortening and angular deformity > 8°.

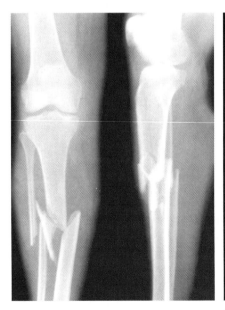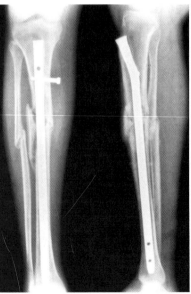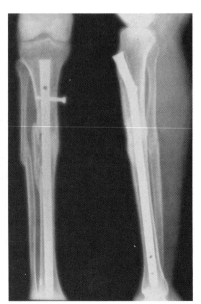

Figs 21.2: Composite radiograph of low-grade open fracture of the tibia and fibula, appropriately treated with an interlocking nail. Distal screws were used but were removed a few weeks later, after intrinsic stability at the fracture site was suspected. The fracture healed uneventfully with very acceptable shortening.

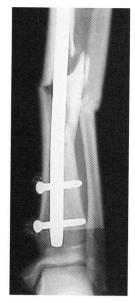

Fig. 21.3: Radiograph illustrating a mild valgus angular deformity that was probably created at the time of surgery, and became worse when the screws broke after the introduction of premature full-weight bearing ambulation. The axially unstable nature of the fracture resulted in the transfer of stresses to the distal screws.

A feature concerning intramedullary nailing which is not sufficiently addressed in the literature is the fact that its use does not always permit early weight bearing ambulation. A nailed fracture with a geometry that resulted in stable bone contact between the two major fragments permits weight bearing at a very early time since the stresses at the fracture site are shared between the bony surfaces and the interlocking screws (Figure 21.3).

However, if the fracture is not intrinsically stable (the major fragments are not in wide contact), weight bearing stresses are not taken by the bone but are transferred to the screws, resulting in their eventual breaking or bending (Figures 21.4 to 21.7).

Not infrequently attempts are made to restore length to a shortened extremity afflicted with a transverse, axially stable fracture. This effort may result in separation between the major fragments in such a manner that when the procedure is completed, a gap remains between the two major fragments (Figures 21.8 and 21.9). If interlocking screws were used and weight bearing is allowed, the weight bearing stresses are transferred to the screws, which eventually fracture, unless the limb is kept from taking major weight until the fracture has formed sufficiently strong callus.

Likewise, an axially unstable fracture (oblique, spiral, comminuted) treated with an interlocking nail, will experience the same phenomenon: the screws will take the stresses of weight bearing leading to their fracture.

It can be concluded that axially unstable fractures and stable transverse fractures that demonstrate a gap between the major fragments, should be protected from premature weight bearing till sufficient intrinsic stability has developed.

Quite often, interlocking screws are used because of fear of development of a rotary deformity. This perception is frequently ill-founded. The interlocking nail for the treatment of femoral fractures was a major contribution, primarily because it made possible to extend the use of intramedullary nailing of metaphyseal fractures. The traditional femoral nail was used only for diaphyseal fractures. When used for diaphyseal fractures, angular and rotary deformities frequently ensued. It was a logical complication, since the cancellous bone

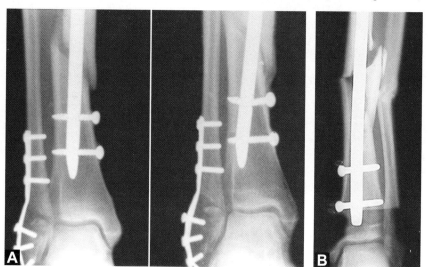

Figs 21.4A and B: (A) Composite photographs of an axial fracture of the distal tibia treated with an interlocking intramedullary nail. Early weight bearing was permitted, resulting in breakage of the screws and a secondary mild and inconsequential varus angular deformity. B) Radiograph of an axially unstable fracture of the distal tibia treated with an interlocking nail. Under weight bearing, a valgus deformity occurred after the screws broke.

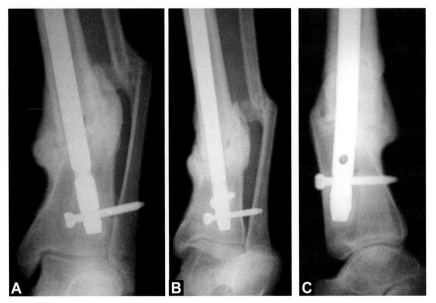

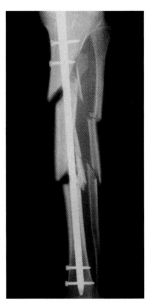

Figs 21.5A to C: (A and B) Antero-posterior and oblique radiographs illustrating a severe varus deformity. Apparently, premature weight bearing produce the deformity and the screw cut into the bone. (C) The lateral view demonstrates the sagittal deformity.

Fig. 21.6: Radiograph of inappropriately nailed segmental fracture of the tibia. Though it is likely that the fracture healed uneventfully, this radiograph demonstrated that anatomical alignment is not always obtained with nailing techniques.

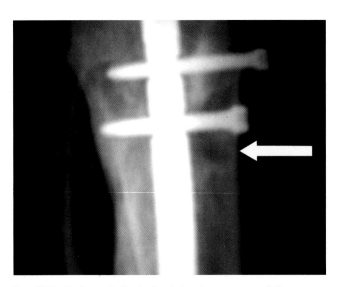

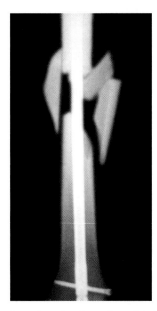

Fig. 21.7: Radiograph illustrating lytic changes around the screws associated with a low-grade infection. Similar changes may be seen from lysis created by metal debris arising at the screw-hole interface.

Fig. 21.8: Illustration of a situation where interlocking screws are necessary to prevent shortening and migration of the nail. However, premature weight bearing easily results in breaking of the screws as the weight bearing stresses are taken by the screws and not by the bone.

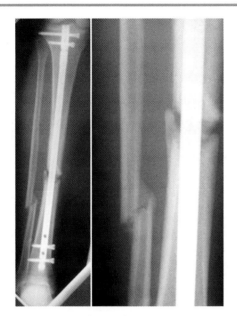

Fig. 21.9: Radiograph illustrating a common phenomenon: While attempting to reduce the fracture using traction, a gap is created between the two major fragments. In this manner, the fibula heals but the gap in the tibia persists, since weight bearing stresses are transferred to the distal screws that either break or perpetuate the gap. In this instance, since the nail is close contact with the cortical bone in both fragments, there is no need to use distal interlocking screws. The tight fit of the nail precludes rotational instability. In addition, the healed fibula fracture will contribute to perpetuating the gap in the tibial fracture.

of the diaphysis was readily cut by the nail when subjected to weight-bearing stresses. A tightly fit nail in the isthmus of the tibia or femur prevents rotation at the fracture site; therefore, the distal interlocking screws are necessary. Furthermore their presence results in an extreme degree of immobilization resulting in delay of fracture healing.

The problem most commonly encountered with non-interlocking nails was the eventual loosening of the nail and its proximal displacement over the greater trochanter, resulting in the development of a bursitis that oftentimes required removal of the nail. The problem most commonly encountered with such nailing was the eventual loosening of the nail and its proximal displacement over the greater trochanter, resulting in the development of a bursitis that oftentimes required removal of the nail.

One can safely extrapolate that transverse, stable diaphyseal fractures do not require interlocking screws distally. They are not needed; quite the contrary, they do harm by preventing the healthy motion that takes place between the fragments and by unloading the fracture site. Screws at both ends are required with metaphyseal fractures and in comminuted diaphyseal fractures.

The technique relatively recently introduced consisting of suprapatellar nailing of proximal fractures of the tibia and for

those associated with a distal femoral appears to be a sound method to address this difficult combination of fractures. However, it should not be taken for granted that it is free from complications. It is likely that during the process of inserting the nail, damage to the articular surface of the distal femur and patella may be produced. Furthermore, the process of recovery is much slower because of associated knee pain. Our concern is due to the fact that the restoration of motion of the knee joint is delayed, but more importantly the possibility of infection at the fracture site could result in extension of the infection into the joint. The prognosis in such an instance is guarded.

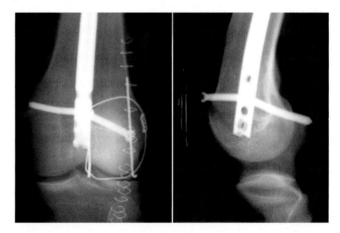

Figs 21.10: Radiograph showing the broken distal interlocking screws, the result of transfer of weight bearing stresses during attempts to bear full weight prior to fracture healing.

REFERENCES

1. Bone LB, Johnson K.D. Treatment of tibial fractures by reaming and intramedullary nailing. J. Bone and Joint Surg. 1986; 68A(6):877-87.
2. Buehler KC, Green J, Woll TS, Duwelius PJ. A technique for intramedullary nailing of proximal-third tibia fractures. J Orthop Trauma. 1997; 11(3):218-223.
3. Court-Brown CM, Keating JF, McQueen MM. Infection after intramedullary nailing of the tibia. Incidence and protocol for management. J Bone Joint Surg Br. 1992; 74-B (5):770-16
4. De Smet K, Mostert AK, De Witte J, De Brauwer V, Verdonk R. Closed intramedullary tibial nailing using the Marchetti-Vicenzi nail. Injury. 2000; 31(8):597-603.
5. Downing ND, Griffin DR, Davis TR. A Comparison of the relative costs of cast treatment and intramedullary nailing for tibial diaphyseal fractures in the UK. Injury. 1997; 28(5-6):373-5.
6. Finkemeier CG, Schmidt AH, Kyle RF, Templeman DC, Varecka TF. A prospective, randomized study of intramedullary nails inserted with and without reaming for the treatment of open and closed fractures of the tibial shafts. J Orthop Trauma. 2000; 14 (3):187-93.
7. Gregory P, Sanders R. The treatment of closed, unstable tibial shaft fractures with unreamed interlocking nails. Clin Orthop Relat Res. 1995; 315:48-55.

8. Habernek H, Kwansy O, Schmid L, Ortner F. Complications of interlocking nailing for lower leg fractures. A three year follow-up of 102 cases. J Trauma. 1992; 33:863-9.

9. Hooper GJ, Keddell RG, Penny ID. Conservative management or closed nailing for tibial shaft fractures. A randomized prospective trial. J Bone and Joint Surg. 1991 Jan; 73B:83-5.

10. Koval KJ, Clapper MF, Elison PS, Poka A, Bathon GH, Burgess AR. Complications of reamed intramedullary nailing of the tibia. J Orthop Trauma. 1991; 5:184-9.

11. Lang GJ, Cohen BE, Bosse MJ, Kellam JF. Proximal-third tibial shaft fractures. Should they be nailed? Clin Orthop. 1995; 315:64-74.

12. Ricciardi-Pollini PT, Falez F. The Treatment of Diaphyseal Fractures by Functional Bracing. Results in 36 Cases. Et al J Orthop Traumatol. 1985 Jun; 11(2):199-205.

13. Templeman D, Varecka T, Kyle R. Exchanged reamed intramedullary nailing for delayed union and nonunion of the tibia. Clin Orthop. 1995; (315):169-75.

14. Toivanen JA, Honkonen SE, Koivisto AM, Jarvinen MJ. Treatment of low-energy tibial shaft fractures. Plaster cast compared with intramedullary nailing. Int Orthop. 2001; 25(2):110-3.

15. Williams J, Gibbons M, Trundle H, Murray D, Worlock P. Complications of nailing in closed tibial fractures. J Orthop Trauma. 1995; 9(6):476-81.

16. Wiss DA, Stetson WB. Unstable fractures of the tibia treated with reamed intramedullary nails. Clin Orthop Relat Res. 1995; 315: 56-63.

17. Court-Brown CM, Will E, Christie J, McQueen M. Reamed or unreamed nailing for closed tibial fractures. J. Bone and Joint Surg. 1996 Jul; 78B:580-3.

18. Court-Brown CM, Christie J, McQueen MM. Closed intramedullary tibial nailing. Its use in closed and Type I open fractures. J Bone Joint Surg Br. 1990; 72B (4):605-11.

19. Bonnevialle P, Bellumore Y, Foucras L, Hezard L, Mansat M. Tibial fractures with intact fibula treated by reamed nailing. Rev Chir Orthop Reparatrice Appar Mot. 2000; 86(1):29-37.

20. Alho A, Ekelan A, Stromsoe K et al. Nonunion of Tibial Shaft Fractures treated with locked intramedullary nailing without bone grafting. J Trauma. 1993; 34(1):62.

21. Alho A, Eckeland A, Stromsoe K, Folleras G, Thorensen B. Locked intramedullary nailing of tibial fractures. J Bone Joint Surg. 1990; 72B:805-11.

22. Hutson J, Zych GA, Cole JD, Johnson KD, Ostermann P, Milne EL, Latta, L. Mechanical failures of intramedullary tibia nails applied without reaming. Clinic Orthop Relat Res. 1995; 315: 129-37.

23. Cole D, Latta LL. Fatigue failure of interlocking tibial nail implants. Orthop Trans Bone Joint Surg. 1992; 16-3A:663.

24. Guilar J, Vazquez P, Ortega M. False aneurysm of the posterior tibial artery complicating fracture of the tibia and fibula. Rev Chir Orthop Reparatrice Appar Mot. 1995; 81(6):546-8.

25. Kyro A. Malunion after intramedullary nailing of tibial shaft fractures. Ann Chir Gynecol. 1997; 86:56-64.

26. Freedman EL, Johnson EE. Radiographic analysis of tibial fracture malalignment following intramedullary nailing. Clin Orthop Relat Res. 1995; 315:25-33.

27. Mawhinney IN, Maginn P, McCoy GF. Tibial compartment syndromes after tibial nailing. J Orthop Trauma. 1994; 8(3): 212-14.

28. Kristensen KD, Kiaer T, Blicher J. No arthrosis of the ankle 20 years after malaligned tibial-shaft fracture. Acta Orthop Scand. 1989:208-9.

29. Lovasz G, Park SH, Ebramzadeh E, Benya PD, Llinas A, Bellyei A, Luck J, Sarmiento A. Characteristic of degeneration in an unstable knee with a coronal surface step-off. J. Bone Joint Br. 2001 Apr; 83(3):428-36.

30. McCollough NC, Vinsant JE, Sarmiento A. Functional Fracture - Bracing of Long-bone Fractures of the Lower Extremity in Children. J Bone Joint Surg. 1978; 60A:314.

31. McKellop HA, Hoffmann R, Sarmiento A, Lu B, Ebramzadeh E. Control of Motion of Tibial Fractures with Use of a Functional Brace or an External Fixator. J Bone & Joint Surg. 1993 Jul; 75A:1019-25.

32. Rankin, EA, Metz CW Jr. Management of delayed union in early weight-bearing treatment of the fractured tibia. J. Trauma. 1970 Sep; 10(9):751-9.

33. Sarmiento A, Latta LL. Functional Bracing in Management of Tibial Fractures. The Intact Fibula. AAOS Symposium on Trauma of the Leg and Its Sequela. Moore TM (Ed). The. C. V. Mosby Company. 1981; 278-98.

34. Sarmiento A, Latta LL. Closed fractures of the middle third of the tibia treated with a functional Brace. Clin Orthop. 2008 Dec; 466:3108-15.

35. Sarmiento A, Latta LL. 450 Closed Fractures of the distal third of the tibia treated with a functional brace. Clin Orthop. 2004; 428: 261-71.

36. Sarmiento A, Latta LL. Closed Functional Treatment of Fractures. Springer-Verlag: Berlin 1981.

37. Sarmiento A. On the behavior of closed tibial fractures: clinical and radiological correlations. J Orthop Trauma. 2000; 14(3):199-205.

38. Sarmiento A. Mechanism of Injury may affect Outcome after Tibial Shaft Fracture. J Bone Joint Surg Am 2003; 85-A(3):571-2.

39. Court-Brown CM, Gustilo T, Shaw AD. Knee pain after intramedullary nailing of proximal third tibia fractures. J Orthop Trauma. 1997; 11:103-5.

40. Keating GJ, Orfaly R, O'Brien PJ: Knee pain after tibial nailing. J Orthop Trauma. 1997; 11:10-3.

41. Olerud S, Dankwardt-Lilliestrom G. Fracture healing in compression osteosynthesis. Acta Orthop Scand Suppl. 1971; 137:1-44.

42. Peter RE, Bachelin P, Fritschy D. Skiers' Lower Leg Shaft Fracture. Outcome in 91 Cases Treated Conservatively with Sarmiento's Brace. Am J Sports Med. 1988 Sep-Oct; 16(5):486-91.

43. Toivanen JA, Vaisto D, Kannus P. Anterior knee pain after intramedullary nailing of fractures of the tibial shaft. A prospective, randomized study comparing two different nail-insertion techniques. J Bone and Joint Surg. 2002; 84A:580-5.

44. Sarmiento A. Medicine and Industry. The Payer, the Piper and the Tune. Royal Canadian Annals of Medicine. 2000; 33(3):144-9.

45. Sarmiento A. Is Socrates dying? J Bone Joint Surg Am. 2008 Mar; 90(3):675-6.

46. Sarmiento A. On the Future of Orthopedics. I am concerned. Journal of Orthopaedic Science (Japan). 2000; 5:425-30.

47. Sarmiento A. Thoughts on the impact of technology on Orthopedics. J Bone Joint Surg. 2000; 82B:942-2.

48. Sarmiento A. The future of our specialty. Acta Orthopedica Scandinavica. 2000; 71(6):574-79.

49. Sarmiento A. On the Education of the Orthopaedic Resident. Clinical Orthopedics. 2002 May; 400:259-63.

50. Sarmiento A. Have we lost Objectivity? J Bone Joint Surg. 2002 Jul; 84-A(7): 1254-58, 447-8.

51. Sarmiento A. The Relationship between Orthopaedic and Industry must be reformed. Clinic Orthop Relat Res. 2003 Jul; (412):38-44.

52. Sarmiento A. Medicine and Industry: The Payer, the Piper and the Tune. Royal Canadian Annals of Medicine. 2000; 33(3):144-9.

53. Sarmiento, A. The future of our specialty. Acta Orthopedica Scandinavica. 2000; 71(6):574-9.

54. Sarmiento A. On the Education of the Orthopaedic Resident. Clin Orthop. 2002 May; 400:259-63.

55. Sarmiento A. Have we lost Objectivity? J Bone Joint Surg. 2002 Jul; 84A(7):1254-58 447-448.

56. Sarmiento A. The Relationship between Orthopaedic and Industry must be reformed. Clin Orthop. 2003 Jul: 412

57. Sarmiento A. Complications and Litigation. Clin Orthop. 2004 Mar; 420:319-20.

58. Sarmineto A. Rise and Decline. J Bone Joint Surg. 2009 Sep; 91:2740-2.

Section

3

The Femoral Shaft Fractures

22

Rationale, Technique and Representative Examples

At this time, the vast majority of femoral shaft fractures are successfully treated by means of intramedullary nailing. This method of treatment has virtually replaced all other modalities. The introduction of the concept of interlocking nails has made possible the surgical treatment of proximal and distal diaphyseal femoral fractures, which the non-interlocking nail does not effectively manage. However, the technology of interlocking nailing is not available in parts of the world where the economic or social resources necessary for its safe implementation are not available.

Even in the environment currently seen in wealthier nations, there are times when for a variety of reasons the surgical treatment is not possible or desirable, such as associated medical conditions that preclude surgery or religious reasons mandating surgery non-permissible. The nonsurgical treatment then becomes an option.[1-21]

Despite increasing popularity of the surgical treatment of femoral fractures in children older than 8 years, there is still a place for the nonsurgical care, which the brace makes a great deal more advantageous; the grown child being a good example.[13,22]

Our experiences with femoral fracture bracing in the 1960s through the 1980s demonstrated that diaphyseal fractures above the middle-third of the bone treated with functional braces have a tendency to angulate into varus.[23-26] Satisfactory results were obtained when the method was used in fractures located in the distal-third of the bone and the brace was applied after intrinsic stability at the fracture site had taken place. This usually requires around 3 to 5 weeks depending on the nature of the fracture. Skeletal traction is used during that time with appropriate radiological follow-up. However, the method is expensive due to the required hospitalization until intrinsic stability of the fracture is demonstrated. Union was rather consistently achieved; the final angular deformity was usually within acceptable degrees; and the ultimate range of motion of the adjacent joints was comparable to that obtained with surgical management. The representative clinical cases we now illustrate were patients who sustained their fractures prior to the introduction of the interlocking nail in the armamentarium of the orthopedic surgeons. Had those fractures occurred during the last 30 years, the vast majority of these patients would have been treated with such a nail.

The following illustrations demonstrate the plastic, custom-made brace and representative examples of fractures that met the desirable requirements for functional bracing at the time of their injuries. The brace can be made of Plaster of Paris, a method with which we first experimented.

TECHNIQUE FOR TREATMENT OF FEMORAL SHAFT FRACTURE

The technique for treatment of femoral shaft fracture is shown in Figures 22.1 to 22.5.

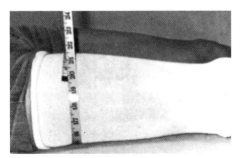 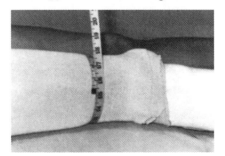 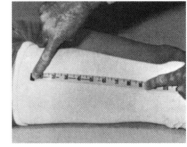

Fig. 22.1: After rolling a stocking, the circumference of the proximal and distal thigh, as well as the distance from the trochanter and the supracondylar points are measured.

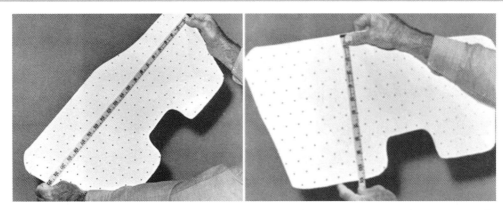

Fig. 22.2: The measurements are transferred to the dry sheet of Orthoplast, and a space is cut to eventually be over the anterior aspect of the thigh.

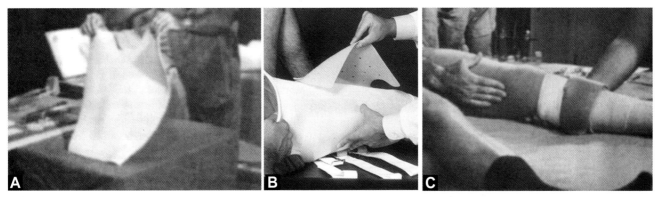

Figs 22.3A to C: (A) The dry sheet of Orthoplast is dipped in hot water for a couple of minutes until the material becomes soft and malleable. (B) It is then snuggly wrapped over the thigh, and its ends overlapped. (C) Over the still malleable material, an elastic bandage is wrapped and the firm molding of the entire structure is carried out.

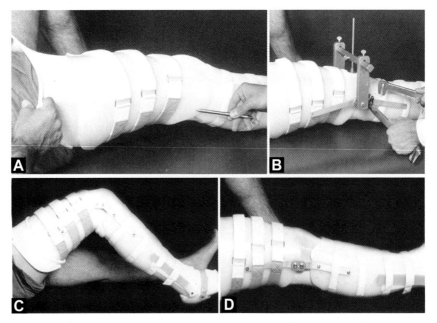

Figs 22.4A to D: (A) The Orthoplast now dry, is split in the anterior aspect of the thigh and its margins brought to overlap slightly. Three or four adjustable Velcro straps are firmly applied. (B) After a cuff of Orthoplast has been wrapped over the distal leg, the metallic hinges are appropriately placed. (C) The distal foot insert is adjusted and the range of motion of the knee is tested. Necessary trimmings of the edges of Orthoplast are conducted. (D) Illustration of the completed brace with the knee in extension.

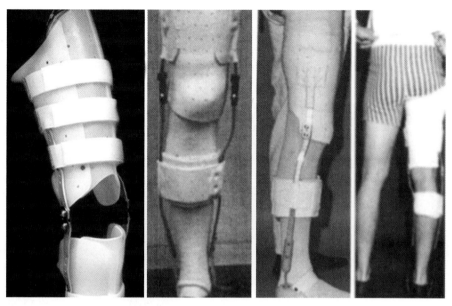

Fig. 22.5: Illustrations of patient wearing the brace.

As stated earlier, intramedullary interlocking nail is the most appropriate treatment for the vast majority of femoral shaft fracture, but that there are times and situations when the surgical treatment is not indicated or the economic, cultural environment does not meet the criteria for surgical intervention. Under those circumstances, the initial traction treatment may be followed by functional bracing—either plaster of Paris or Plastic material—in order to shorten the hospitalization and to restore function at a faster pace. During the traction period, it is essential to maintain knee motion to prevent ultimate limitation of motion of that joint. The initiation of passive motion—permitted by the suspension type of traction—should begin as early as possible and in a gradual manner. Relevent statistics related to fracture of femur have been shown in Table 22.1 to 22.6.

REPRESENTATIVE EXAMPLE

Some of the representative example of fracture of femur are shown in Figures 22.6 to 22.23.

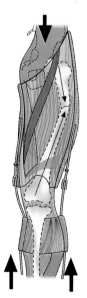

Fig. 22.6: Schematic drawing illustrating the likelihood of varus angular deformity in fractures above the middle-third, particularly in obese patients.

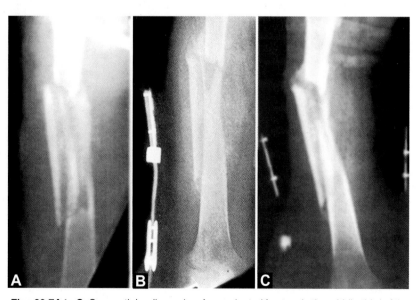

Figs 22.7A to C: Sequential radiographs of comminuted fracture in the middle-third of the femur in an obese patient. Though the alignment was obtained with traction and present at the time of brace application, an angular deformity developed after the introduction of ambulation.

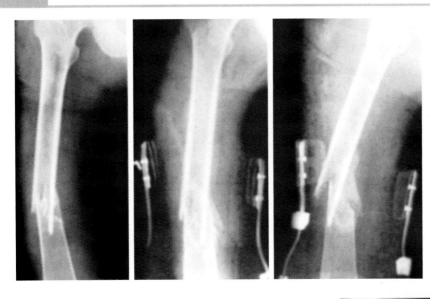

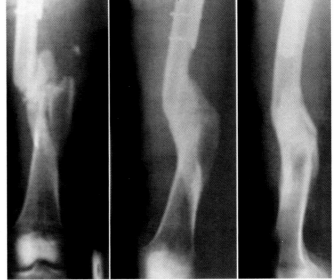

Fig. 22.8: Sequential radiographs of fracture of the femur at the junction of the middle and distal thirds. The patient was obese and the bracing did not prevent the development of an unacceptable varus deformity.

Fig. 22.9: Radiographs of comminuted fracture of the femur in its middle-third. At the time of the injury, an intertrochanteric fracture had occurred, which was treated with open reduction and internal fixation. Because of intra-operative complications, internal fixation of the femur was aborted. The fracture healed after the application of a brace. An angular deformity ensued.

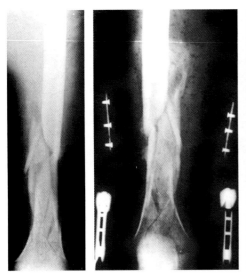

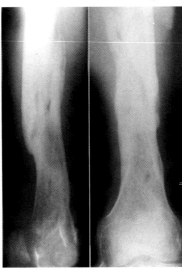

Fig. 22.10: Consecutive radiographs of comminuted fracture of the femur at the junction of the middle and distal thirds illustrating the progressive healing of the fracture and the ultimate acceptable shortening and alignment.

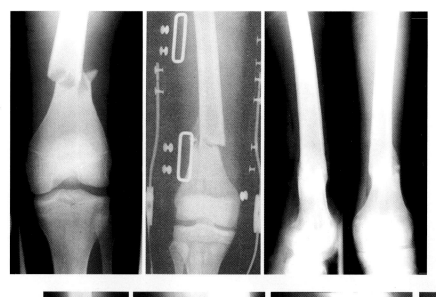

Fig. 22.11: Sequential radiographs of transverse fracture in the distal-third of the femur. The fracture healed with good alignment and without angular deformity.

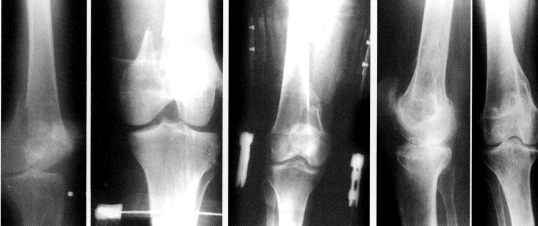

Fig. 22.12: Radiographs of trans-epiphyseal fracture of the distal femur treated successfully with traction followed by brace application and ambulation.

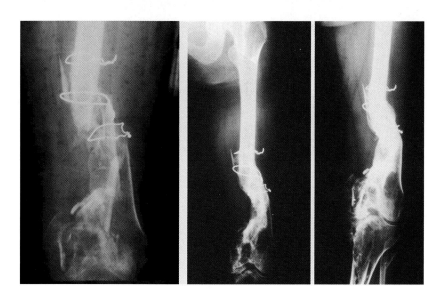

Fig. 22.13: Radiographs of an open, severely comminuted fracture of the distal femur incurred 1 year prior to seeking attention from us. She had been hospitalized for that period of time and finally sought an amputation. Rather than carrying out the ablation procedure, we chose to attempt ambulation with the support of a brace. The fracture healed but the range of motion of the knee was very poor.

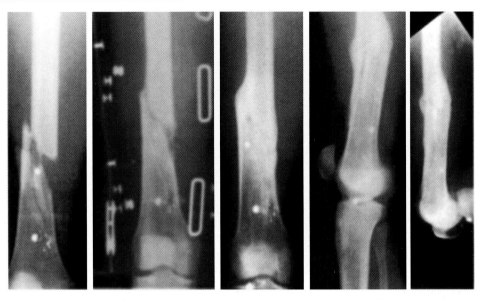

Fig. 22.14: Radiographs of comminuted fracture of the distal femur produce by a low-velocity bullet. The brace was applied 2 weeks after the injury after initial stabilization in traction accompanied with passive traction exercises. The fracture healed with minimal shortening and good alignment.

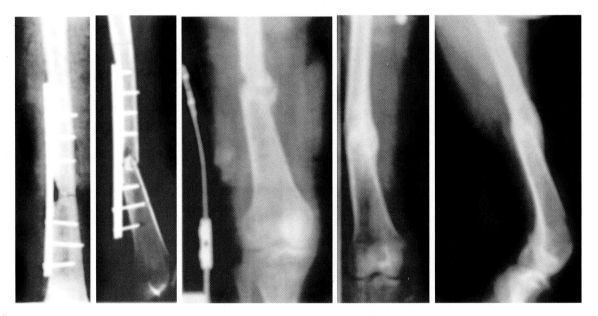

Fig. 22.15: Radiographs of fracture in the middle-third of the femur treated with a plate, which eventually failed to maintain its relationship with the femur. After removal of the plate, a brace was applied and graduated weight bearing ambulation began.

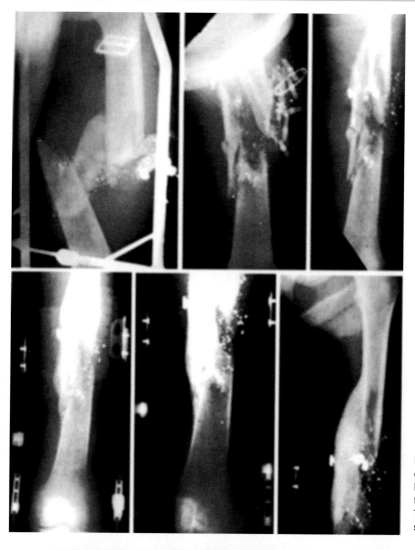

Fig. 22.16: Sequential radiographs of severely comminuted fracture of the femur produced by a high-velocity bullet. After appropriate debridement, traction accompanied with passive exercises began. The fracture healed uneventfully with acceptable shortening and angulation.

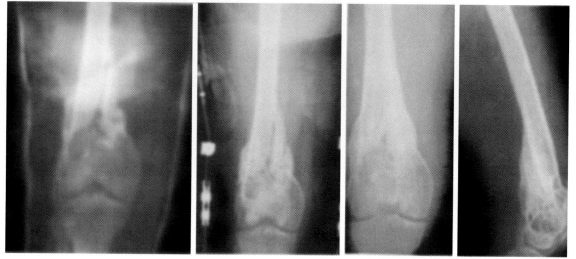

Fig. 22.17: Radiographs of open comminuted fracture of the distal femur sustained in an automobile accident. After a period of stabilization in traction and passive knee range of motion exercises, a brace was applied and ambulation began. The fracture healed with limitation of motion but with acceptable shortening and angulation.

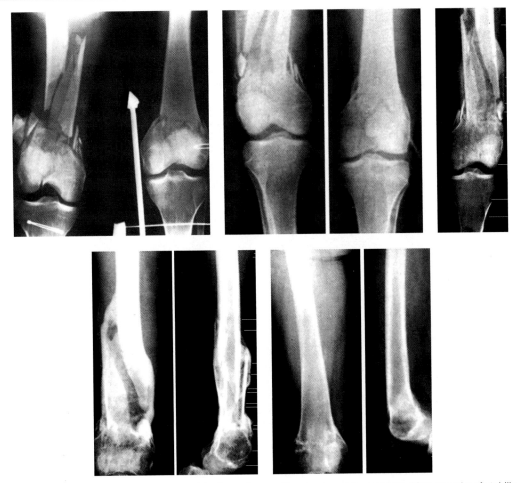

Fig. 22.18: Sequential radiographs of bilateral fractures of the femur incurred in an automobile accident. After 4 weeks of stabilization in traction, accompanied with passive traction exercises, braces were applied. The fractures healed uneventfully. When last seen by us, the patient had a mild residual limitation of motion but ambulated without external support.

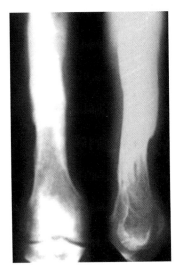

Fig. 22.19: Initial and final radiographs of comminuted fracture in the distal-third of the femur treated with a functional brace. Notice the minimal shortening and the almost perfect alignment.

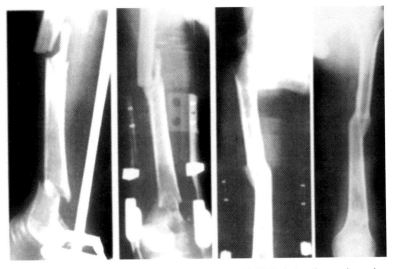

Fig. 22.20: Segmental fracture of the femur treated initially in traction and passive knee exercises, followed by application of a brace. The fracture healed with acceptable shortening and a mild angular deformity.

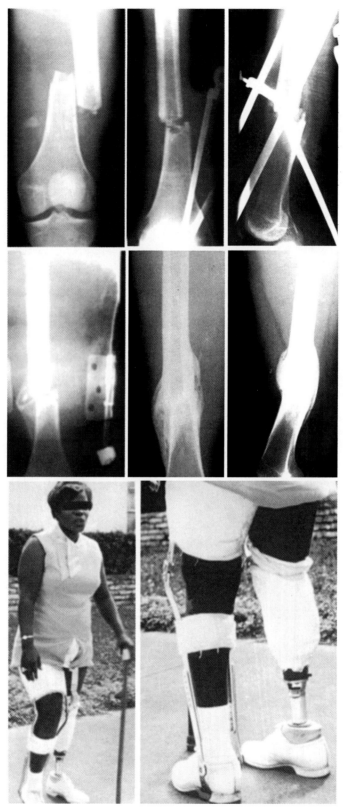

Fig. 22.21: Sequential radiographs of transverse, open fracture in the distal femur sustained in an automobile accident. The mangled right lower extremity was amputated and fit with a temporary below-the-knee Plaster of Paris prosthesis in the operating room immediately after completion of the ablation procedure. The fractured femur on the right was treated in traction, exercises and eventually a brace.

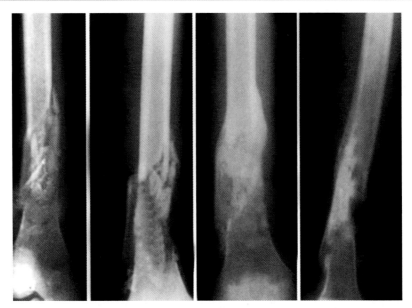

Fig. 22.22: Comminuted fracture of the distal femur, the result of a low-velocity bullet. After 3 weeks of stabilization in traction and accompanying passive exercises, a brace was applied. The fracture healed uneventfully with acceptable shortening and angulation.

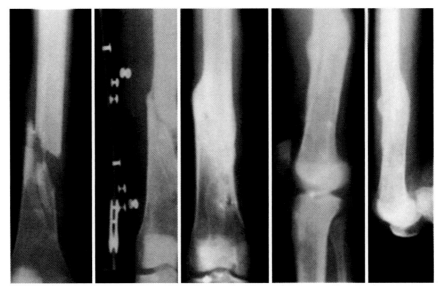

Fig. 22.23: Comminuted fracture of the distal femur produced by a low-velocity bullet. After 3 weeks of stabilization in traction and passive exercises, a functional brace was applied. The fracture healed with minimal shortening and good alignment.

DATA

Table 22.1: Femoral fractures

Total braced in this series	273
Total followed with data collection*	245

Age parameters (years)	
Range	16-98
Median	61
Mode	22; 31; 70
Nature	
Closed	194 (80%)
Open	51 (20%)
Total	245
Location	
Proximal 1/3	18 (7.3%)
Middle 1/3	132 (53.8%)
Distal 1/3	87 (35.5%)
Segmental	8 (3.2%)
Total	245
Type	
Transverse	41 (16.7%)
Short oblique	31 (12.6%)
Spiral	46 (18.7%)
Comminuted	119 (48.5%)
Segmental	8 (3.2%)
Total	245
Delayed unions (longer than 24 weeks) and nonunions	
Delayed union	3 (1.2%)
Nonunion	1 (0.4%)
Total in series	245
Cause	
Passengers (4-wheeled)	98 (40%)
Passengers (2-wheeled)	34 (14%)
Pedestrians	32 (13%)
Gunshot	39 (16%)
Falls	22 (9%)
Other	20 (8%)
Total	245

Table 22.2: Distribution of age parameters by location type of femoral fracture

Location	No. of Cases	Age (years) Range	Med
Proximal 1/3	18	22–78	36
Middle 1/3	132	16–71	28
Distal 1/3	87	31–98	56
Segmental	8	24–48	40
Total	245		
Type			
Transverse	41	16–75	31
Short oblique	31	20–65	34
Spiral	36	21–98	28
Comminuted	119	18–71	36
Segmental	8	24–52	36
Total	245		

Table 22.3: Distribution of age parameters by location type of femoral fracture

Location	No of Cases	Time before bracing (weeks) Average	Time before bracing (weeks) Medium	Time in bracing (weels) Average	Time in bracing (weels) Mediam
Proximal 1/3	18	6	5	10	8.5
Middle 1/3	132	6	4.5	9	8.5
Distal 1/3	87	4	4	8.5	6.5
Segmental	8	6	6	10.5	9.5
Total	245				

Interval between onset of injury and application of brace

Average	5 weeks
Medium	4.5 weeks
Mode	4; 6; 8 weeks

Table 22.4: Associated pathology to femoral fractures

	No. of Cases (%)]
Contralateral femoral fracture	3 (1.2)
Ipsilateral tibial fracture	5 (2.0)
Contralateral tibial fracture	4 (1.6)
Bilateral tibial fracture	3 (1.2)
Abdominal injury	4 (1.6)
Pelvic fracture	2 (0.8)
Femoral neck fracture	1 (0.4)
Upper extremity fracture	5 (0.0)
Other	12 (4.8)

Table 22.5: Degree of residual angulation by type of femoral fracture

Type	No. of Cases	Angulation (%) < 10°	Angulation (%) > 10°
Transverse	41	25 (60)	16 (39)
Short oblique	31	24 (77.4)	7 (22.5)
Spiral	46	39 (84.7)	7 (15.2)
Comminuted	119	103 (86.5)	16 (13.4)
Segmental	8	4 (50)	4 (50)
Total	245	195 (80)	50 (20)

Table 22.6: Residual varus or valgus angulation of more than 10° in Femoral fractures

Location	No. of Cases	Angulation 10° (%) Varus	Valgus	Total
Proximal 1/3	18	10 (55)	–	10 (55)
Middle 1/3	132	23 (17)	5 (4)	28 (21)
Distal 1/3	87	6 (6)	2 (2)	8 (10)
Segmental	8	2 (25)	2 (25)	4 (50)
Total	245	41 (17)	9 (4)	50 (21)

REFERENCES

1. Brown PE, Preston ET. Ambulatory Treatment of Femoral Shaft Fractures with Cast Brace. J. Trauma. 1975; 15:860.
2. Connolly JF, Dehne E, LaFollette B. Closed Reduction and Early Cast Brace Ambulation in the Treatment of Femoral Fractures. J. Bone Joint Surg. 1973; 55A:1581.
3. Connolly JF, Dehne E, LaFollette B. Closed Revision and Early Cast Brace Ambulation in the Treatment of Femoral Fractures. J Bone Joint Surg. 1978; 60A:112.
4. De Lee JC, Clanton TO, Rockwood CA. Closed Treatment of Subtrochanteric Fractures of the Femur in a Modified Cast-brace. J. Bone Joint Surg. 1979; 63A:135.
5. Gross RH, Davidson R, Sullivan JA, Peeples RE, Hufft R. Cast Brace Management of the Femoral Shaft Fracture in Children and Young Adults. J. Ped Orthop. 1983; 3:572.
6. Hackethorm JC, Burkhalter WE, Donley JM, Bailey JD. Review of 156 Open Femoral Fractures. Treatment with Traction and Cast Bracing. J. Bone Joint Surg. 1975; 57A:1029.
7. Hardy AE. Pressure Recordings in Patients with Femoral Fractures in Cast-Braces and Suggestions for Treatment. J Bone Joint Surg. 1979; 61A:365.
8. Hardy AE. Force and Pressure Recordings from Patients with Femoral Fractures Treated by Cast-Brace Application. J Med Engr Tech. 1981; 5:30.
9. Hardy AE. Ipsilateral Fractures of the Femoral and Tibial Diaphyses Treated by Cast-brace Application. J Bone Joint Surg. 1986; 68B:677.
10. Hardy AE. The Treatment of Femoral Fractures by Cast-Brace Application and Early Ambulation - A Prospective Review of One Hundred and Six Patients. J. Bone Joint Surg. 1983; 65A:56.
11. Iwegbu CG. Preliminary Results of Treatment of Fractures of the Femur by Cast-Bracing Using the Zaria Metal Hinge. Injury. 1984; 15:250.
12. Kujat R, Tscherne H. Indications and Technique of Functional Fracture Treatment with the Sarmiento Brace. Zentralbl Chir. 1984; 109:1417.
13. Kumar R. Treatment of Fracture of the Femur in Children by a "Cast Brace." Int. Sug. 1982; 67 (Suppl 4):551.
14. Latta LL, Sarmiento A. The Basic Sciences of fracture healing in a nonsurgical environment. Bruce Browner (Ed), Lippincott. 2007.
15. Linson MA, Lewinnek F, White AA. Ischemic Complications of Femoral Cast-bracing: Report of Two Cases. Clin. Orthop. 1982; 162:189.
16. Meggitt BF, Vaughan-Lane T. Hip Hinge Thigh Brace for Early Mobilization of Proximal Femoral Shaft Fractures. Prosthet Orthot Int. 1980; 4:150.
17. Mooney V, Nickel VL, Harvey JP, Snelson R. Cast-Brace Treatment for Fractures of the Distal Part of the Femur. J Bone Joint Surg. 1970; 52A:1563.
18. Rosa G, Savarese A, Chianca I, Coppola D. Treatment of Fractures of the Lower Limb with Functional Braces. J Orthop Traumat. 1982; 8:301.
19. Thomas TL, Meggitt BF. A Comparative Study of Methods for Treating Fractures of the Distal Half of the Femur. J Bone Joint Surg. 1981; 63B:3.
20. Wardlaw D, McLaughlan J, Pratt DJ, Bowker P. A Biomechanical Study of Cast-Brace Treatment of Femoral Shaft Fractures. J Bone Joint Surg. 1982; 63B:7.
21. Zych GA, Zagorski JB, Latta LL, McCollough NC. Modern Concepts in Functional Fracture Bracing - Lower Limb. In: AAOS Instructional Course Lectures, Chicago IL. Chap. 25, AAOS. 1987; XXXVI.
22. McCollough NC, Vinsant JE, Sarmiento A. Functional Fracture - Bracing of Long-bone Fractures of the Lower Extremity in Children. J Bone Joint Surg. 1978; 60A:314.
23. Sarmiento A. Functional Bracing of Tibial and Femoral Shaft Fractures. Clin Orthop. 1972; 82:2.
24. Sarmiento A. Complications from Functional Fracture Bracing. Complications in Orthopaedic Surgery, Epps C (Ed). J B Lippincott Co. 1994.
25. Sarmiento A, Latta LL. Functional Fracture Bracing. A Manual. Lippincott, Williams and Wilkins. Philadelphia: 2002; 82:147
26. Sarmiento A, Latta LL. Functional fracture bracing. Springer Verlag, Berlin, 1995.

Section

4

The Humeral Shaft Fractures

23

Rationale of Functional Bracing

Humeral shaft fractures are among the ones most likely to respond to non-surgical treatment modalities. It was the first long bone that broke the traditional prescription of immobilization of joints above and below a fracture as a requirement for fracture healing. The "hanging cast" by virtue of the fact that the shoulder was no longer immobilized in a spica cast, readily proved that immobilization of the two adjacent joints was not necessary for uneventful healing.

Following our finding that fractures of the tibial diaphysis, treated with a modified cast (initially mistakenly called the PTB cast) that permitted motion of the knee joint while allowing the gradual introduction of weight bearing ambulation, we subsequently developed a brace, which in addition to allowing motion of the knee, also made possible freedom of the ankle joint. (See Chapter 2)

Several decades of clinical and laboratory experience with fractures of these bones have unequivocally demonstrated that angular deformities of minor or moderate degrees are well tolerated, esthetically and physiologically, in the tibia as well as in the humerus. From the esthetic point of view, an angular deformity in the humerus of 15° in the average weight and height individual is usually unrecognizable to the naked eye. In the moderately or markedly obese individual, more severe angular deformities are acceptable. The opposite is true when dealing with scars left after plate fixation techniques which are visible at all times.

The literature is rich with information that minor angular deformities in the lower extremity are not likely to produce late osteoarthritic changes, and that in those instances where angular deformities and late osteoarthritis are present, the mechanism of injury was of an impacting nature, which probably injured the articular cartilage in an irreversible and permanent manner suggesting that even in the absence of an angular deformity, those fractures are more potentially prone to undergo arthritic changes in the adjacent joints. (See Chapter 2)

Experience with the functional brace for humeral fractures, which permits complete freedom of motion of all joints in the upper extremity, is a simple and uncomplicated apparatus. The brace is usually applied within 1 or 2 weeks following the initial insult. Gradually, following a period of passive exercises to the elbow and shoulder joints, active progressive exercises are introduced.

The system of functional braces of the fractured humerus does not require manipulation of the fragments, a technique we have not carried out in the 4 decades of work with the system. Manipulation is more likely to result in nerve injury. The fact that alignment is improved by the compression of the soft tissues, plus the gravity effects\of the hanging extremity, ensures in the vast majority of instances, the attainment of adequate alignment.

We have divided the subject into three main sections dealing with fractures at the three conventional levels, proximal, middle and distal thirds. A short chapter is devoted to delayed unions and nonunions and to other methods of treatment. Needless to say, the functional brace system is not a panacea, as it is true for all treatment modalities. Complications do occur in a number of situations. The narrative discusses our complications and other important features.

24

Indications and Contraindications

Contrary to long-accepted practices and beliefs regarding the need to immobilize the joints above and below a fracture, the diaphyseal humeral fractures first demonstrated that immobilization of the shoulder was not required in order to achieve union with acceptable alignment in most instances. The popular "hanging cast" that allows free motion of the shoulder joint supports this view. The functional bracing we describe in the text eliminates the need of a heavy cast and allows for unencumbered motion of all joints in the fractured extremity.

INDICATIONS

Most isolated *closed* diaphyseal fractures of the humeral diaphysis, regardless of their geometry can be successfully treated with functional braces.[1-25] However, in order for patients with a humeral fracture to benefit from functional bracing is necessary for them to be able to assume the erect position, to carryout a simple program of exercises, and be capable of adjusting the brace on a regular basis, or to have some one who can provide that service. This, because dependency of the extremity is necessary for restoration of adequate alignment of the fragments, and because during the early days following the injury, the brace needs to be adjusted several times a day as swelling decreases and muscle atrophy takes place.

Even if the uncomplicated treatment protocol is appropriately followed, minor angular deformity can occur due to the anatomy of the arm and chest. Such final radiological deviation from the normal varies according to the type of fracture. Transverse fractures, particularly if non-displaced, are the ones most likely to develop the angular deformity. Weight bearing on the elbow and muscular forces acting on the fracture may produce the deformity. In the case of comminuted or oblique fractures, the muscle contractions produce desirable elastic pistoning at the fracture site without creating permanent deformity (Figures 24.1A and B). Equally, if not more importantly, is the fact that the ubiquitous varus seen in diaphyseal humeral fractures is, in most instances, iatrogenically created during the application of the original cast, and subsequently during the application of the brace. We devote a few paragraphs to this important issue during the description of methodology.

CONTRAINDICATIONS

Bilateral diaphyseal fractures do not necessarily require surgical stabilization even though in most instances surgery is the treatment of choice. There are situations, however, when surgical intervention is not possible or is contraindicated. In such situations, stabilization of the fractures in Velpeau dressing allows for the fractures to become intrinsically stable and in adequate alignment. After a relatively short period of time, the Velpeau dressing is discontinued and the braces applied.

Functional bracing in the treatment of the poly-traumatized patient has limited applications. The same is true for open humeral diaphyseal fractures.

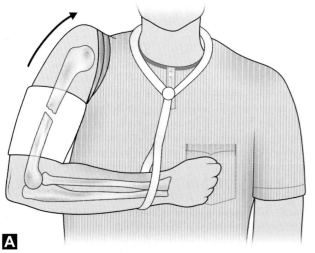
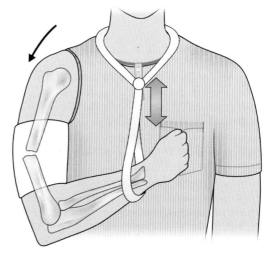

Figs 24.1A and B: (A) At the time of the initial stabilization of the painful extremity, the patient with a fracture of the humerus instinctively shrugs the shoulder. If a sling is applied while the shoulder is shrugged, a deformity occurs (B) Since the elbow flexes and the forearm and hand are displaced proximally, The natural apprehension the patient experiences at the time of application of the original sling prompts him/her to shrug the shoulder. When the shoulder relaxes, a varus angular deformity may occur. It is therefore important to ascertain that the sling is applied after the shoulder is no longer in a shrugged position.

REFERENCES

1. Balfour GW, Mooney V, Ashby ME. Diaphyseal Fractures of the Humerus Treated with a Ready-Made Fracture Brace. J Bone Joint Surg. 1982; 64A:11.

2. Bruggemann H, Kujat R, Tscherne H. Funkionelle Frakturebehandlung nach. Sarmiento an Unterschenkel, Unterarm und Oberarm. Orthopaede, 1983; 12:143.

3. Ekholm R, Tidemark J, Tornkvist H, Adami J, Ponzer S. Outcome after closed treatment of humeral shaft fractures. J Orthop Trauma. 2006 Oct; 20(9):591-6.

4. Ekkernkamp A, Kayser M, Althoff M. Knozept der Funktionellen Therapie am Beispiel des Frischen Geschlossenen Oberarmschaftbruches. Zentralbl Chir. 1989; 114:788.

5. Klestil T, Rangger C, Kathrein B, Huber B, Waldegger M. Sarmiento Bracing of Humeral Shaft Fractures: A comparative study. SOT (Finnish Orthop. Journal. 1997; 2.

6. Latta LL, Sarmiento A, Tarr R. The Rationale of Functional Bracing of Fractures. Clin Orthop. 1980; 146:28-36

7. Latta LL. Sarmiento A. Fracture Casting and Bracing. ASOP Publishing Inc. 2008.

8. Latta LL, Sarmiento A. Functional Bracing of selected Upper Extremity Fractures. AAOS Atlas of Orthoses and Assistive Devices. Mosby Saunders: Philadelphia. 2008: 261-9

9. McMaster WC, Tivnon MC, Waugh TR. Cast Brace for the Upper Extremity. Clin Orthop. 1975; 109:126.

10. Naver L, Aalberg JR. Humeral Shaft Fractures Treated with a Ready-Made Fracture Brace. Arch Orthop Trauma Surg. 1986; 106:20-2.

11. Osterman PAW, Ekkerkamp A, Muhr G. Functional Bracing of Fractures of the Humerus: An analysis of 195 cases. Proc 60th Amer Acad Orthop Surg. 1993; 69.

12. Sarmiento A, Kinman PB, Galvin EG, Schmitt RH, Phillips JG: Functional Bracing of Fractures of the Shaft of the Humerus. J. Bone Joint Surg. 1977; 59A:596.

13. Sarmiento A, Latta LL. Closed Functional Treatment of fractures. Springer-Verlag, Berlin, GFR. 1981.

14. Sarmiento A, Latta LL. Functional Fracture Bracing. Springer-Verlag, Heidelberg, GFR. 1995.

15. Sarmiento A, Zych GA, Zagorski JB, Latta LL. Functional Bracing of Diaphyseal Humeral Fractures. J. Bone Joint Surg, 1999.

16. Sarmiento A, Horowitch A, Aboulafia A, Vangsness CT Jr. Functional Bracing of comminuted extra-articular fractures of the Distal-Third of the Humerus. J Bone Joint Surg. 1990; 72B-2:283-7.

17. Sarmiento A, Zagorski JB, Zych GA, Latta LL, Capps CA. Functional Bracing of Humeral Shaft Fractures. J Bone Joint Surg. 2000; 82A4:478-86

18. Sarmiento A, Latta L, Tarr R. Principles of fracture healing Part II: The effects of function on fracture healing and stability. Amer Acad Orthop Sur Instr Course Lectures. Mosby Saunders: Philadelphia. 1984; XXXIII.

19. Sarmiento A, Waddell JP, Latta LL. Diaphyseal Humeral Fractures: Treatment Options. An Instructional Course. AAOS J Bone and Joint Surg. 1999; 83A(10):1566-79.

20. Sarmiento A, Latta LL. The Evolution of Fracture Bracing J. Bone Joint Surg (B). 2006; 88-8(2):141-8.

21. Sarmiento A, Latta LL. Conservative treatment of humeral shaft fractures. Unfallchirurg. German Trauma Assoc. 2007.

22. Sarmiento A. The functional bracing of fractures. JBJS (A). Classics Techniques. 2007; 89 Suppl 2(2):157-69.

23. Sharma VK, Jain AK, Gupta RK, Tyagi AK, Sethi PK. Non-operative treatment of Humeral Shaft Fracture: A comparative study. J Indian Med Assoc. 1991; 89:157.

24. Wasmer G, Worsdorfer O. Functional Management of Humeral Shaft Fractures with Sarmiento Cast Bracing. Unfallheilkunde, 1984; 87:309.

25. Zagorski JB, Latta LL, Zych G, Finnieston AR. Diaphyseal Fractures of the Humerus. Treatment with pre-fabricated Braces. J Bone Joint Surg. 1988; 70A: 607.

25

Initial Management

It is best to initially stabilize diaphyseal humeral fractures with an above-the-elbow cast or with a coaptation splint (Figures 25.1A and B). These appliances not only provide comfort during the acute stage of the condition, but assist in improving alignment of the fractured fragments. Many prefer the circular cast because it prevents distal edema and perhaps greater comfort to the patient. The elbow should be held at 90 degrees of flexion, the forearm in neutral and the wrist in a few degrees of dorsiflexion. Adding a collar-and-cuff sling is essential. Failure to provide it not only results in increased pain but also may lead to angular deformity at the fracture site.

Under no circumstance should a brace be applied on the day of the injury as the pain and swelling may become more intensive.

At the time of application of the sling, the shoulder must be relaxed. The usually seen shrugging of the shoulder that patients instinctively show in anticipation of pain must be eliminated, otherwise angular deformity is likely to develop (Figures 25.2A and B). Failure to carry-out that precaution is the most common cause of unsightly deformities.

Shortly after the application of the cast, pendulum exercises should be initiated. Initially, they should be performed in a passive manner by holding the injured arm with the normal one. The direction of the pendulum motion should be in the antero-posterior, medio-lateral and circumferential planes in order to prevent eventual limitation of motion of the shoulder. When it is suspected, there is sufficient intrinsic stability at the fracture site, active abduction and elevation exercises may be introduced. Such degree of intrinsic stability is usually suspected when the passive exercises have become totally asymptomatic and the patient "feels" there is no longer motion at the fracture site. If there are any questions regarding "stability," a radiograph demonstrating early bridging callus should confirm the "suspicion." As the active exercise begin, "wall crawling" activities should be carried out.(See Chapter 27)

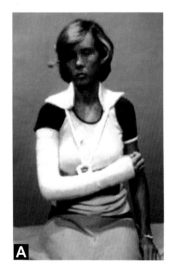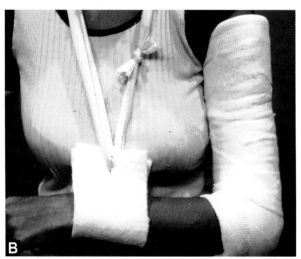

Figs 25.1A and B: Illustrations of an above-the-elbow cast and a cooptation splint used as the initial means of fracture stabilization.

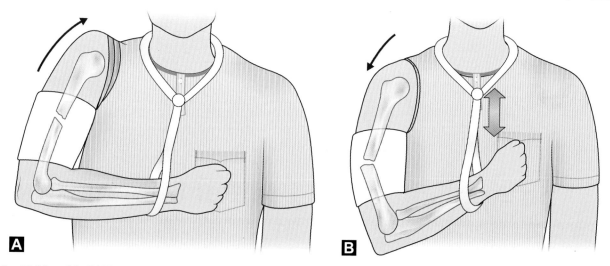

Figs 25.2A and B: (A) The varus deformity can also be created at the time of application of the brace if the shoulder is shrugged during the procedure. (B) If a varus deformity was produced at the time of the application of the original sling, the condition is further aggravated.

26

The Application of the Functional Brace

It is desirable to remove the initial cast when the symptoms are not significant. Otherwise, a few additional days in the cast are recommended. The brace must be adjustable in order to ensure that the soft tissues of the arm can be compressed as swelling decreases and atrophy ensues (Figures 26.1 to 26.3). Frequent tightening of the Velcro straps is necessary during the first 2 weeks. Cylindrical "sleeves" have a ready tendency to slide distally and irritate the antecubital space as physiological changes take place. The brace should extend from approximately 1 inch below the axilla and terminate distally at 1 inch above the humeral condyles. Supra-acromial and supra-condylar humeral extensions are not necessary.

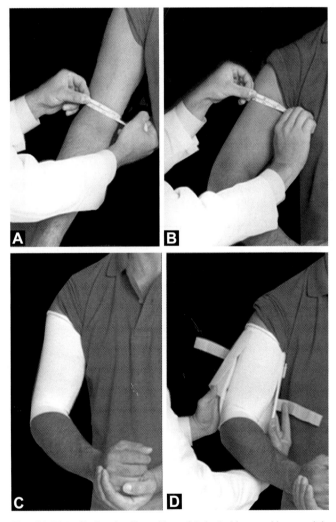

Figs 26.2A to D: If unfamiliar with prefabricated humeral braces, it is best to take measurements to determine the length and girth of the upper arm. The brace once fitted over the arm should not impinge on the axilla or prevent elbow flexion that would result in unhealthy pressure over the antecubital space.

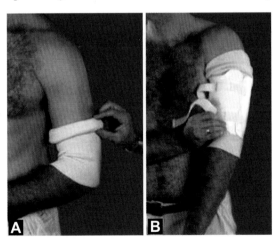

Figs 26.1A and B: The brace should be applied as soon as the acute symptoms have subsided and additional swelling is not anticipated. A layer of stockinette over the skin is desirable. Those familiar with the technique of prefabricated braces do not need to take measurements of the arm in order to select the appropriate size of the brace. What is important is to ascertain that the brace is not too long as to impinge, proximally against the axilla or distally against the anticubital space. Because the swelling present at the time of application of the brace decreases with time and the use of the extremity, it is essential that the brace be adjusted approximately twice a day during the first week, and once a day subsequently.

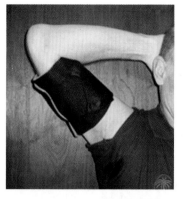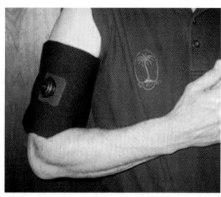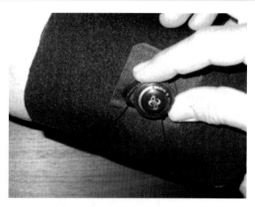

Fig. 26.3: The snugness of the brace (whether prefabricated or custom-made) is easily maintained.

27

Post-bracing Management

The passive exercises of the shoulder, initiated shortly after the application of the initial cast should continue following the application of the brace. The sling should also be held in place. The exercises are of a pendulum nature, combined with adduction/abduction and anterior-posterior directions (Figure 27.1). Initially, the patient holds the injured arm with the opposite hand and in that manner carry out the passive motion of the shoulder. As the symptoms decrease, the need for support with the non-effected hand becomes unnecessary.

During the early period of stabilization of the injured arm in a sling, the patient should, several times a day, temporarily remove the sling and carry-out gradual passive flexion and extension of the elbow. A few days later, the passive motions should be combined with active assistance of the elbow flexors and extensors of the elbow (Figure 27.2). The active contraction of the biceps and triceps assists in correcting the subluxation of the shoulder that is occasionally seen in fractures of the proximal-third of the humerus.

Effort should be made to regain extension of the elbow during the first two weeks following the application of the brace. This should not be done forcefully, simply by gradually extending the elbow through frequent passive exercises.

Once the acute symptoms have subsided and the elbow can be fully extended, the pendulum exercises are then conducted with the elbow in extension. The resulting introduction of gravity forces at the level of the fracture, plus the compression of the soft tissues assist in a major weight to the correction of residual angular deformities (Figures 27.2 to 27.4).

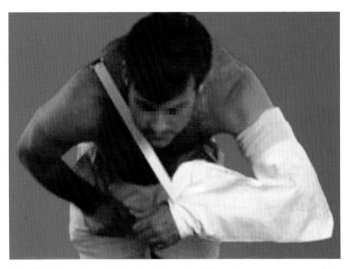

Fig. 27.1: Exercises to the shoulder should begin as soon as possible. Most patients, if properly counseled can start the exercises as early as the second post-injury day. The exercises should consist of pendulum motions in a circular as well as in abduction/adduction, and anterior-posterior motions.

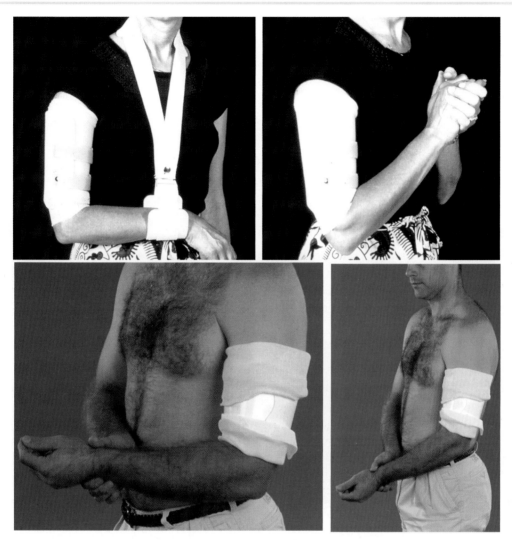

Figs 27.2: The brace should not extend over the humeral condyles or over the acromion. It should simply fit snuggly over the "fleshy" arm. It is wrong to rely on the alleged suspension that a supra-acromial extension provides. The same is true regarding the suspension role that the humeral condyles provide. The addition of a sling is essential in all instances. The exercises must be carried out several times a day and increased in intensity according to symptoms. These exercises should be conducted with sling in place.

Since sleeping may result in loss of the position of adduction of the arm against the body, it is recommended that a shirt or blouse be worn in such a manner that the injured arm is not held inside the garment but buttoned over it. During the waking hours, the need for this protection is no longer necessary (Figure 27.5).

It is best not to instruct patients on the day of application of the brace on the temporary removal and re-application of the brace. The instruction at that time should be limited to the adjustments necessary to prevent and correct the inevitable distal sliding of the appliance, as swelling decreases (Figure 27.6).

Active abduction and elevation of the shoulder prior to intrinsic stability must be forbidden because they may produce angular deformities. Active abduction and elevation may be conducted when intrinsic stability at the fracture is

documented by the presence of early callus and the absence of pain at the fracture site. The force required to actively elevate the arm creates an unfavorable mechanical situation: the long lever arm made by the distal humerus, forearm and hand offsets the shorter lever arm made by the proximal fragment of the fractured humerus. The brace is permanently discontinued when union of the fracture has been documented (Figure 27.7).

Trying to determine intrinsic fracture stability by manipulation of the arm is likely to produce abnormal motions at the fracture site.

Premature introduction of active elevation and abduction of the shoulder is the most common reason for failure of functional bracing of humeral fracture.

Leaning on the elbow is likely to produce varus angulation at the fracture site, a complication that is more likely to develop in transverse, non-displaced fractures

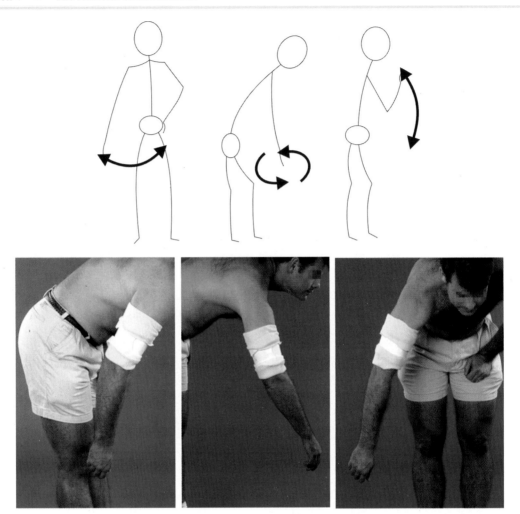

Figs 27.3: Gradually, full extension is regained. In most instances, during the first two post-injury weeks. Once complete extension has been reached and the painful symptoms have disappeared, the exercises can be carried out in that manner. The sling may be discontinued after full extension of the elbow is reached and the pendulum exercises are conducted in that manner. However, confirmation of early intrinsic stability by clinical and radiographic means is necessary before allowing the arm to hang at the side of the body at all times. It is best to use the sling at night during decumbency.

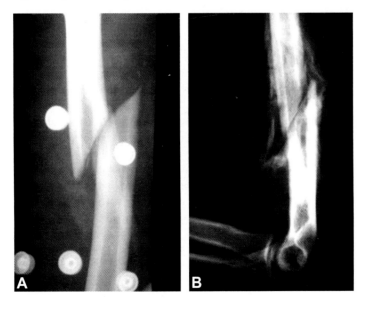

Figs 27.4A and B: (A) Radiograph of an oblique fracture of the humeral diaphysis stabilized in a brace. (B) Later radiograph showing the outline of the forming callus that clearly depicts the motion that occurred during the healing process.

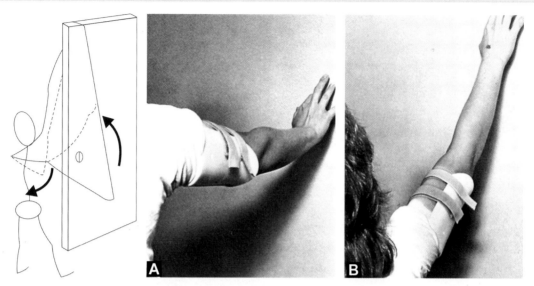

Figs 27.5 A and B: Prior to the beginning of active elevation and abduction of the shoulder, following documentation of intrinsic fracture stability, passive/assisted exercises, such as (A) "towel push and pull" and (B) climbing the wall are most helpful.

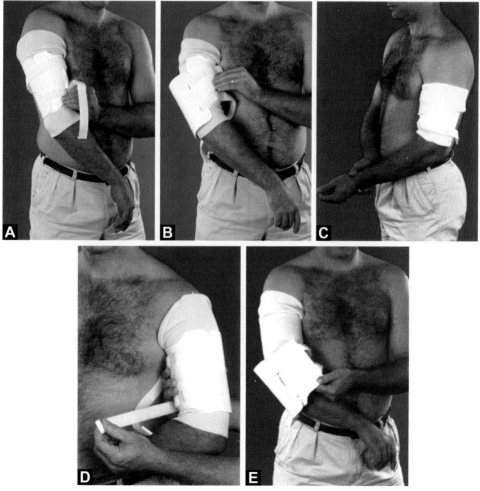

Figs 27.6A to E: The prefabricated brace is easily applied and adjusted by the patient. The Velcro straps are loosened; the brace is pushed superiorly; and the straps tightened again. For hygienic purposes, the brace can be temporarily removed and a clean stockinette applied.

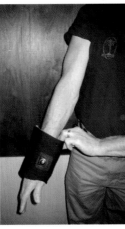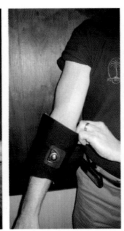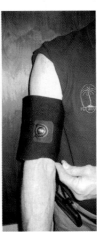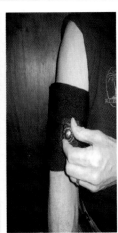

Figs 27.7: Illustrations of a recently introduced brace. The brace is easily applied and its snugness maintained by turning a knob.

28

Cautions and Pitfalls

AXIAL DISTRACTION

Axial distraction between the fragments in a humeral diaphyseal fracture suggests major soft tissue damage. The sudden stripping of supporting musculature from the humeral shaft explains this phenomenon. The marked separation encourages nonunion, particularly if there is an associated nerve injury. In these instances, early internal fixation is frequently indicated. When the nerve injury involves the brachial plexus, the prognosis is usually very serious. In this case, internal fixation or fracture stabilization with a fixator is probably the treatment of choice (Figure 28.1A and B).

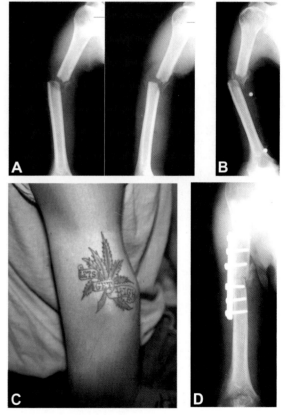

Figs 28.2A to D: (A) Radiograph of transverse fracture in the middle-third of the humerus taken 2 months after the initial insult, showing axial distraction between the fragments. The patient had suffered a radial palsy initially. (B) Radiograph obtained 1 month later showing some peripheral callus. There was however, frank motion at the fracture site. Early return of nerve function was detected at this time. (C) Appearance of the tattooed arm of the 24-year-old "gang" member. (D) Radiograph taken after plating and grafting of the nonunited bone. Patient was lost to follow-up. Even though we have been able to demonstrate that the brace does not necessarily has to cover the fracture site, in this instance it is obvious that the brace was not appropriately held in place and adjusted.

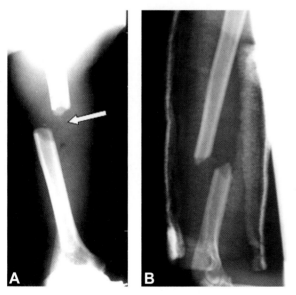

Figs 28.1A and B: Radiographs illustrating marked distraction between the fragments following severe fractures associated with major soft tissue damage, particularly when associated with major nerve injuries. These fractures are usually best treated with plate fixation, if a rapid response to the distraction does not occur following active contractures of the biceps and triceps.

In the absence of nerve palsy, the axial distraction is an invitation to nonunion (Figures 28.1 to 28.3). However, we have witnessed spontaneous reduction of the gap between the fragments following the initiation of active flexion and extension of the elbow. It is likely that contraction of these muscles displaces the distal fragment in a superior direction, while stimulating osteoblastic activity. (See Chapter 12)

There are times when the axial distraction between the major fragments disappears spontaneously within a short period of time. In those instances, functional bracing usually renders good clinical results (Figures 28.4A and B).

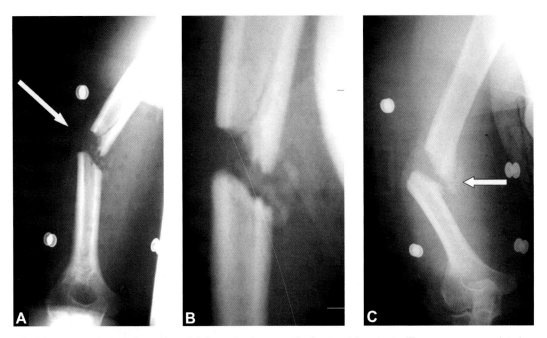

Figs 28.3A to C: (A) Radiograph depicting major axial distraction between the fractured fragments. There was an associated nerve palsy. (B) The fracture was treated with a functional brace. (C) A nonunion developed, necessitating internal plate fixation.

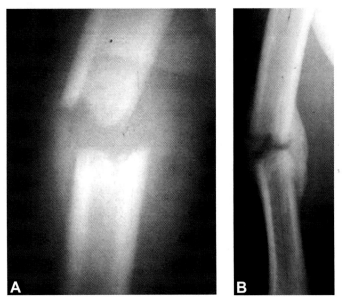

Figs 28.4A and B: (A) Severely distracted fragments in a fracture produced from a high-energy injury. There was no peripheral nerve injury. (B) Despite the separation of the fragments, which frequently lead to nonunion, the fracture united. This radiograph was the last one obtained because the patient never returned for further follow-up.

29

Shoulder Subluxation

Subluxation of the shoulder is common following fractures of the neck of the humerus, but it is not uncommon with diaphyseal fractures. It is best managed by active flexion and extension of the elbow. Since both flexors and extensors muscles have attachments on the scapula and humerus, their contraction forces the humeral head into the glenoid.

Injury to the axillary nerve has been thought to be the responsible cause. This is very unlikely since an axillary nerve injury would be accompanied with a sensory deficit. This situation is extremely rare.

The following case illustrates this rather unusual pathology. The subluxation was accompanied with a definitive area of anesthesia over the territory of the axillary nerve. The head relocated itself readily when active contractions of the biceps and triceps were instituted (Figures 29.1A to 29.2I).

Though this text does not include fractures of the humeral neck, and we are not recommending functional bracing as the treatment for these fracture, we would be remised if were to remain silent of the issue, since a number of clinical experiences have suggested that many such fractures, currently treated by surgical means, can be very appropriately managed non-surgically.

It is appropriate to suggest that if the following fractures of the humeral head had been treated by means of open reduction and internal fixation, the final outcome would have been inferior, because of greater final limitation of motion. That has been our experience.

Many of the diaphyseal fractures discussed in the text had associated subluxation of the humeral head, and responded well to a simple protocol of active flexion and extension of the elbow, beginning a few days after the onset of the disability.

Regardless of the real pathophysiological process, the most effective way to correct the subluxation is with active flexion and extension of the elbow. Attempts to relocate the joint with early active exercises of the deltoid are painful and even harmful. In the case of a diaphyseal fracture, contraction of the shoulder abductors precipitates the development of varus angular deformities.

The claim that a contraction of the deltoid muscle is responsible for the commonly seen abduction of the proximal fragment cannot be supported scientifically for it is likely that the deltoid muscle, immediately following a fracture, is not in a state of spasticity. Under such state of flaccidity, the muscle cannot create a deformity (Figure 29.3).

This situation is similar to the one we observed a number of years ago regarding the varus deformity that femoral neck and intertrochanteric fractures usually experience. It is commonly believed that the shortening of the limb following the fracture is brought about by the painful contraction of a spastic gluteus medius, which is the major muscle attached to the greater trochanter.

We demonstrated with electromyography that the gluteus medius is in a stage of flaccidity, but the adductors are in a stage of spasticity. They are the ones to create the deformity (Figures 29.4 to 29.7).

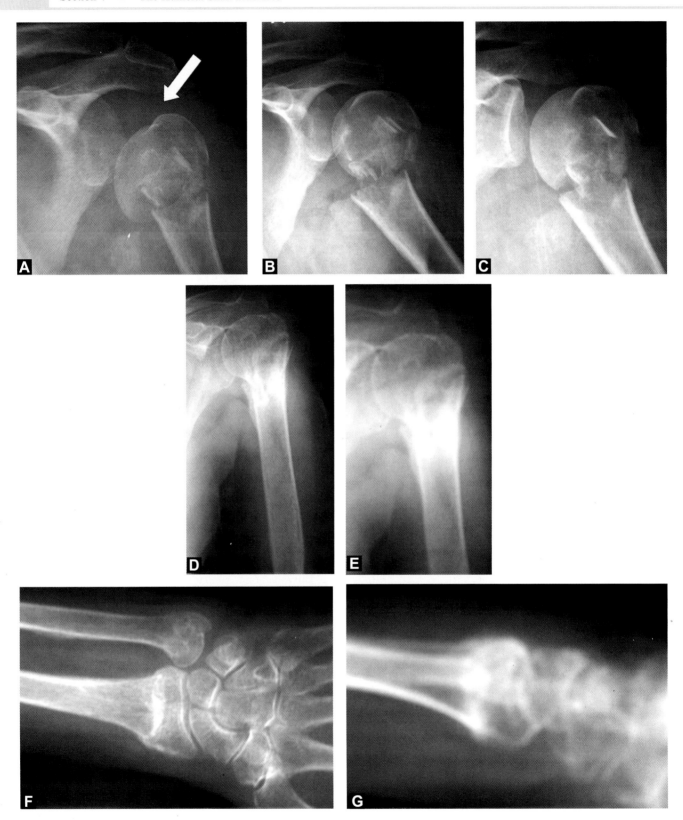

Figs 29.1A to G

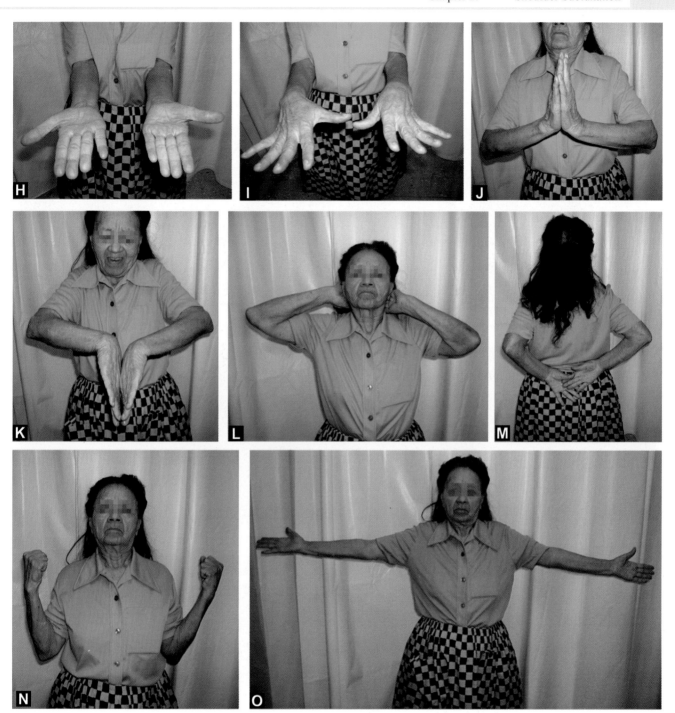

Figs 29.1H to O

Figs 29.1A to O: (A) Radiograph of fracture of the neck of the humerus with associated subluxation of the humeral head. (B) Radiograph obtained a few days later after a functional brace was applied and active flexion and extension exercises were introduced. Within a few days, the head began to show improvement of the subluxation. (C) Two weeks after the injury, the relationship of the humeral head with the glenoid fossa was normal. (D and E) Radiographs obtained 5 and 8 weeks after the initial insult. The fracture had not shown evidence of radiological union, but the patient was asymptomatic and had regained normal motion, minus the last few degrees of external rotation and elevation. (F and G) The patient had also sustained a fracture of the distal radius, that healed following manipulation. The normal volar tilt was lost as well as some of the length of the radius. These minor deviations from the normal are inconsequential as the patient demonstrates on figures H to K. The minimal limitation of wrist motion present 2 months after the injury will eventually disappear. (I to O) Patient demonstrates the asymptomatic range of motion of her upper extremities.

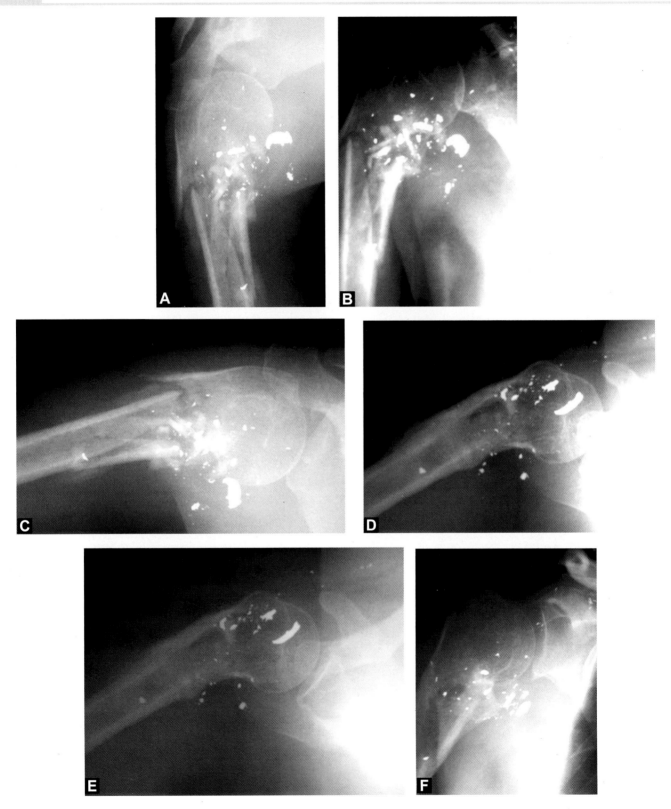

Figs 29.2A to F

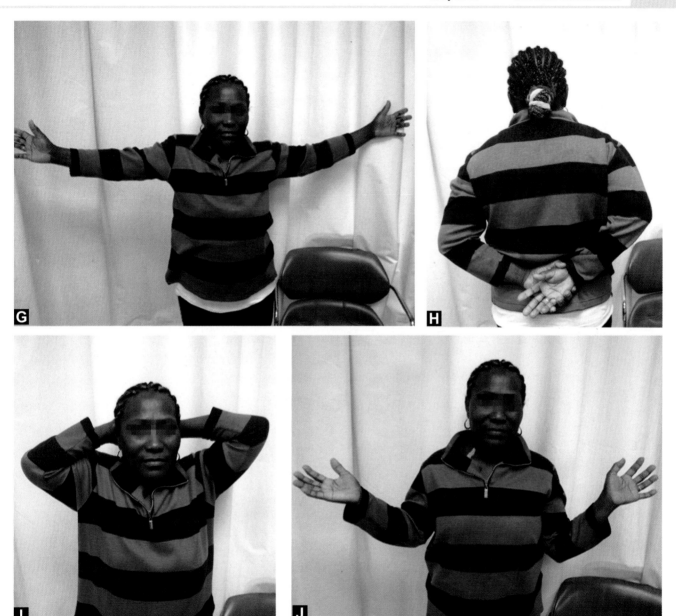

Figs 29.2G to J

Figs 29.2A to J: (A and B) Comminuted fracture of the very proximal humerus secondary to a bullet wound. (C and D) The fracture was treated with a functional brace and early introduction of active flexion and extension of the elbow, and passive exercises of the shoulder joint. The subluxation of the shoulder subsided rapidly. (E) Radiograph obtained three months after the initial injury showing anatomical alignment of the fragments. (F and G) Radiographs obtained 5 months after the initial injury. (H to J) The range of motion of the shoulder was limited in the last degrees of external rotation and elevation. It is anticipated that continued use of the extremity will eliminate the residual limitation of motion.

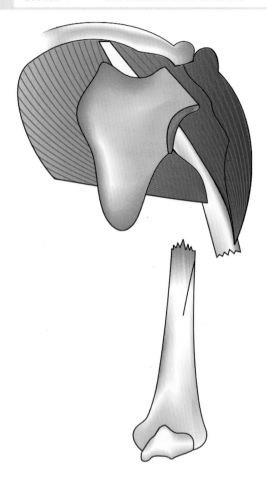

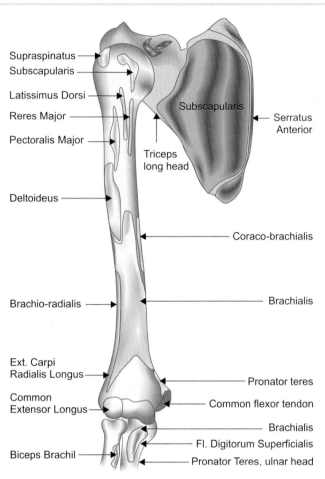

Supraspinatus
Subscapularis
Latissimus Dorsi
Reres Major
Pectoralis Major
Deltoideus
Brachio-radialis
Ext. Carpi Radialis Longus
Common Extensor Longus
Biceps Brachil

Subscapularis
Serratus Anterior
Triceps long head
Coraco-brachialis
Brachialis
Pronator teres
Common flexor tendon
Brachialis
Fl. Digitorum Superficialis
Pronator Teres, ulnar head

Fig. 29.3: Illustration suggesting that the deltoid muscle in a state of spasticity (brought about by the pain associated with the injury) abducts the proximal humeral fragment. This is an unlikely possibility since the muscle is in a stage of flaccidity and therefore incapable of producing the abduction deformity.

Fig. 29.4: The biceps and triceps muscles have origins and attachments on the scapula and humeral shaft. Their contractions during active flexion and extension of the elbow move the subluxated head into the glenoid.

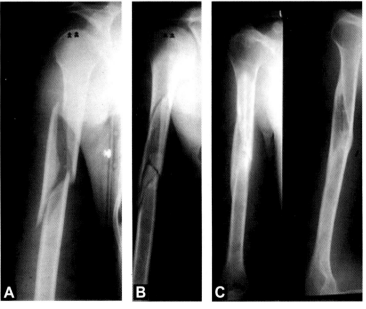

Figs 29.5A to C: (A and B) Radiographs of comminuted fracture of the proximal humerus demonstrating the alignment of the fragment in the functional brace and the subluxation of the shoulder, which disappeared within a very short period of time, following the introduction of active flexion and extension of the elbow. (C) Radiographs obtained after completion of healing.

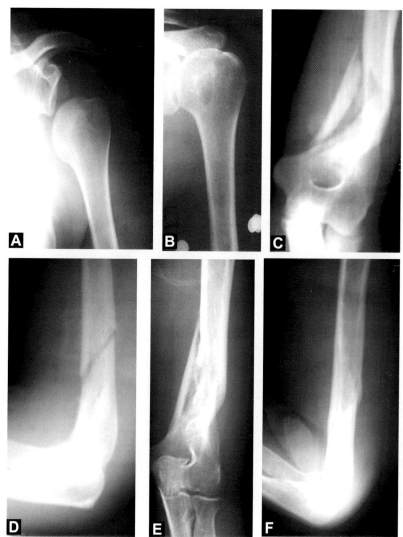

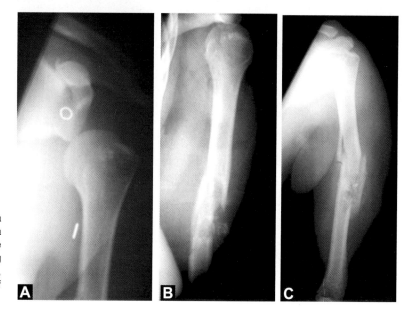

Figs 29.6A to F: (A) Radiograph of subluxated humeral head of a patient who had sustained a closed fracture of the distal humerus. (B) Radiograph taken 2 weeks after the initiation of a program of active flexion and extension of the elbow. The contractions of the biceps and triceps brought about the reduction of the suluxation. (C and D) Radiographs of the initial fracture of the distal humerus. (E and F) Radiographs taken after completion of healing.

Figs 29.7A to C: (A) Radiograph illustrating a severe degree of subluxation in the presence of a diaphyseal fracture. (B) Radiograph showing the diaphyseal fracture. (C) Radiograph demonstrating the spontaneous reduction of the subluxation, which was expedited by the early introduction of active flexion and extension of the elbow.

30

Associated Nerve Palsy

NERVE PALSY

Most closed fractures with associated radial palsy can be treated with functional bracing in anticipation of spontaneous recovery when the nerve palsy develops immediately after the injury.[1-19] A dorsal cock-up wrist splint is not usually necessary if no contraindications exist for early extension of the elbow. Once the elbow is extended, the partially paralyzed wrist spontaneously extends, preventing, in that manner, the development of a flexion contracture of the joint.

If the palsy appears at a later day, the prognosis is more guarded and suggesting encroachment of the nerve by the forming callus. MRI and electrical studies should be conducted to rule out the possibility of serious pathology. If identified, surgical exploration is necessary. Following the repair of the nerve, the fractured humerus should be stabilized with either an external fixator or a plate.

Fractures of the humerus associated with brachial plexus injuries have a guarded prognosis. Nonunion is common. Surgical stabilization is the treatment of choice.

Open fractures with major soft tissue damage preclude successful management with functional bracing particularly if there is an associated peripheral nerve injury. Other treatment modalities are more appropriate (Figures 30.1 and 30.2).

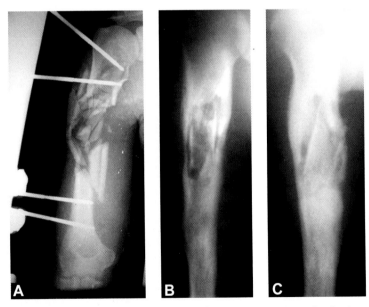

Figs 30.1A to C: (A) Radiographs of severely comminuted fracture produced by a high-velocity projectile. An associated multi-nerve palsy was present. The fracture was treated with open debridement and stabilization with an external fixator. (B and C) Radiographs illustrating the healed fracture, however, associated with an infection that required multiple surgical debridement procedures.

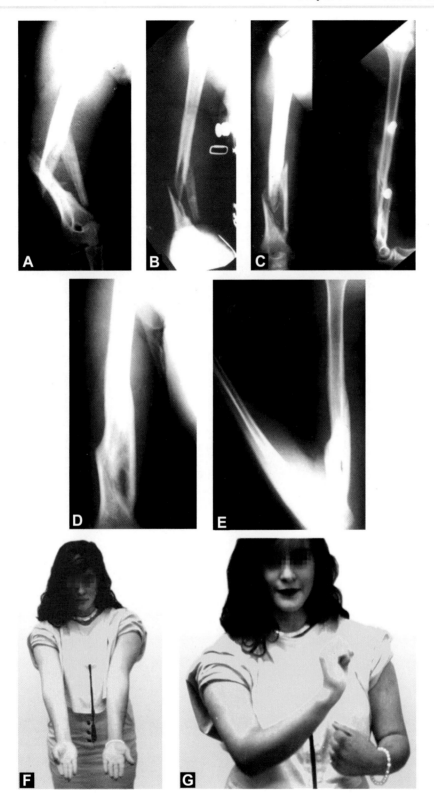

Figs 30.2A to G: (A) Radiograph of fracture of the distal end of the humerus in a 22-year-old girl illustrating the frequently seen medial free fragment. (B) Radiograph taken 9 days after the initial injury, following the application of the functional brace. (C) Radiograph taken 3 months after the injury showing callus at the fracture site. (D and E) Last radiographs illustrating solid union of the fracture and full flexion of the elbow. (F and G) Patients demonstrates the full extension of the elbow and the recovered radial palsy that occurred at the time of the injury.

REFERENCES

1. Aiken GK, Rorabeck CH. Distal humeral fractures in the adult. Clin Orthop Relat Res. 1986; 207:191-7.
2. Balfour GW, Mooney V, Ashby ME. Diaphyseal Fractures of the Humerus Treated with a Ready-Made Fracture Brace. J Bone Joint Surg. 1982; 64A:11.
3. Bleeker WA, Nijsten MW, ten Duis HJ. Treatment of humeral shaft fractures related to associated injuries: A retrospective study of 237 patients. Acta Orthop Scand. 1991; 62(2):148-53.
4. Bruggemann H, Kujat R, Tscherne H. Funkionelle Frakturebehandlung nach. Sarmiento an Unterschenkel, Unterarm und Oberarm. Orthopaede, 1983; 12:143.
5. Ekholm R, Adami J, Tidemark K, Hansson K, Tornkvist H, Ponzer S. Fractures of the shaft of the humerus: An epidemiological study of 401 fractures. J Bone Joint Surg Br. 2006 Nov; 88(11);1469-73.
6. Ekkernkamp A, Kayser M, Althoff M. Knozept der Funktionellen Therapie am Beispiel des Frischen Geschlossenen Oberarmschaftbruches. Zentralbl Chir. 1989; 114:788
7. McMaster WC, Tivnon MC, Waugh TR. Cast Brace for the Upper Extremity. Clin Orthop. 1975; 109:126.
8. Naver L, Aalberg JR. Humeral Shaft Fractures Treated with a Ready-Made Fracture Brace. Arch Orthop Trauma Surg. 1986; 106:20-2.
9. Osterman PAW, Ekkerkamp A, Muhr G. Functional Bracing of Fractures of the Humerus: An analysis of 195 cases. Proc 60th Amer Acad Orthop Surg. 1993; 69.
10. Sarmiento A, Kinman PB, Galvin EG, Schmitt RH, Phillips JG: Functional Bracing of Fractures of the Shaft of the Humerus. J. Bone Joint Surg. 1977; 59A:596.
11. Sarmiento A, Latta LL. Closed Functional Treatment of fractures. Springer-Verlag, Berlin, GFR. 1981.
12. Sarmiento A, Latta LL. Functional Fracture Bracing. Springer-Verlag, Heidelberg, GFR. 1995.
13. Sarmiento A, Zych GA, Zagorski JB, Latta LL. Functional Bracing of Diaphyseal Humeral Fractures. J. Bone Joint Surg, 1999.
14. Sarmiento A, Horowitch A, Aboulafia A, Vangsness CT Jr. Functional Bracing of comminuted extra-articular fractures of the Distal-Third of the Humerus. J. Bone Joint Surg. 1990; 72B-2:283-7.
15. Sarmiento A, Latta LL. Functional Fracture Bracing. A review Article Journal AAOS. 1999; 7(1):66-78.
16. Sarmiento A, Zagorski JB, Zych GA, Latta LL, Capps CA. Functional Bracing of Humeral Shaft Fractures. J. Bone Joint Surg. 2000; 82A4:478-86
17. Sarmiento A, Waddell JP, Latta LL. Diaphyseal Humeral Fractures: Treatment Options. An Instructional Course. AAOS J Bone and Joint Surg. 1999; 83A(10):1566-79.
18. Sarmiento A, Latta LL. Conservative treatment of humeral shaft fractures. Unfallchirurg. German Trauma Assoc. 2007.
19. Sharma VK, Jain AK, Gupta RK, Tyagi AK, Sethi PK. Non-operative treatment of Humeral Shaft Fracture: A comparative study. J Indian Med Assoc. 1991; 89:157.

31

Obesity

Obesity in itself is not a contraindication. However, angular deformities are more severe in obese patients due to the fact that since the injured arm must be held against the chest for a period of time, the obese chest and arm places a varus inducing force at the fracture site. However, the larger amount of adipose tissue camouflages the deformities quite effectively. The same can be contemplated from the following illustrations as shown in Figures 31.1 to 31.5.

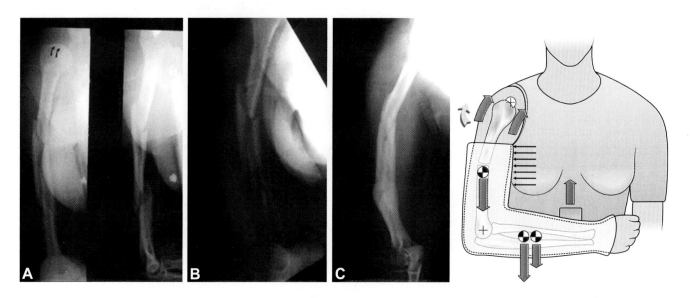

Figs 31.1A to C

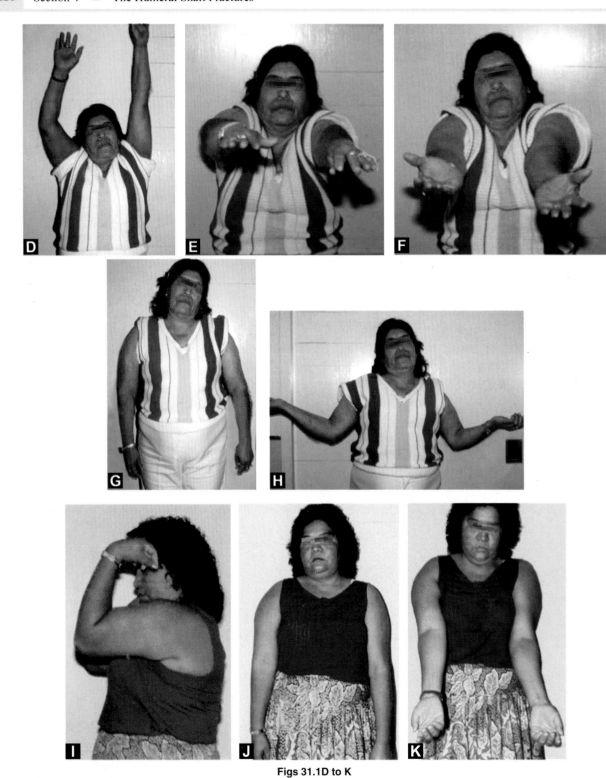

Figs 31.1D to K

Figs 31.1A to K: (A) Radiograph of double segmental fracture of the humerus sustained in an automobile accident by an obese woman. Notice the subluxation of the shoulder. (B) Radiograph obtained after application of the brace 10 days after the initial injury. An angular deformity is already apparent. Her large adipose tissues created a fulcrum leading to the angulation. (C) Radiograph obtained approximately 1 year after the initial injury. The subluxation had corrected after the initiation of active elbow exercises. The angular deformity remained unchanged. (D to H) The obese patient demonstrates the overall appearance of her fractured arm and the function of the shoulder and elbow. These photos were taken 3 months after the initial insult. (I to K) Photos of patient showing the cosmetic appearance of her arms and the degree of flexion of her elbows.

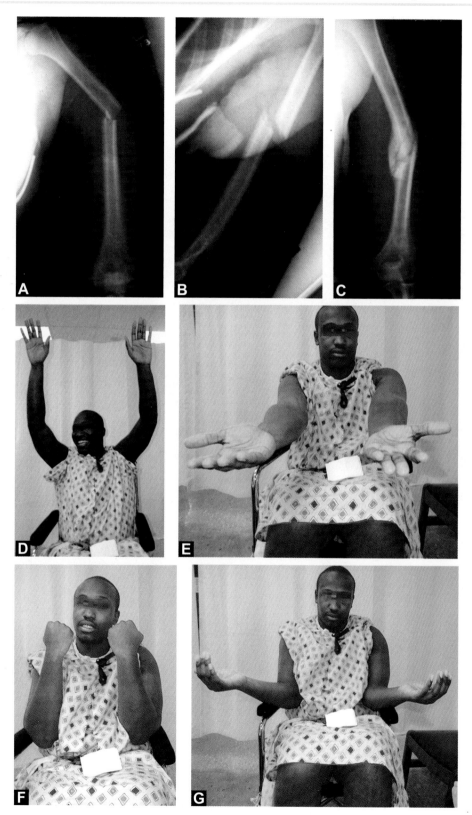

Figs 31.2A to G: (A to C) Radiographs of transverse, displaced fracture of the humeral shaft treated with a functional brace. The fracture healed with a varus angulation, probably secondary to lack of patient cooperation. (D to G) Photographs of the patient, a prisoner, showing the range of motion of his shoulders and elbows 2½ months after the initial injury. He still was in prison at that time.

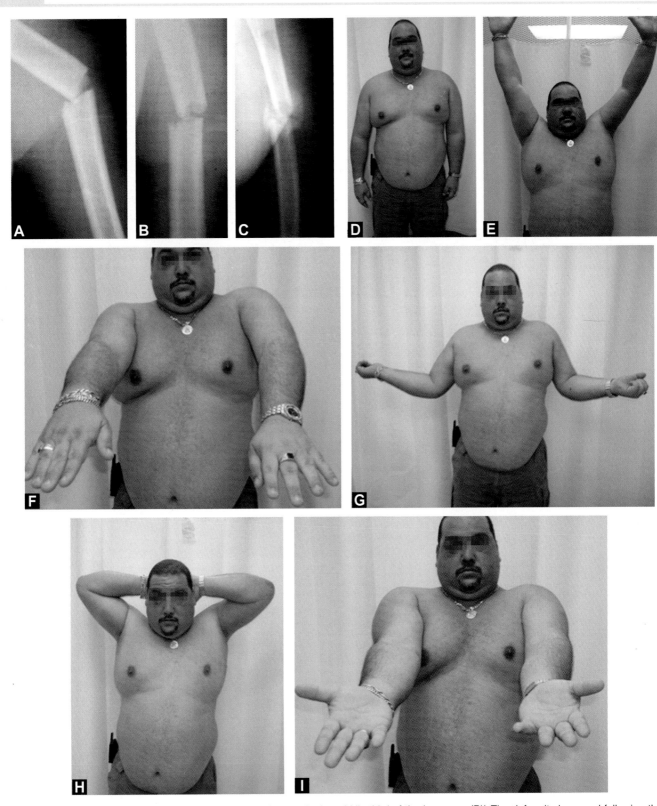

Figs 31.3A to I: (A) Radiograph of severely angulated fracture in the middle-third of the humerus. (B)) The deformity improved following the application of the functional brace and subsequent dependency of the extremity. (C) Radiograph obtained 2½ months following the injury. Early callus was present. The patient failed to return to further follow-up. (D to I) Clinical photographs illustrating the range of motion of the patient's arms.

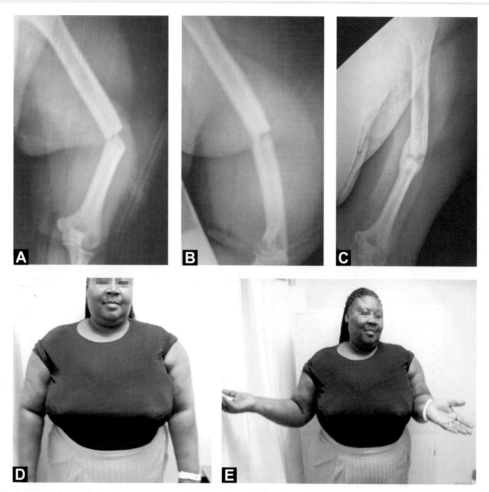

Figs 31.4A to E: (A) Initial radiograph of transverse, angulated fracture in the middle-third of the humerus. (B) Radiograph after application of the brace. (C) Final radiograph obtained after union of the fracture. Notice the final angular deformity. (D) Patient shows the overall appearance of her upper extremities. (E) Patient shows the still limited external rotation of her shoulder.

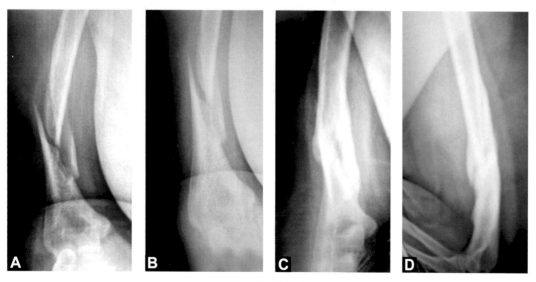

Figs 31.5A to D

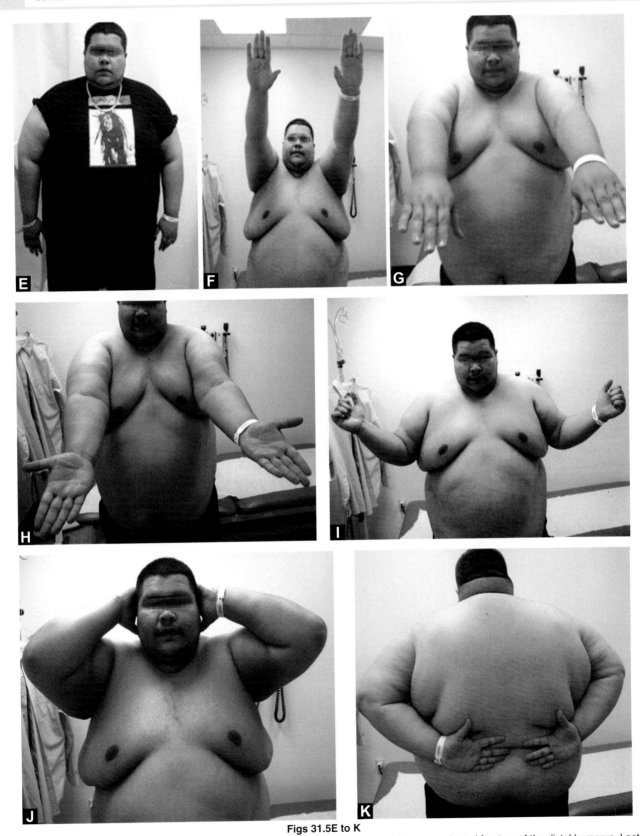

Figs 31.5E to K

Figs 31.5A to K: Radiographs and clinical pictures of a morbidly obese young man with a comminuted fracture of the distal humerus. Last photos were taken 4 months after the initial injury.

32

Malrotation

Final malrotation deformity in diaphyseal humeral fractures is rare, despite the fact that it is assumed such problem should be a common one, since it is customary to stabilize the injured extremity in a position of internal rotation of the shoulder. One might assume that in that manner, the proximal fragment would take a neutral or external rotation position, while the distal one would be forced into internal rotation. This assumption is either ill-founded or the coiling of the muscles around the bone–created at the time of the fracture—uncoil the malrotated bone as muscular forces are reintroduced (Figures 32.1A and B).

This theory of ours may not be able to withstand scientific scrutiny since the absence of malrotation seems to be present in instances when early introduction of corrective uncoiling muscular forces were not introduced before intrinsic fracture stability developed.

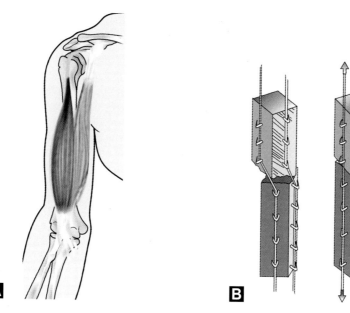

Figs 32.1A and B: Drawing depicting the origin and insertion of the elbow flexors. At the time of the fracture, the muscle fibers coil as the bony fragments rotate. Their subsequent contraction uncoils the muscle, correcting the rotary bony deformity.

33

Angular Deformities

MALALIGNMENT

Most angular deformities encountered with functional bracing of humeral shaft fractures are those of varus.

Manipulation of a diaphyseal fracture of the humerus is strongly criticized because of the danger of producing nerve damage.

Most angular deformities correct spontaneously as the brace compresses the soft tissues and the weight of the arm assists in improving alignment (Figures 33.1A to E). Most angular deformities are physiologically and cosmetically tolerated. If the conservative approach fails to provide the desired alignment of the fragments, a surgical intervention is required. This is a very unlikely event.

It took us a long time to fully realize that the ubiquitous angular deformity seen initially in the fractured humerus is iatrogenically induced. This angular deformity cannot be produced by muscle deforming forces since when a fracture occurs, the potential deforming muscles are in a state of flaccidity. If they were rendered spastic by the pain the fracture produces, then the deformity could be explained on the contraction of the generated forces. But since this is not the case, we have concluded that the deformity is produced when the arm is placed in a sling that supports the arm by covering the forearm and wraps over the patient's neck. Normally, the patient with an acute fracture of the humerus instinctively shrugs the shoulder. Since the sling is not elastic and it usually attempts to hold the elbow at 90° of flexion, once the shrugging is relaxed, the resulting forces produce the angular deformity (Figures 33.2A to 33.3).

This phenomenon strongly suggests that every possible effort should be made to ascertain, at the time of application of the original sling, and subsequently during the application of the cast, and later the brace, that shrugging be prevented (Figures 33.4A and B).

In addition to taking the above-described precautions against angular deformity, residual angulation can be corrected, if not in its entirety, by applying gentle pressure at the apex of the deformity and counter-pressure over the medial aspect of the elbow as the brace straps are tightened (Figures 33.5A to C).

As it is true for all situations in medicine, the degree of acceptability of angular deformity should be individualized. For example, an obese patient with a deformity of 30° heals the fracture in such a manner that visual examination will not demonstrate a deformity, and the function of the elbow and shoulder will be normal. I have emphasized "woman" simply because women, in general, as they grow older show a fat distribution quite different from that of men. Women's fat tends to deposit primarily in their arms and legs; in men in the abdomen. Fat camouflages deformities effectively. The same rule applies to men with large musculature.

In order to detect varus deformity of the humerus—the most common deformity—it is best to examine the patient with both arms flexed to approximately 80°, with the forearms in pronation and supination. The pronated position makes identification of deformity easier (Figures 33.6A to C).

It should be obvious to the reader that a sleeve that cover only portion of the upper arm cannot possibly immobilize the fractured fragments. In actuality, no matter how much a sleeve covered the fracture site, immobilization is never obtained, simply stabilization. Regardless of the length of the sleeve —firmly compressing the soft tissue surrounding the bone— stiffens the body segment in a manner that significantly reduces motion at the fracture site and contributes to the alignment of the fragments. We have chosen to explain this mechanism by comparing the fractured humerus covered by a relatively stiff sleeve with the sausage or the "hot dog." In the case of the two examples, soft meat is rendered stiff by its compression by a thin and relatively inelastic membrane. Under bending forces, the structure deforms but upon

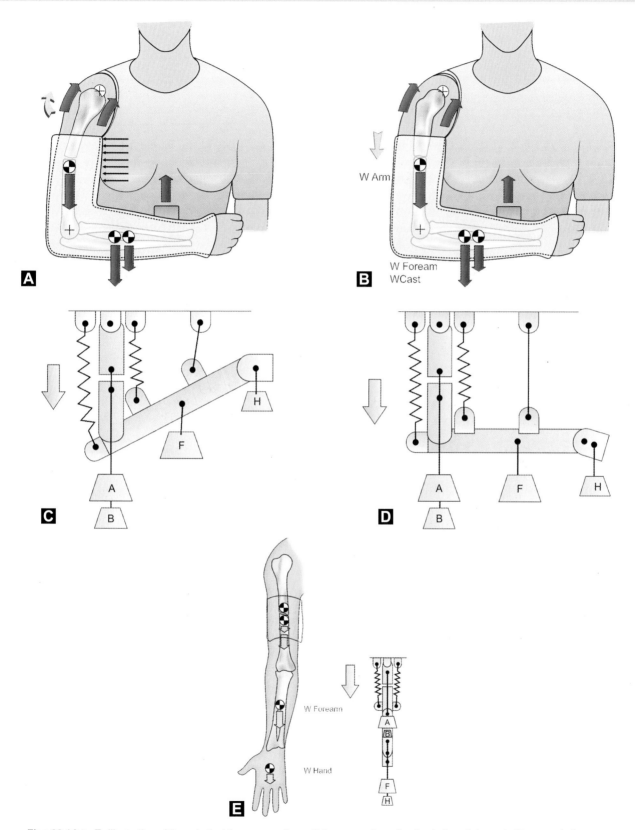

Figs 33.1A to E: Illustration of the role that the surrounding soft tissues and gravity play in the attainment of improved alignment.

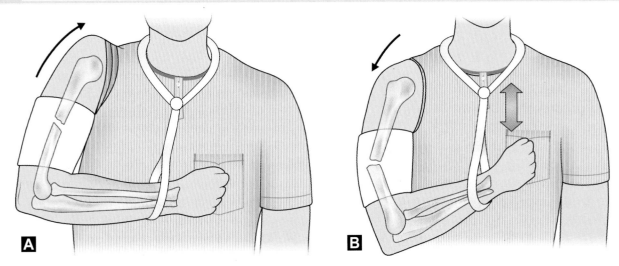

Figs 33.2A and B: (A) At the time of the initial stabilization of the painful extremity, the patient with a fracture of the humerus instinctively shrugs the shoulder. If a sling is applied while the shoulder is shrugged, a deformity occurs (B) since the elbow flexes and the forearm and hand are displaced proximally. The natural apprehension the patient experiences at the time of application of the original sling prompts him/her to shrug the shoulder. When the shoulder relaxes, a varus angular deformity may occur. It is therefore important to ascertain that the sling is applied after the shoulder is no longer in a shrugged position.

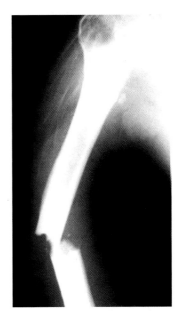

Fig. 33.3: The varus deformity at the fracture site, usually observed radiologically after the initial sling is applied, is iatrogenically created by the sling that flexes the elbow of the painful arm.

relaxation of the forces it returns to the original shape. This is probably the way the fractured humerus behaves when stabilized with a brace. Experimental studies have indicated that the thickness and rigidity of the surrounding material is relatively unimportant. A thin sleeve of paper provides stiffness that is sufficient to create adequate stability. Increasing the stiffness of the material enhances stiffness of the composite by only two fold (Figures 33.7A to F).

The varus deformity observed from the improper application of the sling is the same one produced by leaning on the elbow after it has been stabilized in a brace. Therefore, strict avoidance of weight bearing on the elbow is essential (Figures 33.8A to D).

The adjustable brace should be removed every day for hygienic purposes and reapplied snuggly. Patients should avoid active elevation or abduction of the shoulder before clear evidence of sufficient intrinsic stability at the fracture site has been diagnosed clinically and radiographically. The premature performance of those exercises lead to the development of a varus deformity. If the patient leans forward during the pendulum and abduction-adduction swinging exercises, he or she is flexing and abducting to 90° without subjecting the fracture site to excessive varus deforming forces.

It is for similar reasons that leaning on the elbow should be forbidden. The resulting varus forces brought about by the weight of the upper body can produce a varus deformity. This varus deformity is more likely to occur if the fracture is transverse, and even more so, if the fragments are in contact with one another. If the fracture is comminuted or oblique, weight bearing provokes elastic pistoning between the fragments, a motion that is conducive to osteogenesis. It is not necessary for the patient to sleep in the sitting position. All is needed is the suspension of the arm in the sling. It is most desirable to regain extension of the elbow in preference to flexion as it is anticipated that with the necessary activities of daily living, spontaneous gain of flexion will take place. Regaining extension early is important because once full

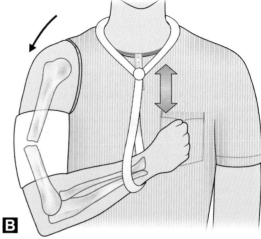
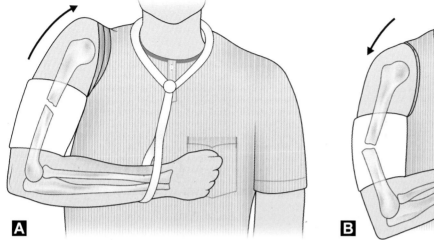

Figs 33.4A and B: (A) The varus deformity can also be created at the time of application of the brace if the shoulder is shrugged during the procedure. (B) If a varus deformity was produced at the time of the application of the original sling, the condition is further aggravated.

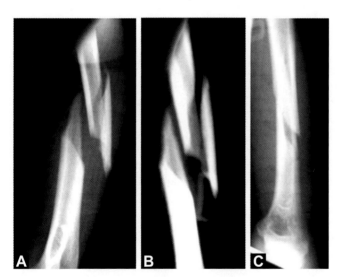

Figs 33.5A to C: (A) Initial radiograph illustrating the frequently observed varus angulation at the fracture site. (B and C) Radiographs obtained immediately after the application of the brace. The deformity was corrected by gentle pressure on the apex of the fracture, with opposite counter-pressure over the medial aspect of the elbow. Subsequent dependency of the extremity and compression of the soft tissues by the brace usually ensure maintenance of the corrected deformity.

extension of the elbow is reached the patient can, after an additional period of time for the fracture to gain intrinsic stability, discontinue the use of the sling and walk with the swing of the arm in a normal way. The weight of the distal arm can now further assist in improving the ubiquitous varus angulation seen in humeral diaphyseal fractures.

In addition, the extension of the elbow eliminates the fulcrum-effect created by the chest when the arm rests over protruding muscular tissues or large breasts (Figures 33.9A to 33.11K). It is well known that large-breasted women have a greater tendency to develop varus deformities as a result of the alleged fulcrum-effect.

Most final angulations seen in humeral fractures managed by functional bracing is of a varus nature. Valgus deformity is rarely seen. The residual varus deformity implies a loss of the carrying angle of the upper arm. We have not seen any impairment of function resulting from the loss of the few degrees of carrying angle the normal humerus has (Figures 33.12A to 3.13G).

The transverse/nondisplaced fracture has a greater tendency to angulate into varus, secondary to leaning on the elbow or from premature strong contraction of the flexors and extensor of the elbow. In this instance (Figure 33.14) good alignment was maintained.

Initial overriding of the fragments is a desirable feature. Distraction in the vertical plane may lead to nonunion.

The desirable motion at the fracture site, when the fracture is not reduced, is of an elastic type. On the other hand, when the fracture is transverse and nondisplaced, the motions at the fracture site are of a bending nature, and capable of creating permanent angular deformities.

Women with large breasts also have a tendency to develop a varus deformity as a result of the fact that during the early stages of treatment, when the arm held in a sling that forces it into adduction, the breast functions as a fulcrum. This is why it is important to reduce as much as possible the length of usage of the sling, for as long as the arm is held against the

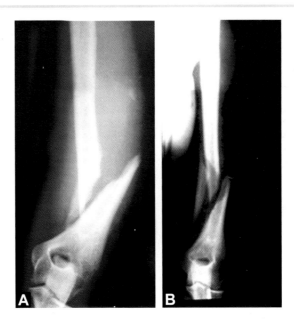

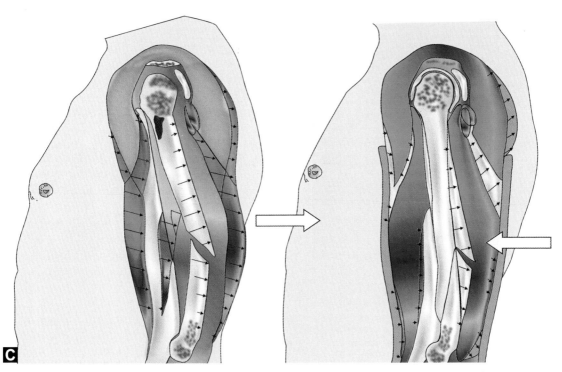

Figs 33.6A to C: (A) Radiograph obtained 24 hours after the initial insult. The fractured extremity had been stabilized in a sling that held the elbow at 90°. It is likely that the sling was applied while the shoulder was shrugged, and upon relaxation of the scapular elevators the angular deformity was either created or aggravated. (B) As soon as full extension of the elbow was accomplished approximately 1 week later, the severe varus angular deformity corrected spontaneously. The weight of the arm and the compression of the soft tissue by the brace, made the correction possible. (C) The compression of the soft tissues, which is maintained through frequent tightening of the Velcro straps, assists in the correction of deformities.

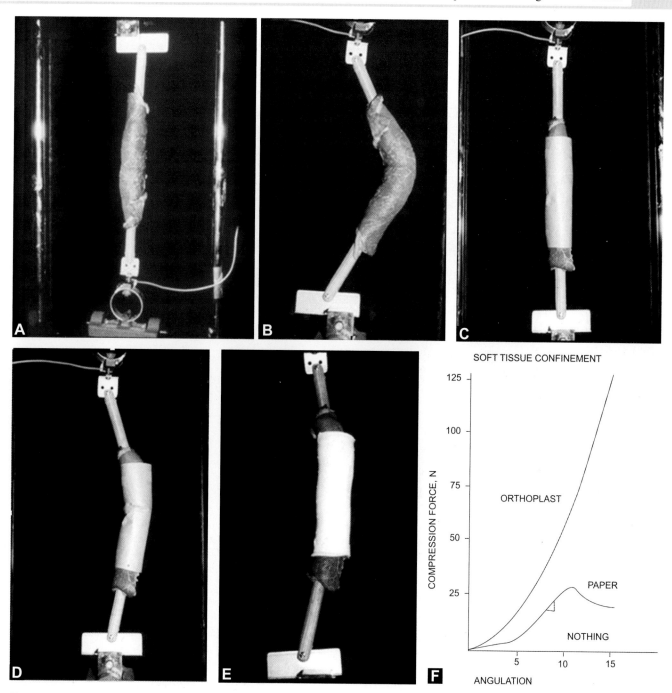

Figs 33.7A to F: (A) In an effort to measure the effect of soft tissue compression, a piece of meat was wrapped around a "broom stick" model of a fracture to simulate a fracture in a single bone limb segment. (B) The resistance to bending was measured when an axial load was applied (C) Then the soft tissue was compressed by wrapping with brown paper, similar to the manner in which a butcher wraps meat. (D) (This was done to simulate the description of the senior author about the apparent increase in rigidity one can observe when a butcher rolls and wraps a piece of meat tightly with a simple piece of brown paper). The construct was again loaded and the resistance measured. (E) Finally, the meat was wrapped with Orthoplast® and the soft tissue compressed to simulate a fracture brace applied to the construct, the compression of the soft tissue with brown paper raised the resistance to bending by 96X. Compression with Orthoplast® only increased the resistance by 2X over that of the brown paper. (F) So the rigidity of the wrapping material was much less important than the compression of the soft tissue in providing resistance to bending.

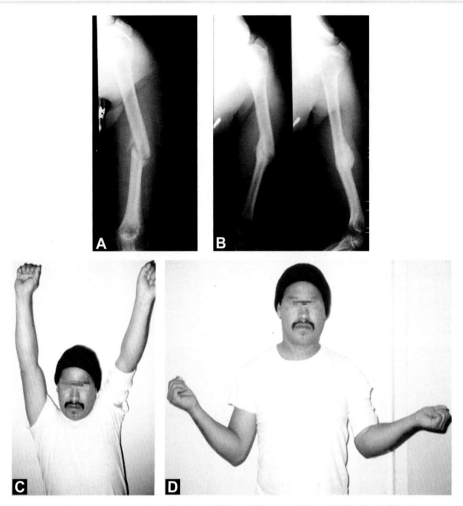

Figs 33.8A to D: (A) Radiograph of transverse, angulated but non-displaced fracture in the middle-third of the humerus seen approximately 4 weeks after the initial insult. The angular deformity was probably produced from premature pressure of the elbow against the patient's lap or on hard surfaces. (B) The fracture healed with the residual angular deformity shown in the film. (C and D) Patient demonstrates the function of his fractured arm while still in the brace. Notice the limitation of external rotation which, most likely, disappeared upon resumption of activities of daily living.

chest in an internal rotation attitude, the fulcrum phenomenon will exist. However, when the elbow is extended and the pendulum exercises can be conducted in that manner, the arm falls behind the fulcrum-producing breast. Usually the loss of the "carrying angle" from the varus-angular deformity goes undetectable with no adverse clinical consequences. It is very likely that the deformity was the result of leaning on the elbow during the early stages of treatment.

The humeral diaphysis tolerates, functionally and cosmetically, angular deformities of degrees that most other long bones do not tolerate. Arms with either large musculature or excessive adipose tissues camouflage deformity quite well. Loss of the "carrying angle" of the elbow is very common,

particularly in fractures of the distal-third of the bone. Since women are more likely to have valgus elbows, a varus deformity of 15 of 20° is difficult to recognize.

Leaning on the elbow should be strongly discouraged, since it produces angular deformities. This may occur during the initial period of cast immobilization, but more likely after the application of the brace.

Antero-posterior deformities can also develop and are more likely to be seen in transverse, non-displaced fractures. A delay in reaching extension of the elbow may aggravate an angulation with an anterior apex. The "stiff elbow" creates abnormal stresses at the fracture site when the arm finally hangs over the side of the body.

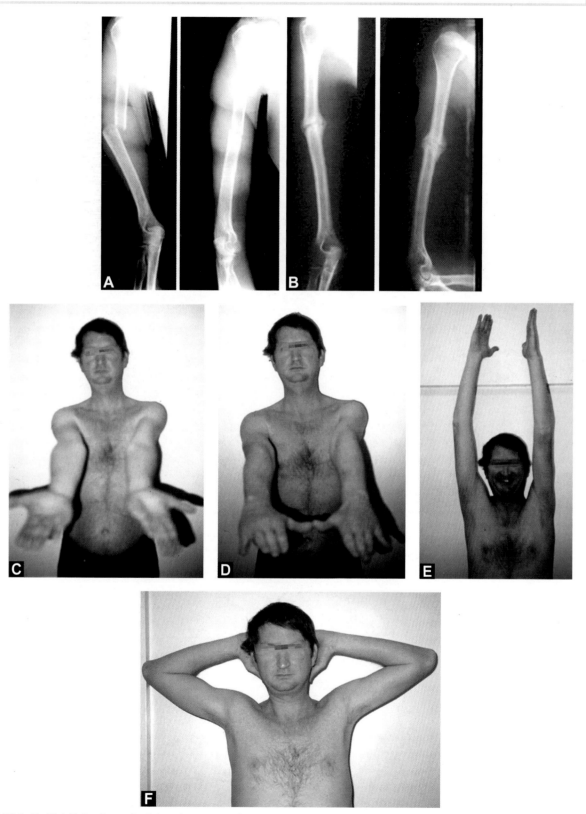

Figs 33.9A to F: (A) Initial radiograph of closed transverse fracture in the middle-third of the diaphysis. (B) The compression of the soft tissues by the brace and the extension of the elbow within a few days after the initial injury aligned the fragments in an almost anatomical position. The fracture healed uneventfully. (C to F) Patient demonstrate the range of motion of his upper extremity on the day the brace was discontinued.

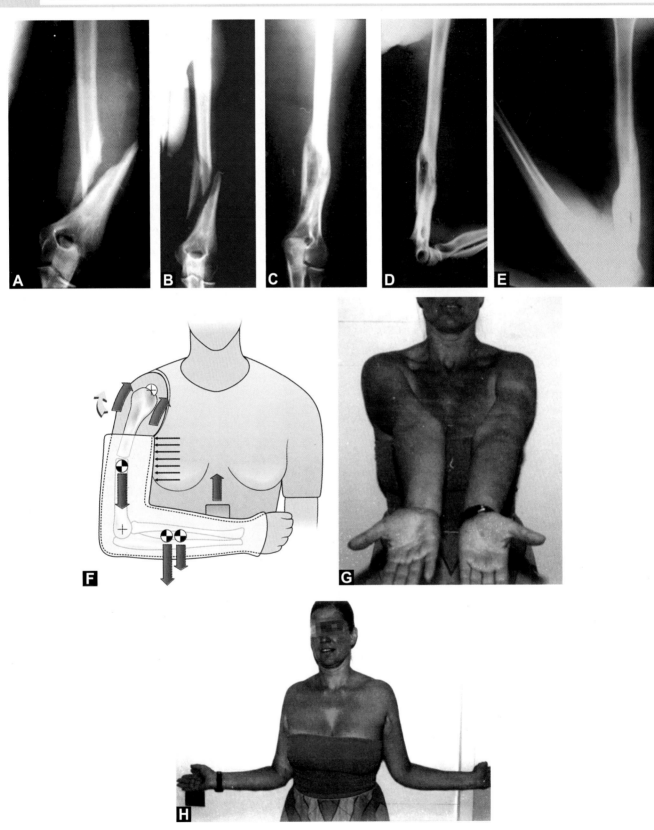

Figs 33.10A to G

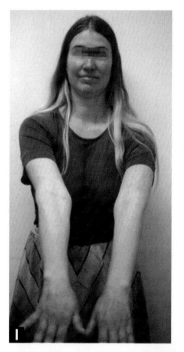

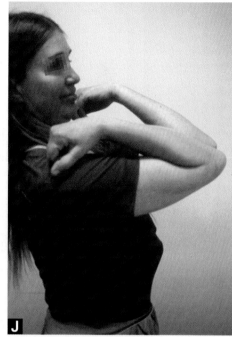

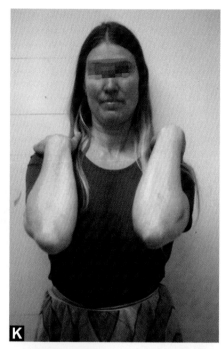

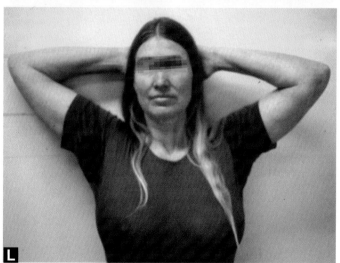

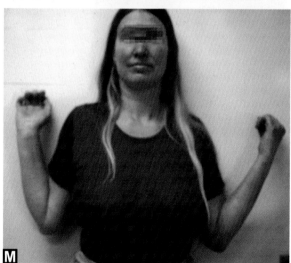

Figs 33.10 I to M

Figs 33.10A to M: (A to F) Radiological and clinical photographs of an extra-articular fracture of the left distal humerus. Notice the frequently seen free medial fragment, which is most likely iatrogenically produced when the sling is applied. The shoulder is shrugged during the sling application, but when the shoulder relaxes, the inelastic sling forces the fractured humerus into a varus position. Gravity and compression of the tissues by the snuggly held brace restored alignment to an acceptable degree. The patient's large breasts functioned as a fulcrum during the time the arm was held in a sling. The loss of the "carrying angle" of the left arm can best be detected when the elbows are in extension and the forearms in pronation. The original clinical photos (G and H) were taken shortly after the fracture healed, and (I to M) the last ones 9 months after the injury.

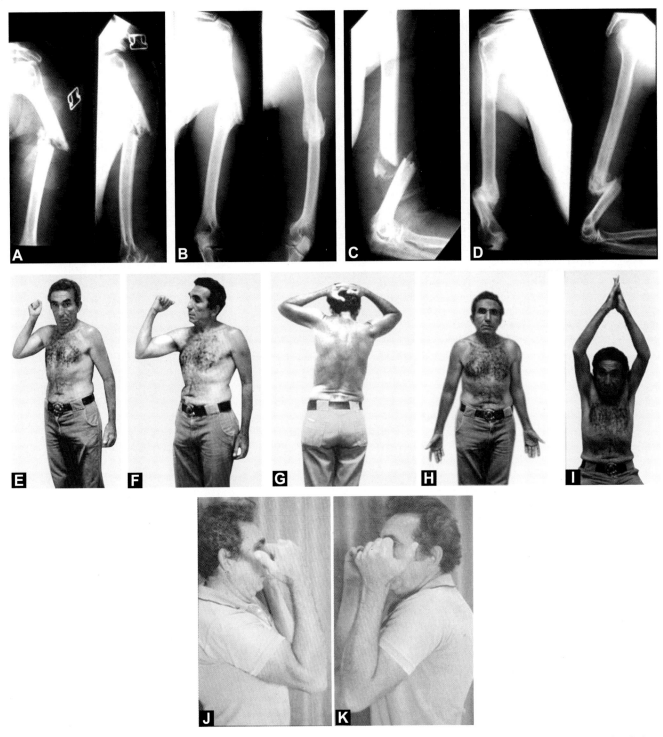

Figs 33.11A to K: (A to D) Radiographs of bilateral humeral fractures sustained in an automobile accident. The patient had associated chest injury. When first seen by us, 3 weeks had already elapsed. The fractures healed with marked angular deformities. (E to I) Patient demonstrates the range of motion of his shoulders and elbows 6 months after the initial insult. (J and K) Photographs taken a year later. Notice the acceptable cosmetic appearance of his arms and the further improved function. (See bilateral fractures)

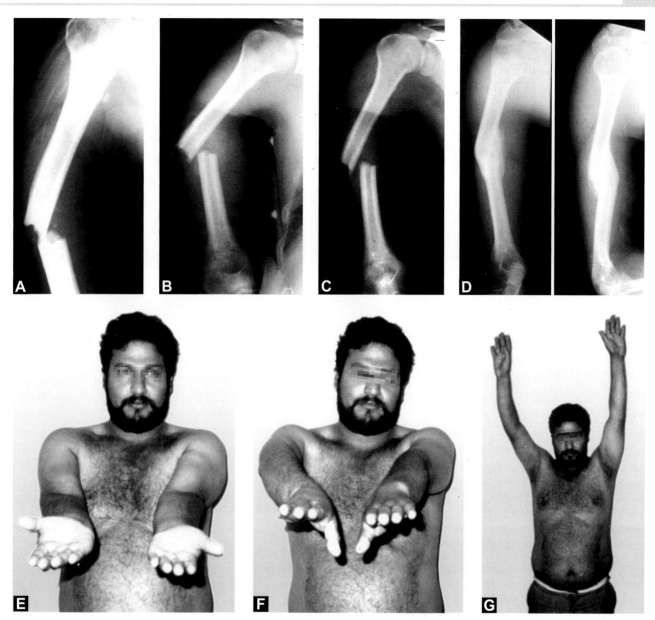

Figs 33.12A to G: (A) Radiograph of closed, transverse fracture of the humeral shaft. (B and C) Patient was seen by us three weeks later with a severe varus deformity. We elected to accept the elbow the angular deformity improved. (D) The fracture healed solidly with a varus deformity. (E to G) Patient demonstrates the acceptable cosmetic of his right arm and the range of motion of his shoulders. Notice that with the shoulder slightly internally rotated and the forearm in pronation, the deformity is more easily recognized.

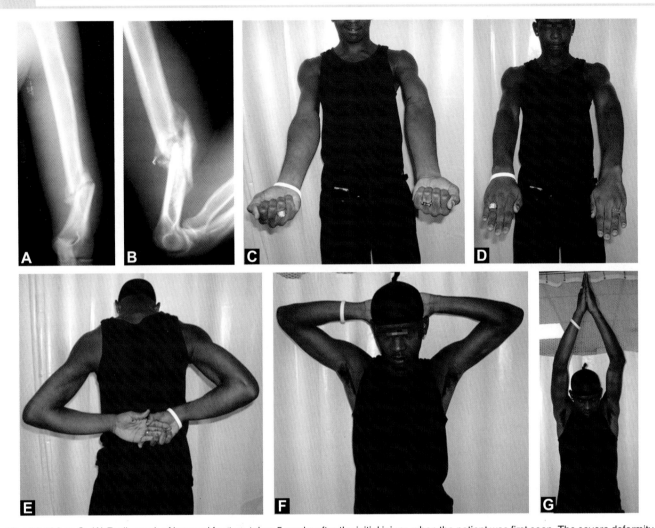

Figs 33.13A to G: (A) Radiograph of humeral fracture taken 5 weeks after the initial injury, when the patient was first seen. The severe deformity in the coronal plane is easily recognized. Notice the large amount of callus that formed in 5 weeks. Patient had discarded the brace 2 weeks after the injury. (B) Lateral radiographs illustrating the severe sagittal deformity. (C to G) Multiple photographs obtained 5 weeks after the initial fracture demonstrating the recognizable deformity and the range of motion of the patient's elbows and shoulders. Patient was lost to further follow-up.

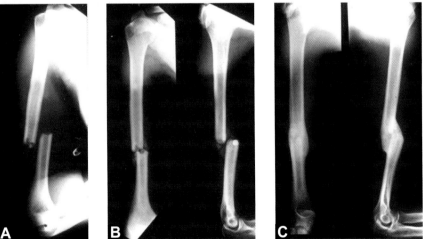

Figs 33.14A to C: (A) Initial radiographs of transverse/laterally displaced fracture in the middle-third of the humerus. (B) Radiograph obtained in the brace. Early callus may be seen 4 weeks after the injury. (C) The fracture healed with good alignment of the fragments.

34

Skin Problems

Complications related to the skin are rare, but have been observed. When they occur, are likely to be secondary to the patient failure to adjust the brace on a frequent basis during the early stages of management. Since the brace is usually applied while the arm still undergoing a reduction of swelling, it is logical that if the straps of the brace are not tightened regularly, the brace would slip distally and compress the antecubital space (Figures 34.1A to C). The other reason is maceration of the tissues under the stockinette due to failure to cleanse the extremity on a regular basis.

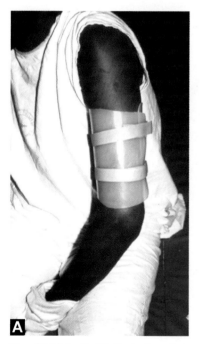 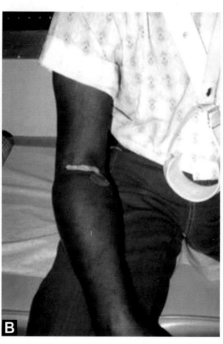 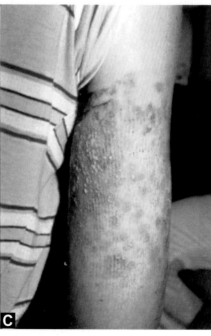

Figs 34.1A to C: (A) Illustration of an experimental brace extending too far distally. As the swelling decreased and no effort was made to maintain the highest position of the brace against the fleshy arm, it began to press against the antecubital space. (B) The constant pressure of the distal sleeve over the antecubital space cuts into the skin. (C) Illustration of skin rash in a patient who as a result of misinformation failed to remove the brace and clean the extremity for 2 weeks.

35

The Polytraumatized Patient

Polytraumatized patients who are unable to ambulate are best treated by surgical means if the medical condition permits a safe intervention. Functional bracing is likely to result in unacceptable angular deformities because of the patient's inability to assume the erect position. However, the approach we have recommended in the case of the bilateral fractures can apply to the polytraumatized patient (Figures 35.1A to G). The literature is rich with data concerning the results from the surgical treatment of the polytraumatized patients, which in general are most satisfactory.[1-6]

Fractures associated with vascular injuries that require surgical repair and stabilization of the fracture, should not be braced early. If surgical stabilization is not carried out at the time the injured vessels are surgically repaired, delayed bracing can be carried out.

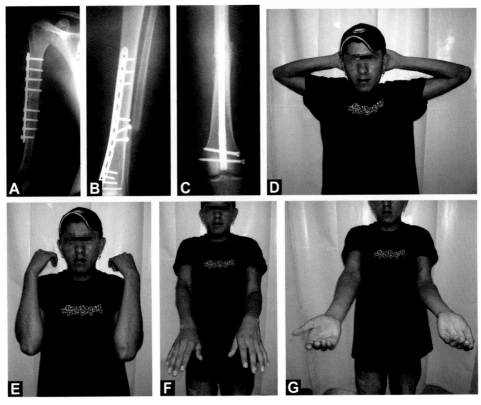

Figs 35.1A to G: (A to C) Radiograph of appropriately surgically treated fractured humerus, tibia and femur. The young patient had sustained multiple fractures in an automobile accident. (D to G) Patient demonstrates very good range of motion of his left upper extremity, lacking only the last few degrees of elbow extension. Photos were taken 4 months postoperatively.

REFERENCES

1. Bleeker WA, Nijsten MW, ten Duis HJ. Treatment of humeral shaft fractures related to associated injuries: A retrospective study of 237 patients. Acta Orthop Scand. 1991; 62(2):148-53.
2. Crates J, Whittle AP. Antegrade interlocking nailing of acute humeral shaft fractures. Clin Orthop. 1998; 350:40-50.
3. Heim D, Herkert F, Hess P, Regazzoni P. Surgical treatment of humeral shaft fractures - the Basel experience. J Trauma. 1993; 35(2):226-32.
4. Liebergall M, Jaber S, Laster M, Aub-Snieneh K, Mattan Y, Segal D. Ender nailing of acute humeral shaft fractures in multiple injuries. Injury. 1997; 28(9-10):577-80.
5. Sarmiento A, Waddell JP, Latta LL. Diaphyseal Humeral Fractures: Treatment Options. An Instructional Course. AAOS J Bone and Joint Surg. 1999; 83A(10):1566-79.
6. Ward EF, Savoie FH, Hughes JL. Fractures of the diaphyseal humerus. In: Browner, Jupiter, Levine, Trafton (Eds). Skeletal Trauma. WB Saunders. 1992; 2:1177-200.

36

The Open Fracture

Although the place for functional bracing of humeral fractures is primarily in closed fractures, open fractures which are not associated with major soft tissue damage may be successfully treated with the bracing technique. Those open fractures with major soft tissue damage may be successfully braced following a period of rest after the necessary debridement of the damaged tissue has been completed. When external fixators are used as the initial means of stabilization, the risk of nonunion is greater, because the apparatus rigidly holds the fragments; therefore discouraging osteogenesis. Despite this potential disadvantage, external fixation is today a preferred method of treatment for these fractures, especially if there is an associated peripheral nerve or vascular injury.[1-4]

Many surgeons prefer plating, particularly if the fracture is associated with a nerve or vessel injury.[5-16] Intramedullary nailing may also be an appropriate treatment under those circumstances, though the complication rate from nailing is high.[3,17-30]

However, if the soft tissue damage is not major and there is no vertical distraction between the main fragments, functional bracing may effectively be used. Low velocity gunshot-produced fractures are usually associated with some comminution, but the degree of soft tissue pathology is usually mild. Therefore, the healing of these fractures takes place at a pace comparable to that of closed fractures. Oftentimes the lateral displacement of the comminuted fragments enlarges the diameter of the callus resulting in an ultimately very strong bone at the level of the old fracture. The initially enlarged diameter of the bone at the level of the fracture, spontaneously decreases, from the compression of the soft tissues by the functional sleeve and the gravity effect at the fracture site (Figures 36.1 to 36.5).

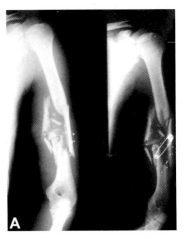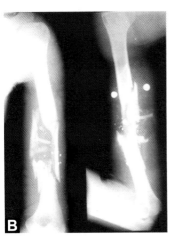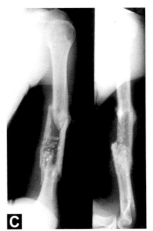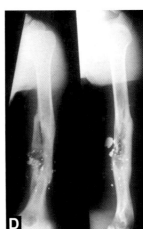

Figs 36.1A to D: (A) Radiograph of comminuted fracture of the humerus produced by a low-velocity projectile. (B) Radiograph obtained 2 weeks after the injury. (C) Radiographs obtained 2½ months after the accident. Notice the desirable enlarged diameter of the bone at the level of the fracture. (D) Final radiographs taken 4 months after the initial injury.

We have not used functional bracing in the management of intra-articular fractures of the distal humerus, since it is very likely that the clinical and radiological results would be unsatisfactory in too many instances. The resulting articular cartilage incongruity could be of a degree greater than the one normally tolerated. We recognize the fact that internal fixation of these fractures can be accomplished in most instances with varying degrees of success. Early range of motion following surgery gives the best functional results; however, residual limitation of motion is not uncommon, particularly extension in the last few degrees.

Had this fracture been treated with conventional surgical methods, it is likely that the ultimate result may have not been better. Internal fixation of these fractures oftentimes leave residual limitation of motion. The residual articular incongruity that this fracture experienced may not be of importance, since instability is not present. The cartilage probably remodeled.

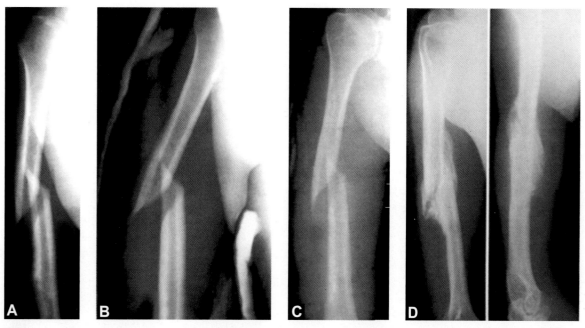

Figs 36.2A to D: Sequential radiographs of diaphyseal fracture produced by a low-velocity bullet. Notice the spontaneous alignment of the fragments following application of the brace.

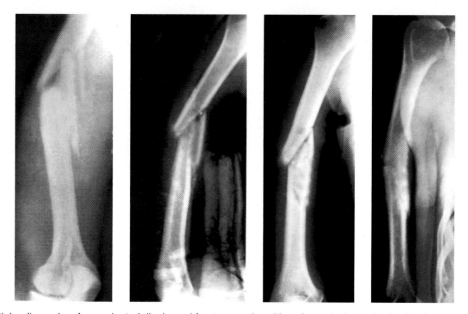

Fig. 36.3: Sequential radiographs of comminuted diaphyseal fracture produced by a low-velocity projectile. The fracture healed uneventfully.

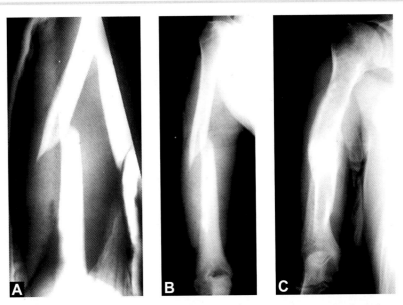

Figs 36.4A to C: (A) Radiograph of open fracture produced by a low-velocity bullet. (B)) Radiograph taken after application of the brace. (C) Radiograph obtained 6 months after the initial insult. The bullet fragments had been removed upon patient's request.

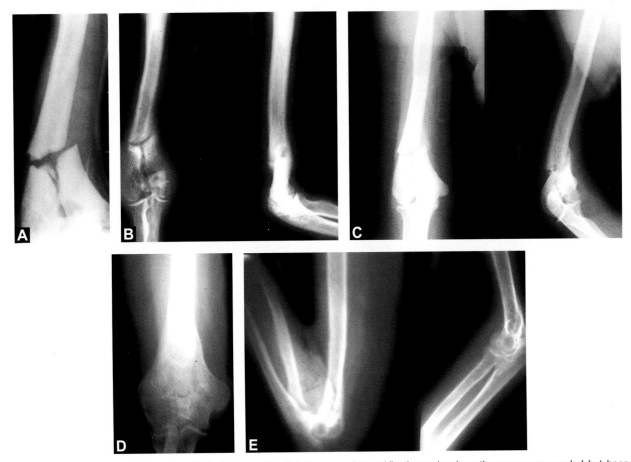

Figs 36.5A to E: (A) Low-grade open intra-articular fracture of the distal humerus. Internal fixation and early motion was recommended, but, because of the patient's religious reasons against surgery, the fracture was treated with a brace. (B) Radiograph taken through the brace demonstrating adequate alignment of the fragments. (C) The fracture demonstrating further healing and limitation of extension. (D) Radiograph obtained 2 months later showing solid union of the fracture. (E) Radiographs demonstrating the range of motion at that time. Patient was lost to follow-up.

REFERENCES

1. Bleeker WA, Nijsten MW, ten Duis HJ. Treatment of humeral shaft fractures related to associated injuries: A retrospective study of 237 patients. Acta Orthop Scand. 1991; 62(2):148-53.

2. Joshi A, Labbe M, Lindsey RW. Humeral fracture secondary to civilian gunshot injury. Injury. 1998; 29 Suppl 1:SA13-17.

3. Liebergall M, Jaber S, Laster M, Aub-Snieneh K, Mattan Y, Segal D. Ender nailing of acute humeral shaft fractures in multiple injuries. Injury. 1997; 28(9-10):577-80.

4. Wisniewski TF, Radziejowski MJ. Gunshot fractures of the humeral shaft treated with external fixation. J Orthop Trauma. 1996; 10(4):273-87.

5. Aiken GK, Rorabeck CH. Distal humeral fractures in the adult. Clin Orthop Relat Res. 1986; 207:191-7.

6. Gill DR, Torchia ME. The spiral compression plate for proximal humeral shaft nonunion: A case report and description of a new technique. J Orthop Trauma. 1999; 13(2):141-4.

7. Ekholm R, Adami J, Tidemark K, Hansson K, Tornkvist H, Ponzer S. Fractures of the shaft of the humerus: An epidemiological study of 401 fractures. J Bone Joint Surg Br. 2006 Nov; 88(11):1469-73.

8. Gardner MJ, Voos JE, Wanich T, Helfet DL, Lorich DG. Vascular complications of minimally invasive plating of proximal humeral fractures. J Orthop Trauma. 2006 Oct; 20(9):602.

9. Heim D, Herkert F, Hess P, Regazzoni P. Surgical treatment of humeral shaft fractures - the Basel experience. J Trauma. 1993; 35(2):226-32.

10. Jawa A, McCarthy P, Doornberg J, Harris M, Ring D. Extra-articular distal-third diaphyseal fractures of the humerus. J Bone and Joint. 2006; 88A(11):2343-7.

11. Joshi A, Labbe M, Lindsey RW. Humeral fracture secondary to civilian gunshot injury. Injury. 1998; 29 Suppl 1:SA13-17.

12. Olerud S, Dankwardt-Lilliestrom G. Fracture healing in compression osteosynthesis. Acta Orthop Scand Suppl. 1971; 137:1-44.

13. Perren SM. Physical and biological aspects of fracture healing with special reference to internal fixation. Clin Orthop Relat Res. 1979; 138:175.

14. Perren SM, Rahn B. Biomechanics of fracture healing I: Historical review and mechanical aspects of internal fixation. Orthop Surg. 1978; 2:108.

15. Ring D, Perey BH, Jupiter JB. The functional outcome of operative treatment of ununited fractures of the humeral diaphysis in older patients. J Bone Joint Surg. 1999; 81A(2):177-19.

16. Wasmer G, Worsdorfer O. Functional Management of Humeral Shaft Fractures with Sarmiento Cast Bracing. Unfallheilkunde, 1984; 87:309.

17. Crates J, Whittle AP. Antegrade interlocking nailing of acute humeral shaft fractures. Clin Orthop. 1998; 350:40-50.

18. Emmerson KP, Sher JL. A method of treatment of nonunion of humeral shaft fractures following treatment by locked intramedullary nail: A report of three cases. Injury. 1998; 29(7):550-2.

19. Flinkkila T, Hyvonen P, Lakovaara M, Linden T, Ristiniemi J, Hamalainen M. Intramedullary nailing of humeral shaft fractures: A retrospective study of 126 cases. Acta Orthop Scand. 1999; 70(2):133-6.

20. Hems TE, Bhuller TP. Interlocking nailing of humeral shaft fractures: The Oxford experience 1991 to 1994. Injury. 1996; 27(7):485-9.

21. Lin J, Hou SM: Antegrade locking nailing for humeral shaft fractures. Clin Orthop. 1999; 365:201-10.

22. Lin J, Inoue N, Valdevit A, Hang YS, Hou SM, Chao EY. Biomechanical comparison of antegrade and retrograde nailing of humeral shaft fracture. Clin Orthop. 1998; 351:203-13.

23. Lin J. Treatment of humeral shaft fractures with humeral locked nail and comparison with plate fixation. J Trauma. 1998; 44(5): 859-64.

24. Moran MC. Distal interlocking during intramedullary nailing of the humerus. Clin Orthop. 1995; 317:215-8.

25. Rommens PM, Blum J, Runkel M. Retrograde nailing of humeral shaft fractures. Clin Orthop. 1998; 350:26-39.

26. Rodriguez-Merchan EC. Hackethal nailing in closed transverse humeral shaft fractures after failed manipulation. Int. Orthop. 1996; 20(3):134-6.

27. Rupp RE, Chrissos MG, Ebraheim NA. The risk of neurovascular injury with distal locking screws of humeral intramedullary nails. Orthopedics. 1996; 19(7):593-5.

28. Svend-Hansen H, Skettrup M, Rathcke MW. Complications using the Seidel intramedullary humeral nail: outcome in 31 patients. Acta Orthop Belgica. 1998; 64(3):291-5.

29. Thomsen NOB, Mikkelsen JB, Svendsen RN, Skovgaard N, Jensen CH, Jorgensen U. Interlocking nailing of humeral shaft fractures. J Orthop Sci. 1998; 3(4):199-203.

30. Wu CC, Shih CH. Treatment of nonunion of the shaft of the humerus: Comparison of plates and Seidel interlocking nails. Comments. Canadian J Surg. 1992; 35(6):576.

37

The Proximal-third Fractures and Representative Examples

The level of the fracture does not appear to have an influence on the ultimate result since fractures at various levels seem to heal at the same speed and with similar degrees of angulation. The brace does not have to fully cover very proximal or distal fragments is irrelevant (Figure 37.1A to C).

As long as the soft tissues of the extremity are compressed by the adjustable brace and the arm hangs freely at the side of the body, the desirable environment for healing is present.

Some of the representative examples illustrating fractures in proximal-third of the humerus are shown in Figures 37.2 to 37.13.

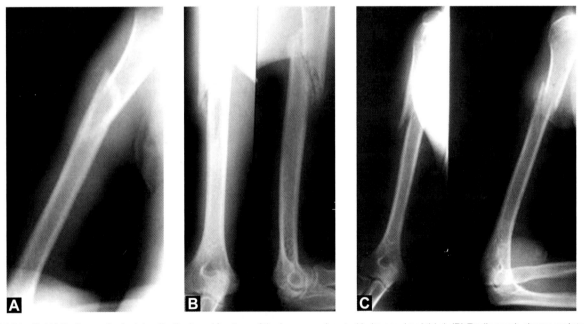

Figs 37.1A to C: (A) Radiograph of minimally displaced fracture of the humerus, located in its proximal third. (B) Radiograph shows maintenance of good alignment, and early callus formation. Notice that the brace does not fully cover the fracture site. (C) The fracture healed uneventfully. Notice that the brace does not cover the fracture site. However, the compression of the tissues by the brace provides the necessary stability to allow uneventful healing.

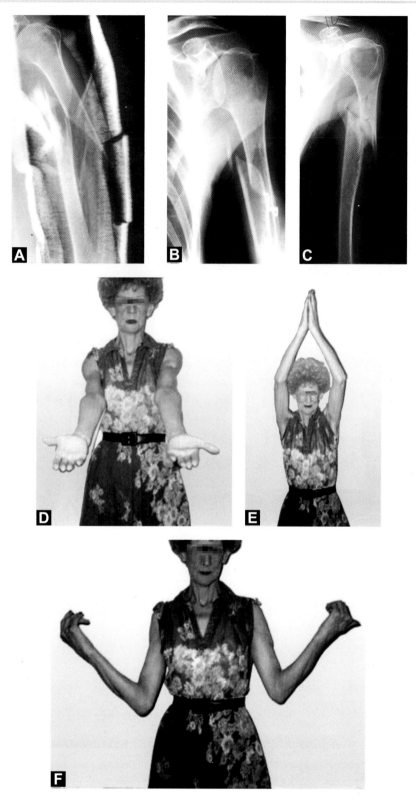

Figs 37.2A to F:(A) Oblique fracture of the proximal humerus. (B) Spontaneous correction of the initial deformity obtained through the compression of the soft tissues by the adjustable brace, and the effect of gravity. (C) The fracture healed in good alignment. (D to F) Patient demonstrates the functional range of motion of the shoulder and the aesthetic appearance of the extremity.

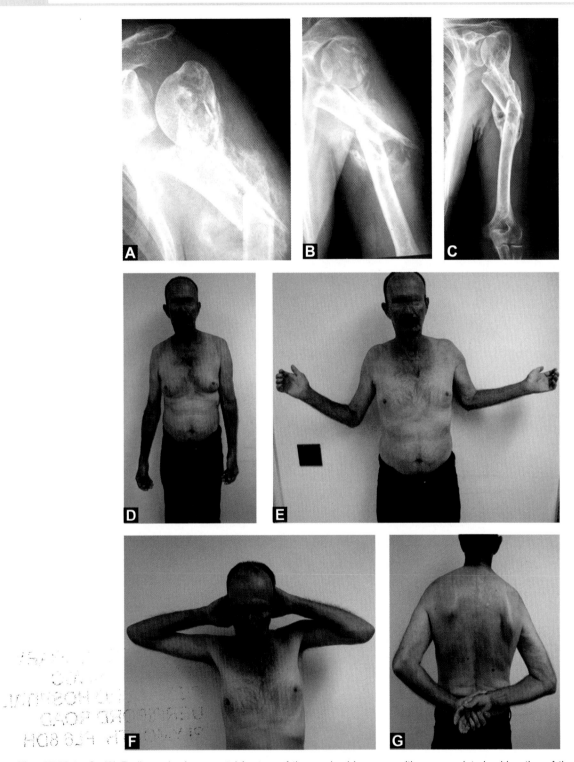

Figs 37.3A to G: (A) Radiograph of segmental fracture of the proximal humerus with an associated subluxation of the humeral head. The patient had been injured when hit by a moving vehicle. For unknown reasons, he spent 4 weeks in a nursing home without receiving care for his fractured humerus. When seen by us at that time, there was already evidence of callus formation. Plans to handle the condition nonsurgically at first and then to carry out surgery if necessary were accepted by the patient. Notice the subluxated humeral head. (B) Radiograph obtained 3 weeks later after a program of active flexion and extension of the elbow. Notice the re-positioning of the humeral head in the glenoid. (C) Radiographs taken 6 months post-injury. (D to G) Patient demonstrates, 6 months after the fracture occurred, the range of motion of this injured extremity. The shoulder is painless and motion is improving gradually.

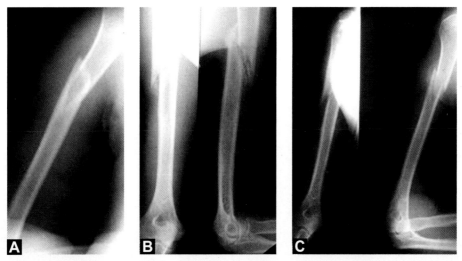

Figs 37.4A to C: (A) Radiograph of minimally displaced fracture of the humerus, located in its proximal-third. (B) Radiograph shows maintenance of good alignment, and early callus formation. (C) The fracture healed uneventfully.

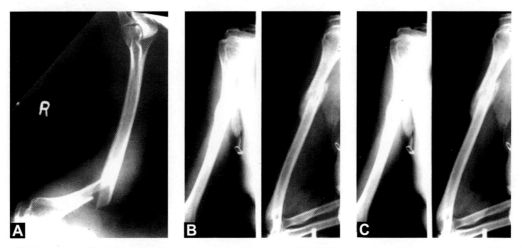

Figs 37.5A to C: (A) Radiograph illustrating an oblique fracture in the proximal-third of the humerus with severe angular deformity. The valgus deformity present in this instance is most unusual. When found, it is usually in fractures of the proximal-third of the diaphysis. (B and C) By simply allowing the extremity to hang over the side of the body, the deformity corrects spontaneously. Under no circumstances should angular deformities be corrected through forceful manipulation.

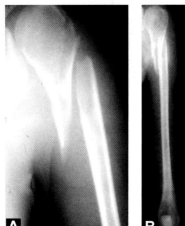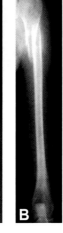

Figs 37.6A and B: (A) Radiograph of oblique fracture in the proximal-third of the humerus. (B) Radiograph taken 4 weeks after the injury. A brace had been applied on the 7th day post injury. Patient was then lost to follow-up.

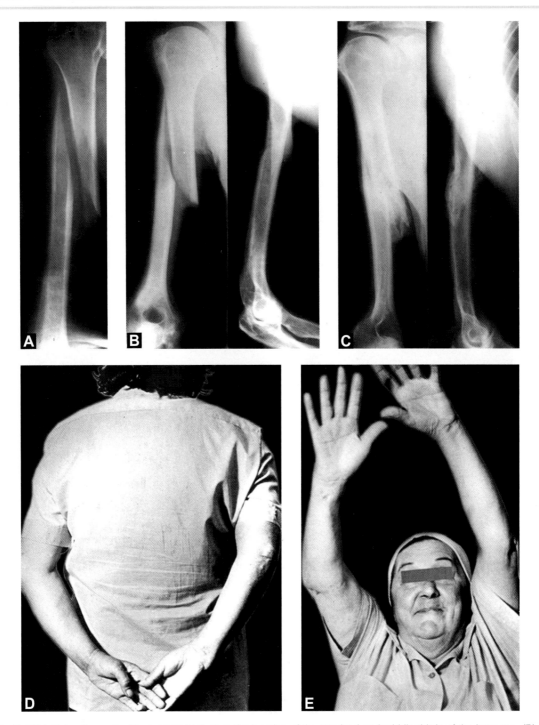

Figs 37.7A to E: (A) Initial radiograph of long spiral fracture at the junction of the proximal and middle-thirds of the humerus. (B) Radiograph obtained approximately 2 weeks after application of the brace. (C) Radiograph taken 10 weeks after the initial injury. The fracture healed uneventfully. The initial shortening improved when the arm was allowed to hang freely at the side of the body. (D and E) Patient demonstrates elevation and internal rotation of the shoulders.

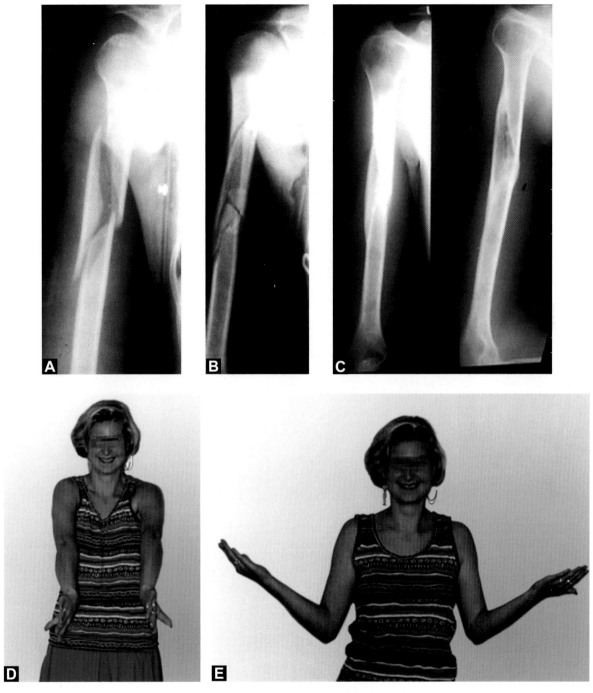

Figs 37.8A to E: (A) Radiograph of fracture in the proximal-third of the humerus. Notice the subluxation of the humeral head. (B) Radiograph obtained after stabilization of the fracture in a brace. (C) Following completion of healing, notice the relocated humeral head through the conduct of early flexion and extension of the elbow. The contracting biceps, brachialis and triceps-all with insertions on the scapula and humerus shaft-gradually push the shaft superiorly and reduce the subluxation. (D and E) Patient demonstrating the range of motion of her injured shoulder upon completion of healing.

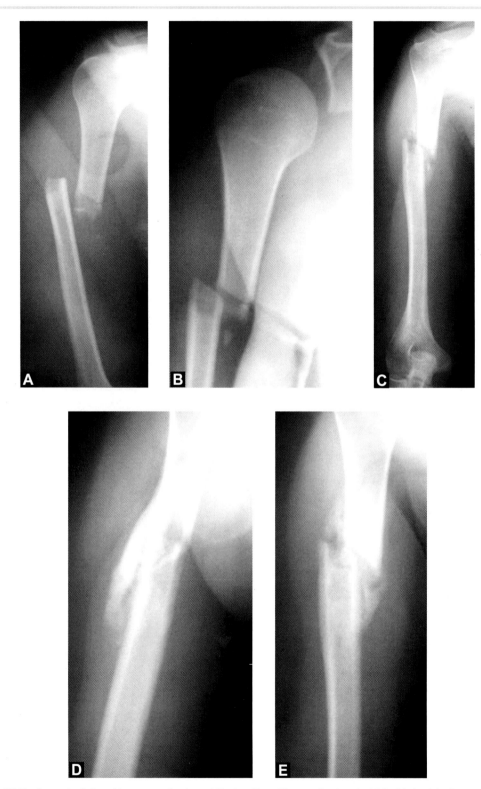

Figs 37.9A to E: (A) Radiograph of closed transverse fracture at the junction of the proximal and middle thirds of the humeral diaphysis. (B) The initial severe displacement improved spontaneously after the application of the brace. Notice the secondary subluxation of the humeral head. (C to E) Radiographs illustrating the continued improvement in the alignment of the fragments and progressive healing. The alignment of the fragment was very good. The brace was discontinued at this time. The motion of the shoulder was limited in the last few degrees of external rotation, which as anticipated will be overcome within the next few weeks. The patient was lost to follow-up.

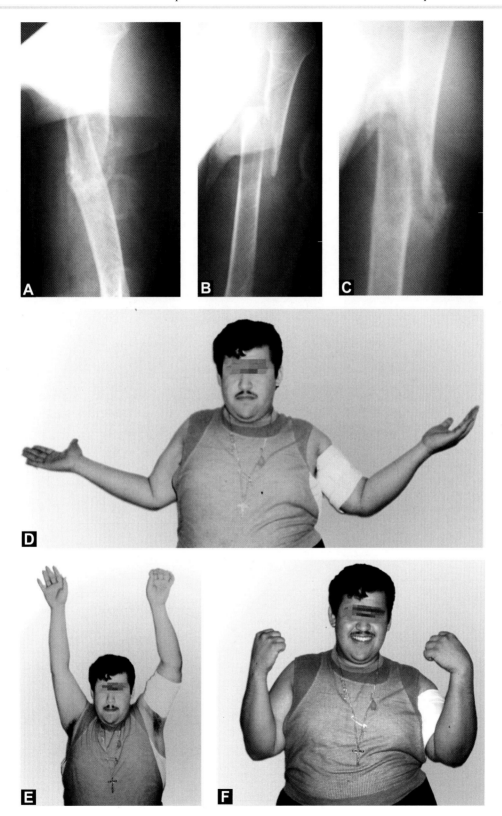

Figs 37.10A to F: (A) Radiograph of oblique fracture in the proximal-third of the humerus. (B) Radiograph taken 4 weeks later. (C) Radiograph obtained 2½ months after the initial injury. The brace was discontinued at this time. (D to F) Patient demonstrates the range of motion of this shoulder and elbow joints.

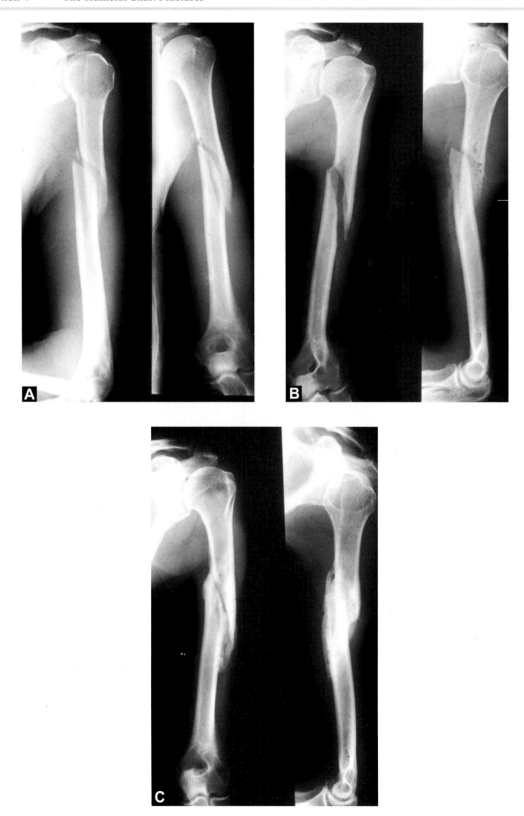

Figs 37.11A to C: (A) Radiograph of long-oblique fracture demonstrates the minimal shortening and acceptable alignment of the fragments. (B) Radiograph obtained 2½ days after the initial injury. Notice that the sleeve does not cover the fracture. (C) Radiograph taken 8 months after the initial fracture. The alignment of the fragments is very acceptable.

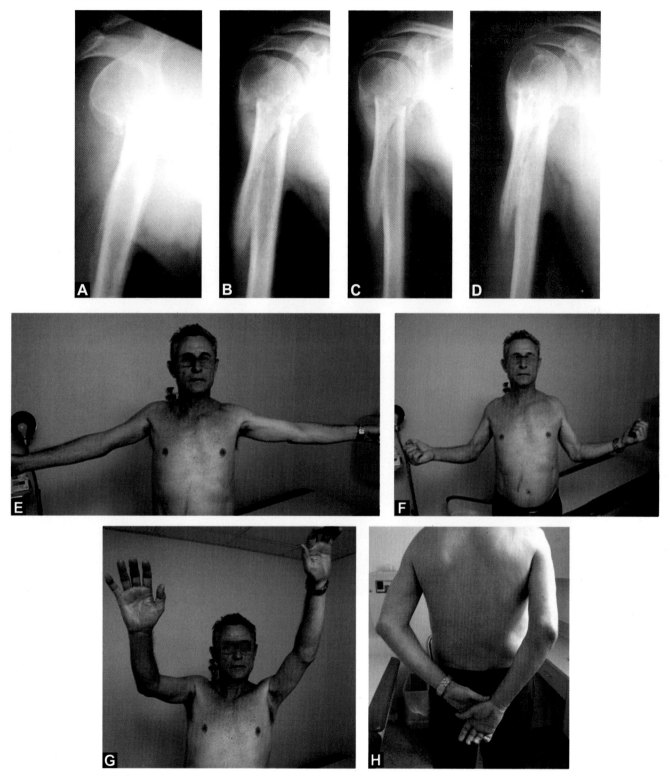

Figs 37.12A to H: (A) Radiograph of fracture of the proximal humerus. This radiograph failed to show the more complex nature of the fracture as depicted in subsequent radiographs. (B) Radiograph obtained after application of the brace showing the comminution of the fracture and its extension into the humeral shaft. (C) Radiograph obtained 3 weeks after bracing. (D) Radiograph taken 7 weeks after the initial injury. (E to H) Patient demonstrates the range of motion of his injured upper extremity 7 weeks after the initial insult. Though motion of the shoulder is still limited, improvement was taking place when his last photos were taken 7 weeks post-injury.

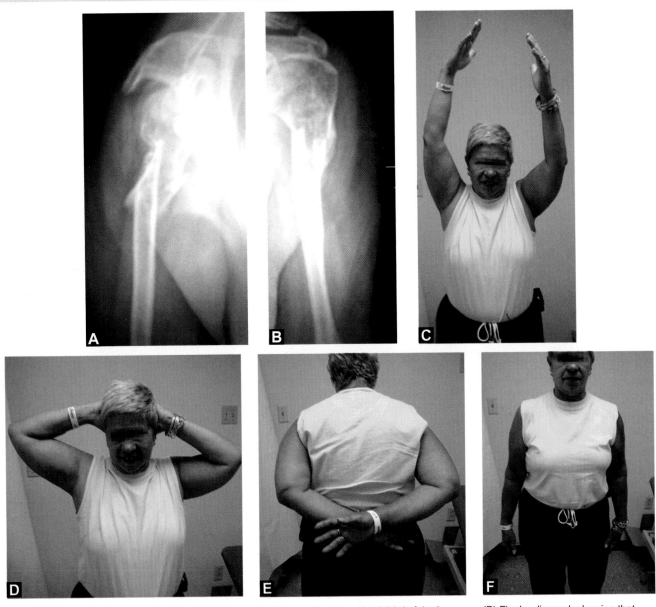

Figs 37.13A to F: (A) Initial radiograph of comminuted fracture in the proximal-third of the humerus. (B) Final radiograph showing that the fracture healed in good alignment. (C to F) Patient demonstrates the range of motion of her shoulders.

38

The Middle-third Fractures and Representative Examples

The majority of humeral diaphyseal fractures occur in its middle-third, and most frequently from a fall to the ground, in which case the fracture is usually of a transverse nature. Elderly osteoporotic patients frequently experience this type of fracture. A twisting injury produces fractures which are either comminuted, oblique or spiral. An associated radial palsy is rather common. In our series, the incidence is 11%.

Fractures, the result of severe injuries, associated with significant soft tissue damage, are prone to show distal separation between the major fragments. This separation oftentimes leads to nonunion of the fracture. In such cases, surgical stabilization may be the treatment of choice. If associated nerve palsy is present, the prognosis is seriously guarded.

Some of the representative samples illustrating middle-third fractures of humerus are shown in Figures 38.1 to 38.28.

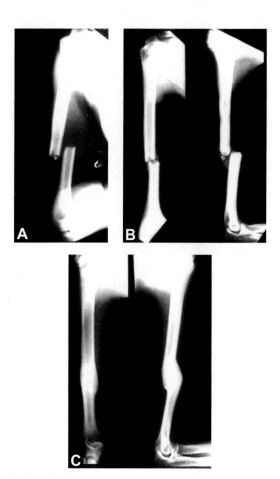

Figs 38.2A to C: (A) Radiograph of transverses fracture of the humeral diaphysis demonstrating overriding of the fragments. (B) Radiograph obtained through the brace showing spontaneous alignment of the fragments, but with persistence of reduced overriding. (C) The fracture healed uneventfully with very good alignment. Transverse fractures showing overriding have a good prognosis, since the desirable motion that takes place at the fracture site is of a pistoning, elastic nature. Angular deformity under this circumstance is easily prevented. On the other hand, transverse, non-displaced fractures are prone to varus angulation.

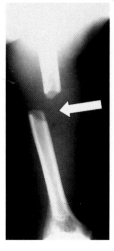

Fig. 38.1: Radiograph of transverse fracture in the middle-third of the humeral diaphysis, the result of a severe injury. The distal separation between the fragments suggests major soft tissue damage. An associated radial palsy makes the prognosis poor and the treatment consists of brace stabilization. Plate fixation is usually the treatment of choice.

Contrary to popular belief, transverse nondisplaced fractures are not the ones with the best prognosis. They tend to angulate if premature active elevation or abduction of the shoulder is done, prior to the development of intrinsic fracture stability. The displaced fracture has a better prognosis; and the best prognosis is for the oblique or comminuted fractures. They heal with abundant peripheral callus, and are subjected to healthy pistoning motion at the fracture site.

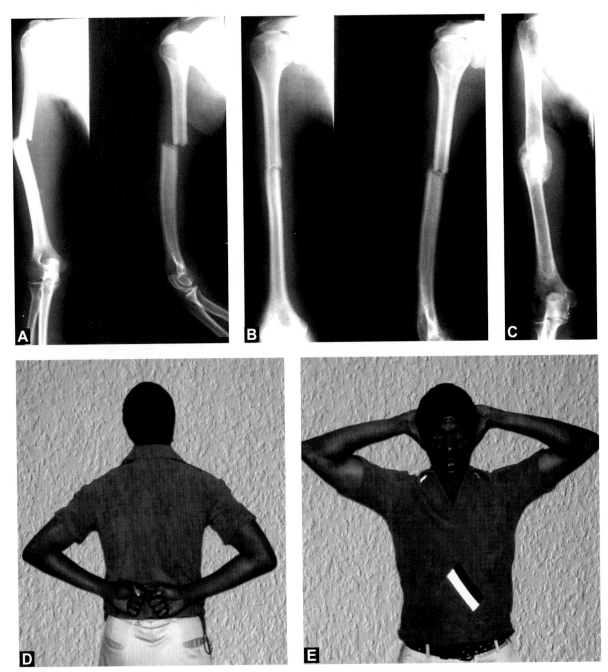

Figs 38.3A to E: (A) Radiograph of transverse fracture of the humeral diaphysis showing a varus angulation and mild displacement of the fragments. (B) The brace, which compresses the soft tissues, plus the weight of the arm, spontaneously aligned the fragments almost anatomically. (C) The fracture healed with abundant callus. (D and E) Patient demonstrates the function of his elbows and shoulder.

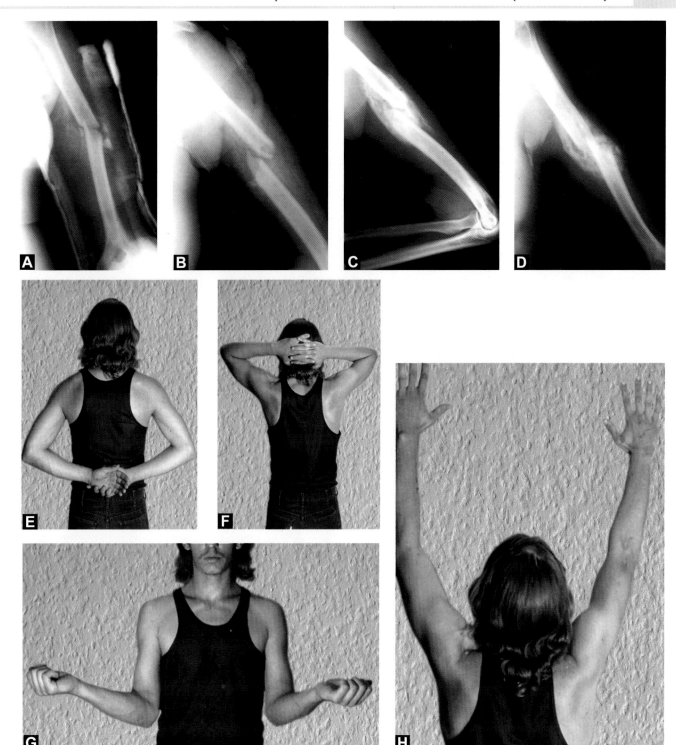

Figs 38.4A to H: (A to D) Radiographs of fracture in the middle-third of the humeral shaft treated with a functional brace. The fracture healed with acceptable alignment. (E to H) Photographs of patient demonstrating the range of motion of his upper extremities. Notice the residual limitation of external rotation, which is likely to improve with use of the extremity.

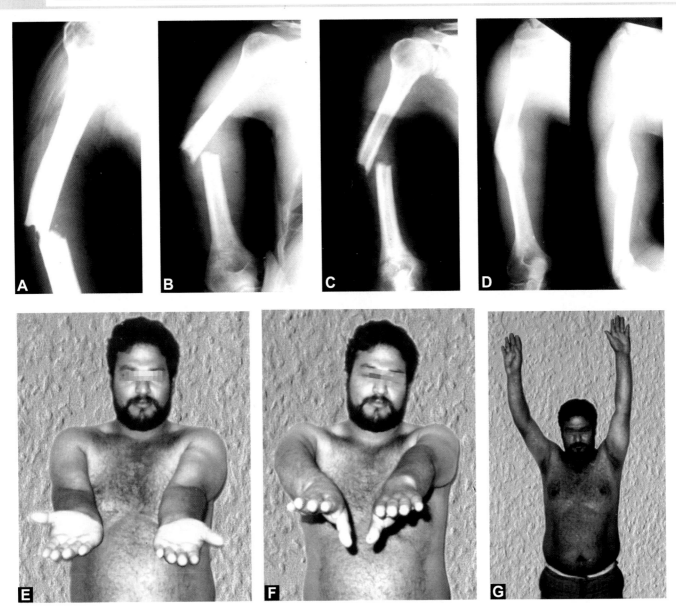

Figs 38.5A to G: (A to D) Radiograph of transverse fracture of the humeral diaphysis showing a severe varus angular deformity. (B) The patient was first seen 23 days after the initial injury. The initial deformity had been made worse by a sling that forced the elbow into extreme flexion. (C) Radiograph taken through the brace showing mild correction of the deformity from the compression of the tissues provided by the adjustable brace and the dependency of the extremity. (D) Radiograph taken after union of the fracture had taken place. Notice that the ultimate deformity, though less than the original one, improved significantly. (E to G) The patient demonstrates the acceptable appearance of the extremity and the range of motion of the elbow and shoulder. Notice that with the shoulder in internal rotation and the forearm in pronation, the deformity is more easily recognized.

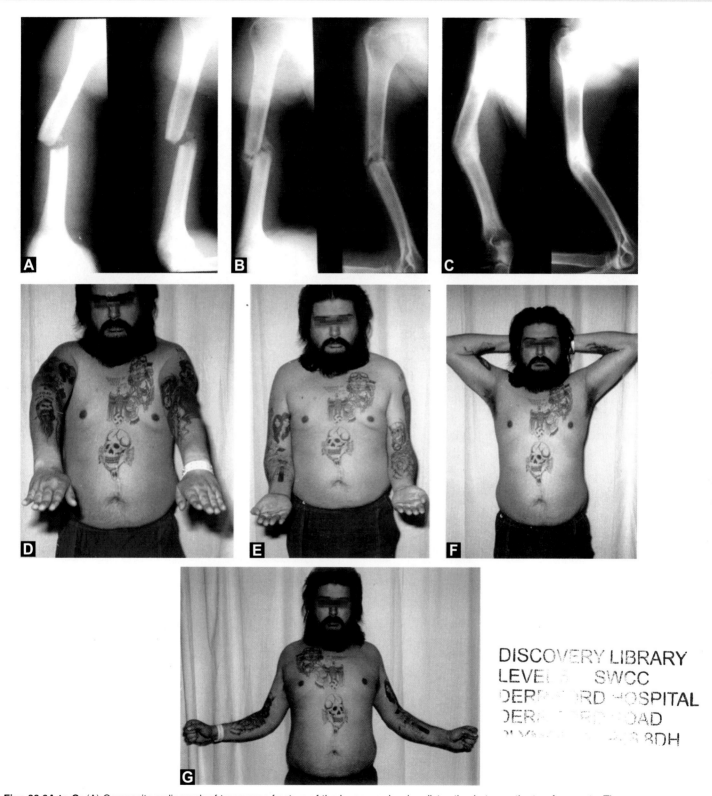

Figs 38.6A to G: (A) Composite radiograph of transverse fracture of the humerus showing distraction between the two fragments. The x-rays were taken through the brace. (B) Two months later, there was evidence of early callus and a varus deformity. (C) The patient failed to return for follow up. When finally convinced to have new x-rays taken, the films demonstrated a severe deformity. (D to G) Patient, a motorcyclist, demonstrates the appearance of the extremities and the range of motion of the elbows and shoulders.

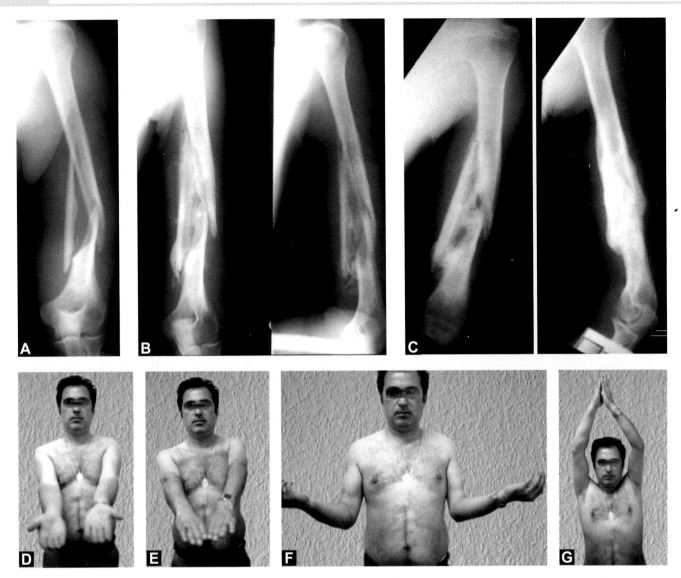

Figs 38.7A to G: (A) Radiograph of comminuted fracture of the humeral diaphysis illustrating severe coronal separation between the fragments. (B) Radiograph taken through the brace demonstrating spontaneous improved alignment of the fragments and early callus. (C) Final radiograph showing a solidly united fracture with a mild varus angular deformity. (D to G) Patient demonstrates the appearance of the extremities and the range of motion of his shoulders. Notice that the varus deformity is always best demonstrated when the shoulder is in neutral rotation, but the forearm is in pronation.

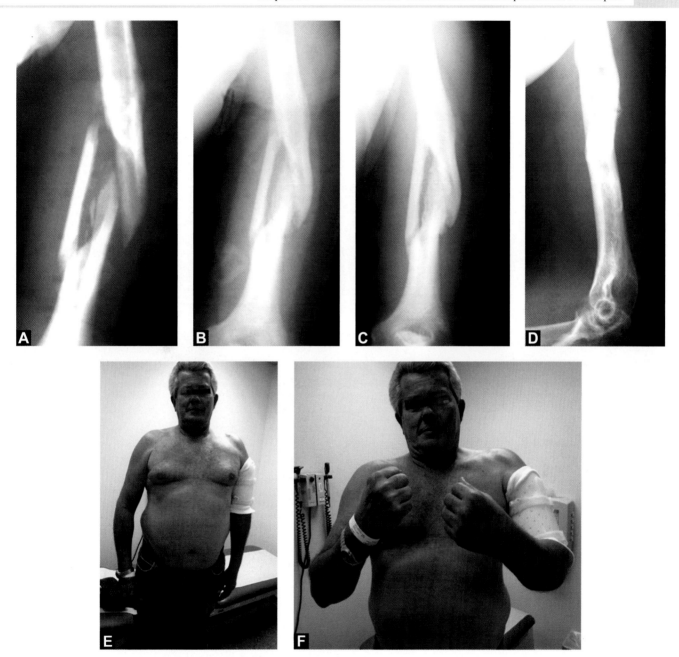

Figs 38.8A to F: (A) Radiograph of comminuted fracture, the result of an automobile accident. (B) Radiograph obtained 3 months post-injury showing peripheral healing. (C and D) Radiographs obtained 4½ months after the initial injury. (E and F) Clinical photos taken 3 months after the accident, showing the range of motion of his elbows. The brace was discontinued at that time.

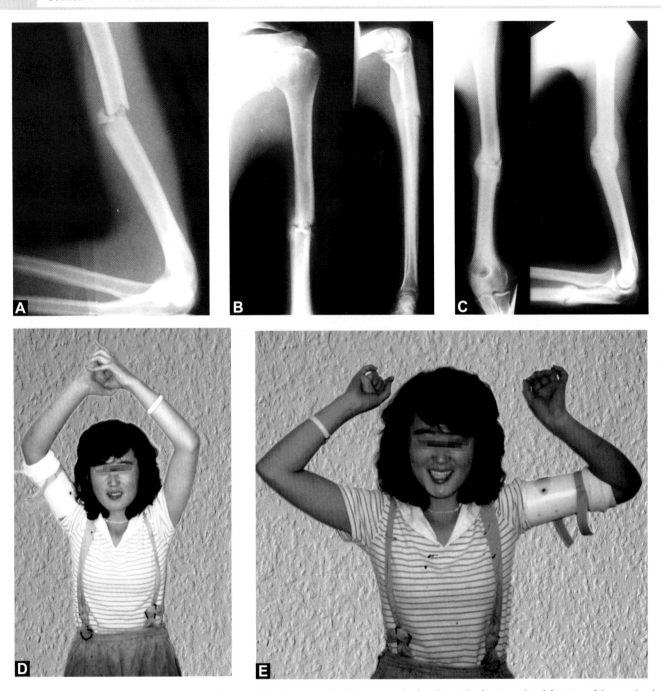

Figs 38.9A to E: (A) Radiograph of transverse fracture of the humerus showing an anterior bowing at the fracture site. A fracture of the proximal ulna was also present. (B) Radiograph taken through the brace showing early callus in the humeral and ulnar fractures. The ulna was treated with a functional sleeve. (C) Radiographs demonstrating solid union of the humeral and ulnar fractures. The original anterior bowing of the humerus became slightly worse. Failure to mobilize the elbow early to regain full extension may aggravate the angular deformity. As the elbow is extended, the weight of the distal arm forces the fracture to angulate in that manner. (D and E) Photographs of patient demonstrating range of motion of her elbows and shoulders.

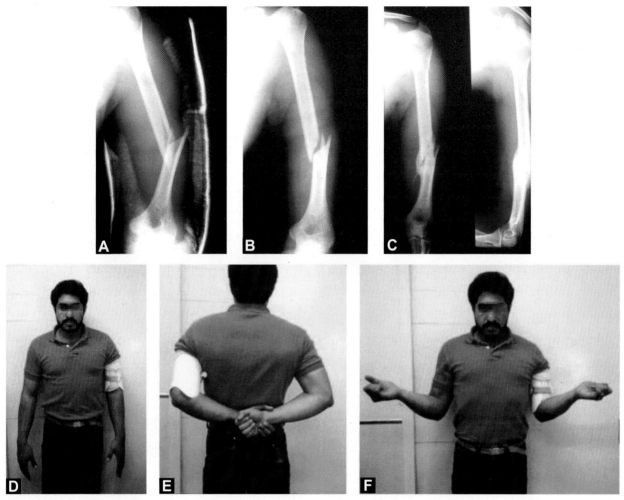

Figs 38.10A to F: (A to C) Radiograph of oblique fracture showing a severe varus angulation. The angulation was probably created by the sling applied immediately after the injury. The sling places pressure over the forearm distally and over the shoulder proximally. This pressure is aggravated when the sling is applied while the patient's shoulder is shrugged. When the shoulder relaxes, the pressure over the shoulder and forearm is increased. (D to F) The patient demonstrates the range of motion of his shoulder and forearm.

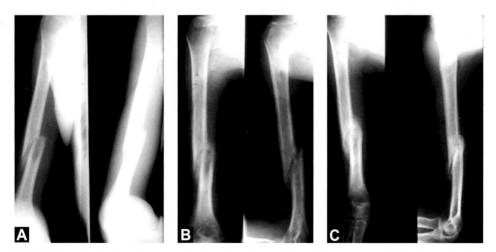

Figs 38.11A to C: (A) Radiograph of oblique fracture showing minimal overriding of the fragments. (B) Radiograph taken 2 weeks after the initial insult. (C) Radiograph obtained approximately 5 months after the injury.

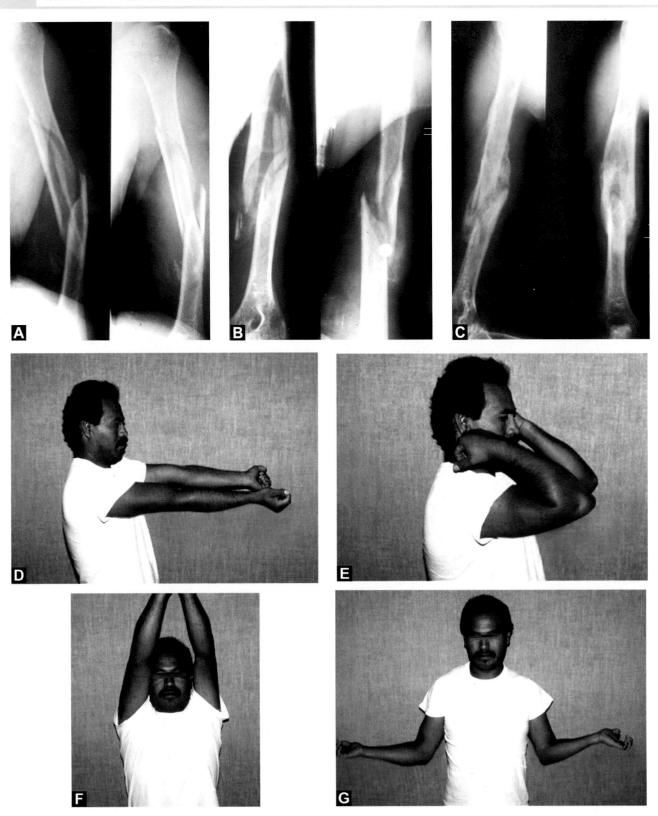

Figs 38.12A to G: (A) Radiograph of comminuted fracture of the humeral diaphysis. (B) Radiograph taken 5 weeks following the initial injury. Notice the abundant peripheral callus. (C) Radiograph obtained 10 weeks after the application of the brace. (D to G) Patient demonstrates the range of motion of his arms.

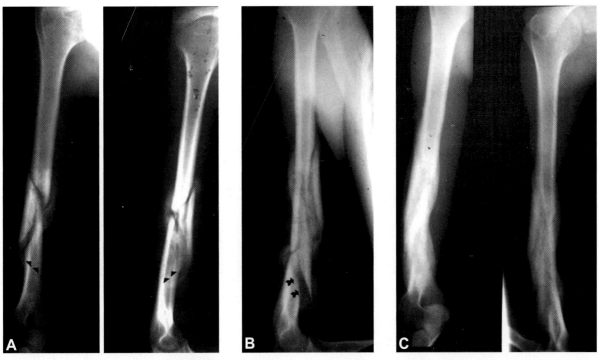

Figs 38.13A to C: (A) Radiograph of comminuted fracture obtained 5 weeks after the initial injury. (B) Patient was lost to follow-up, but returned after sustaining a new injury that produced a fracture below the old one. (C) The brace was reapplied and the fracture healed uneventfully.

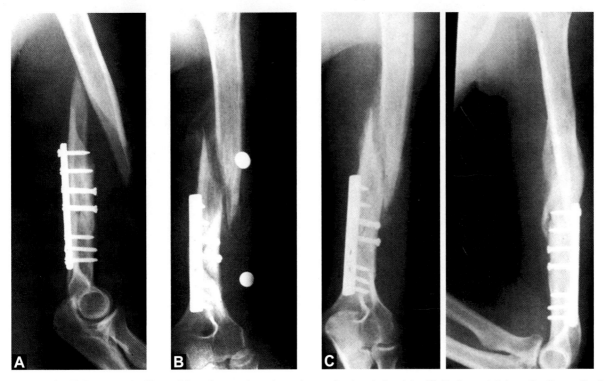

Figs 38.14A to C: (A) Radiograph of long oblique fracture just above the proximal end of a plate. (B) Radiograph taken after the application of the functional brace. (C) Radiograph taken 6 weeks later. Notice the early bridging callus.

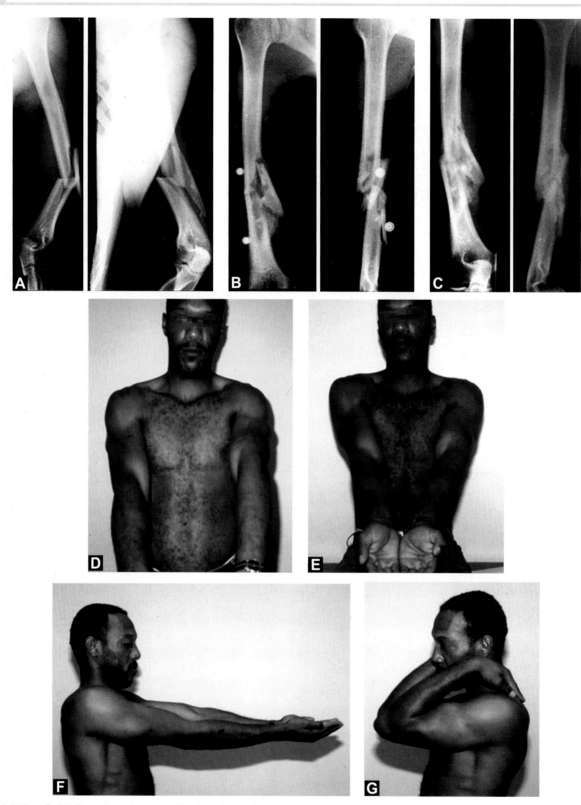

Figs 38.15A to G: (A) Comminuted fracture showing a lateral free fragment. Usually the fragment is located in the medial side. (B) Radiograph obtained after the brace was applied. The compression of the soft tissues by the brace and the weight of the extremity after extension of the elbow was regained, resulted in appropriate re-alignment of the bone. (C) Radiograph showing solid healing of the bone. (D to G) Patient demonstrates the normal range of motion of his arms.

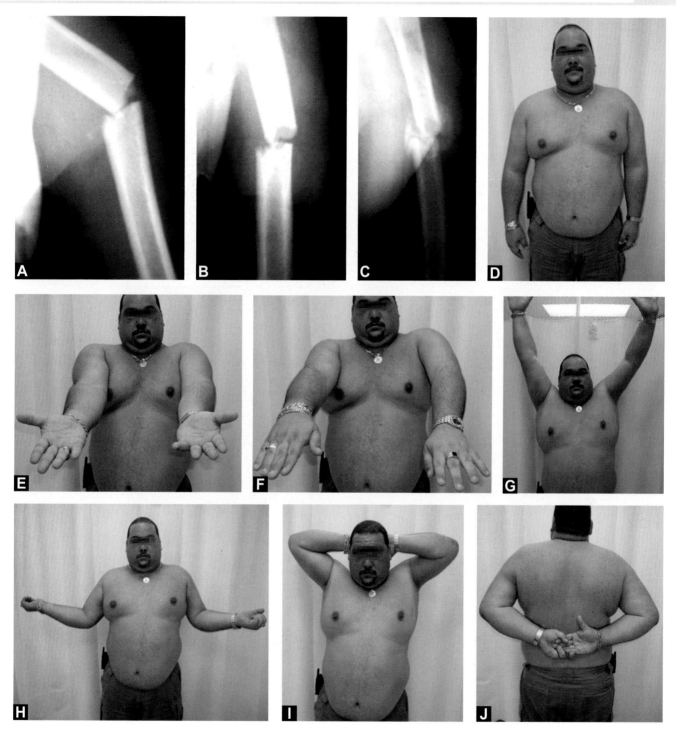

Figs 38.16A to J: (A) Radiograph of transverse fracture of the humerus showing the typical varus deformity. (B) Following the application of the brace 1 week after the injury, the alignment of the bone was restored. (C) Radiograph obtained 6 weeks after the initial injury. This was the last time the patient was seen. Notice the early callus. (D to J) The following photographs were taken the same day illustrating excellent range of motion.

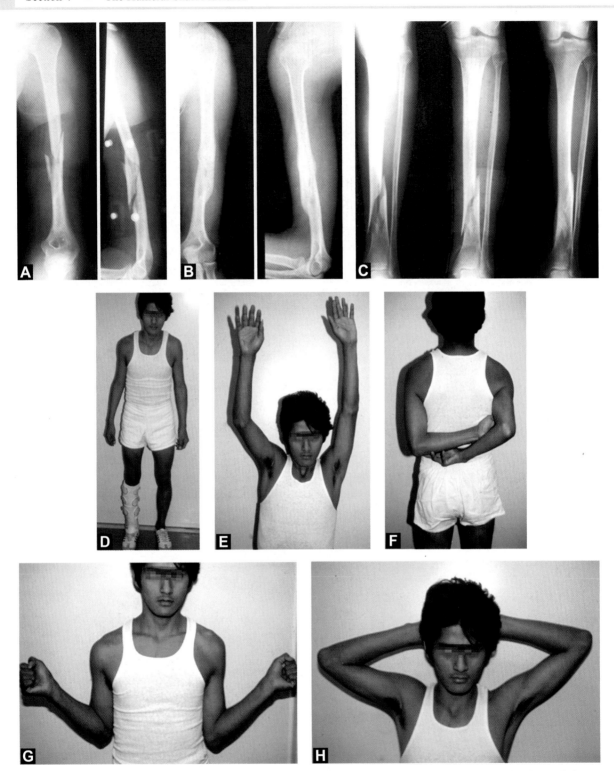

Figs 38.17A to H: (A) Radiograph of comminuted fracture of the right humerus obtained through a functional brace. (B) Radiograph demonstrating solid union of the fracture and acceptable alignment. (C) Composite radiograph of the patient's tibia showing progression of healing and ultimate shortening and alignment. As anticipated, his closed fracture healed with exactly the same shortening it had experienced at the time of the initial insult, despite the fact that graduated weight bearing ambulation was encouraged early. (D) Photo of patient showing the right leg stabilized in a below-the-knee functional brace after removal of the humeral brace. (E to H) Patient demonstrating the range of motion of his upper extremities. Notice the still present limitation of shoulder elevation and external rotation. It is anticipated that complete range of motion was regained within the ensuing months.

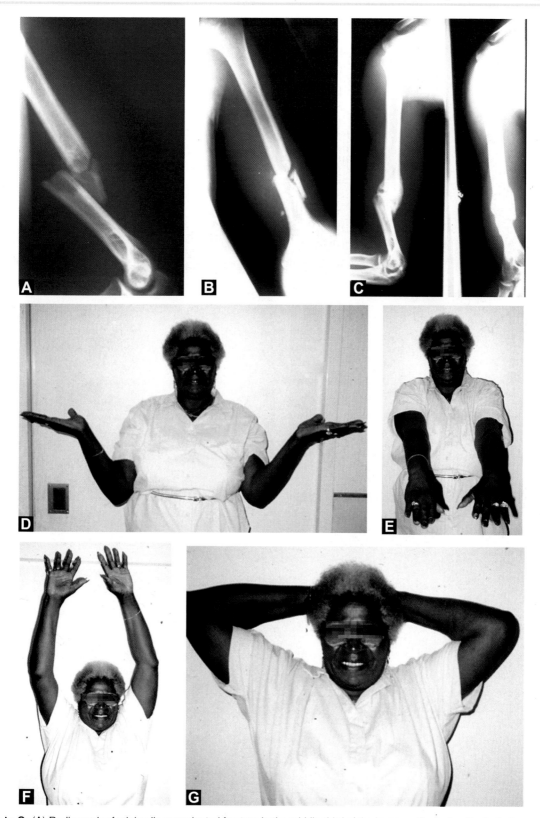

Figs 38.18A to G: (A) Radiograph of minimally comminuted fracture in the middle-third of the humerus illustrating the typical varus angulation, which is likely to be produced by the sling applied after the injury. (B and C) Sequential radiographs illustrating progression of healing with abundant peripheral callus. (D to G) Photos of patient demonstrating the range of motion of her shoulders and elbows.

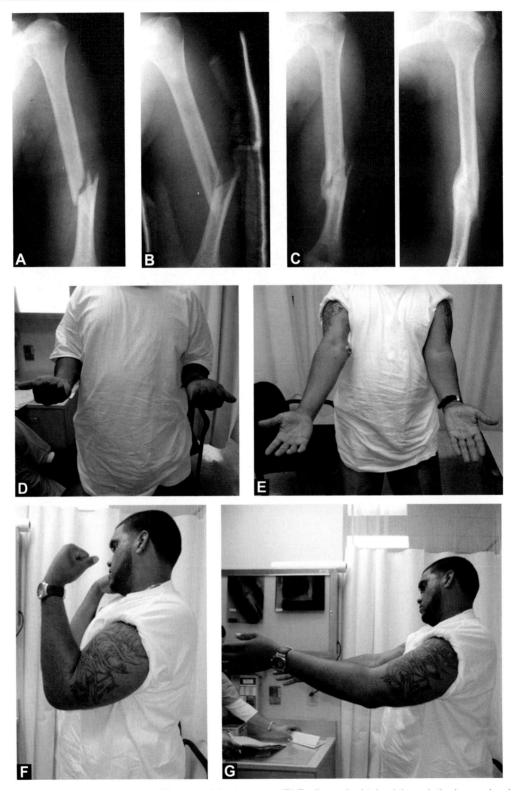

Figs 38.19A to G: (A) Radiograph of comminuted fracture of the humerus. (B) Radiograph obtained through the brace showing good antero-posterior alignment. (C) Radiograph illustrating the solidly healed fracture and the residual lateral angular deformity, most likely secondary to delayed attempts to regain elbow extension. The radiological deformity is functionally inconsequential and represents simply a mild deviation from the normal. (D to G) Patient demonstrates the range of motion of his shoulders and elbows.

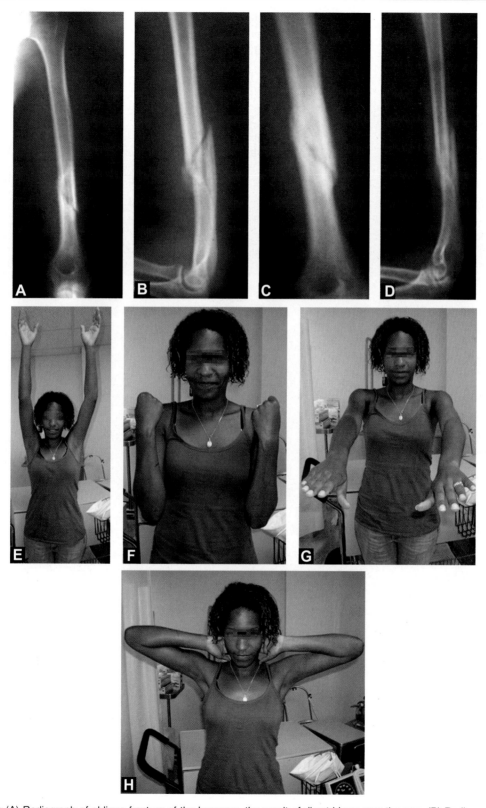

Figs 38.20A to H: (A) Radiograph of oblique fracture of the humerus, the result of direct blows over the arm. (B) Radiograph taken through the functional brace 3 weeks post-injury. Notice the early callus formation. (C and D) Radiograph showing solid union of the fracture and very acceptable alignment 3 months after the injury. (E to H) Patient demonstrating the appearance of her arms and the range of motion of her elbows and shoulders 2½ months after the initial accident.

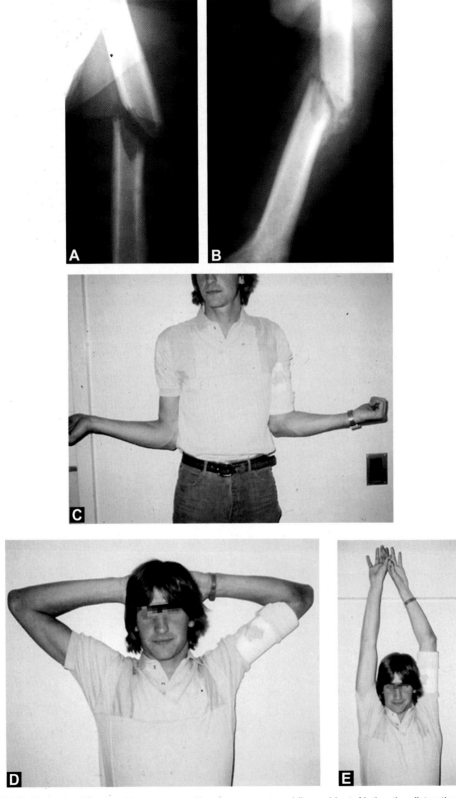

Figs 38.21A to E: (A) Radiograph of fractured humerus resulting from an automobile accident. Notice the distraction of the fragments; an ominous sign that frequently leads to nonunion. (B) Radiograph taken 6 weeks after the initial injury. Notice the early callus formation. (C to E) Patient demonstrates the range of motion of her shoulders and elbows at 6 weeks post injury. Patient was then lost to follow-up.

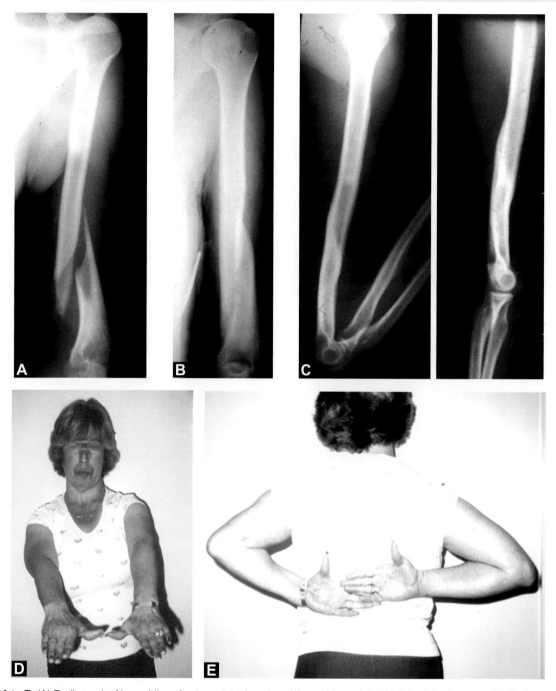

Figs 38.22A to E: (A) Radiograph of long oblique fracture at the junction of the middle and distal thirds of the humerus. (B) Radiograph showing the fracture solidly healed. (C) Radiographs illustrating the full flexion and extension of the elbow. (D and E) Patient demonstrates the range of motion of her elbows and shoulders.

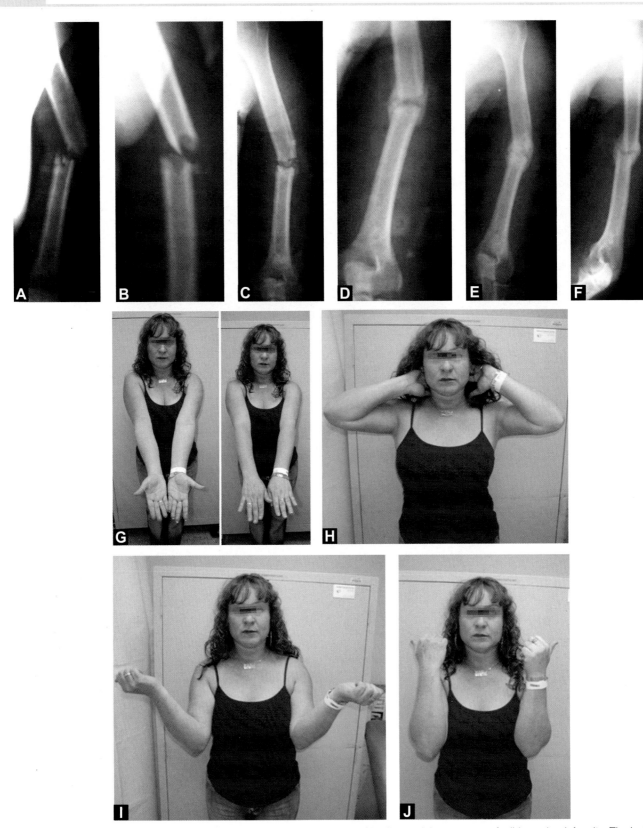

Figs 38.23A to J: (A to F) Radiographs illustrating the gradual progression of healing and the presence of mild angular deformity. The last film was obtained 2½ months after the initial injury. (G to J) Clinical demonstration of the range of motion present in the shoulder and elbow on the day the brace was removed 2½ months after the fracture occurred.

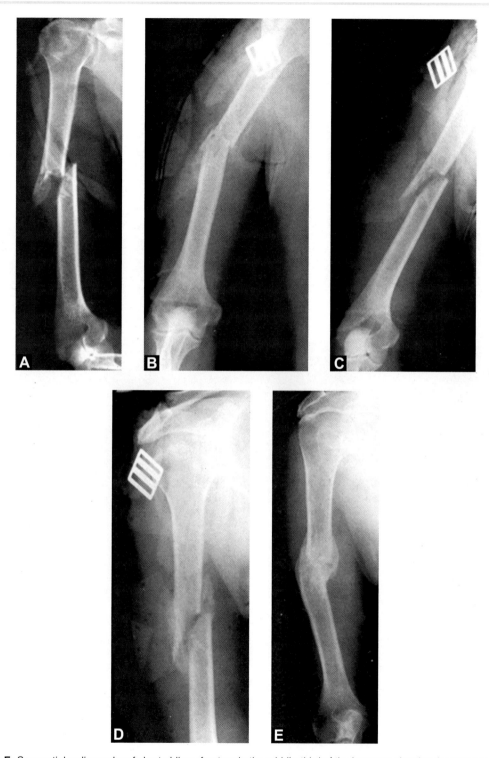

Figs 38.24A to E: Sequential radiographs of short oblique fracture in the middle-third of the humerus showing the presence and then the disappearance of a varus deformity. The fracture healed with abundant callus.

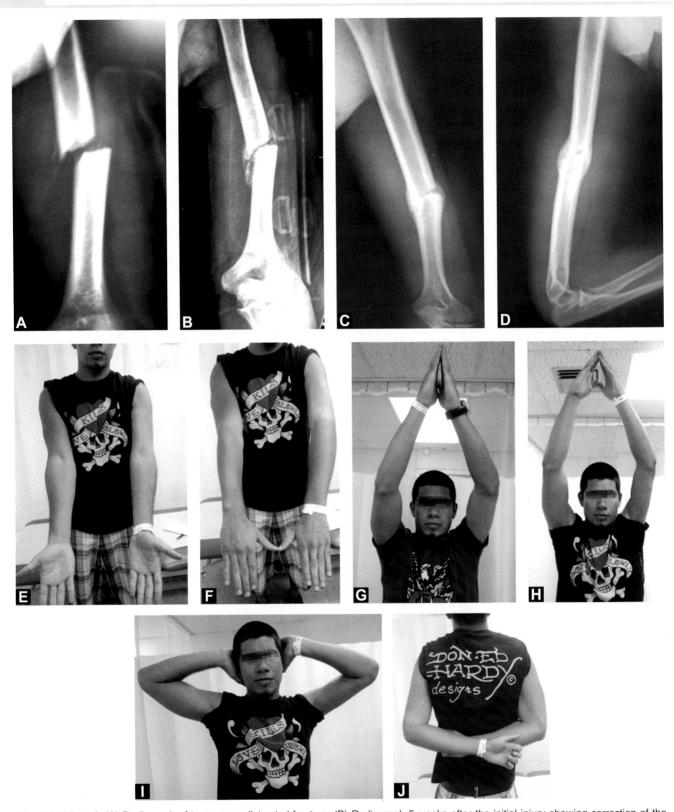

Figs 38.25A to J: (A) Radiograph of transverse, distracted fracture. (B) Radiograph 5 weeks after the initial injury showing correction of the distraction and the presence of early callus. (C and D) Radiographs showing the fracture united with acceptable alignment. (E to J) Patient demonstrates the range of motion of his shoulders on the day the brace was removed 2½ weeks after the initial insult.

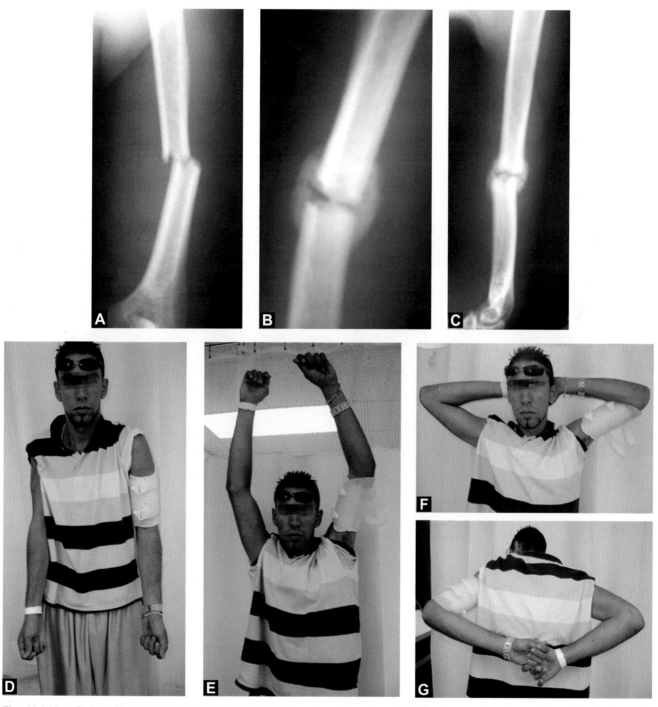

Figs 38.26A to G: (A to C) Initial radiograph of humeral fracture produced when the patient's bicycle was struck by an automobile. Radiographs obtained 2 months after the initial injury. Notice the peripheral callus and the mild angular deformity. (D to G) Clinical photographs of the patient demonstrating the range of motion of his shoulders and elbows, while still in the brace. He was lost to follow-up. Notice the residual, though most likely temporary loss of internal rotation.

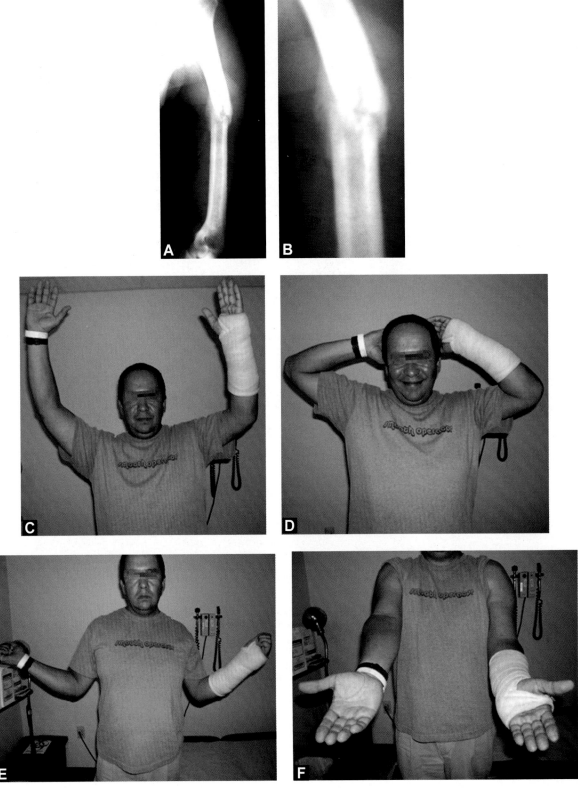

Figs 38.27A to F: (A) Radiograph obtained 4 weeks after an injury sustained during a motorcycle accident that also produced a fracture of the wrist. (B) Radiograph taken 5 weeks later. Notice the immature callus and the mild varus deformity. (C to F) Patient demonstrates the range of motion of his shoulders and elbows 2½ months after the initial insult.

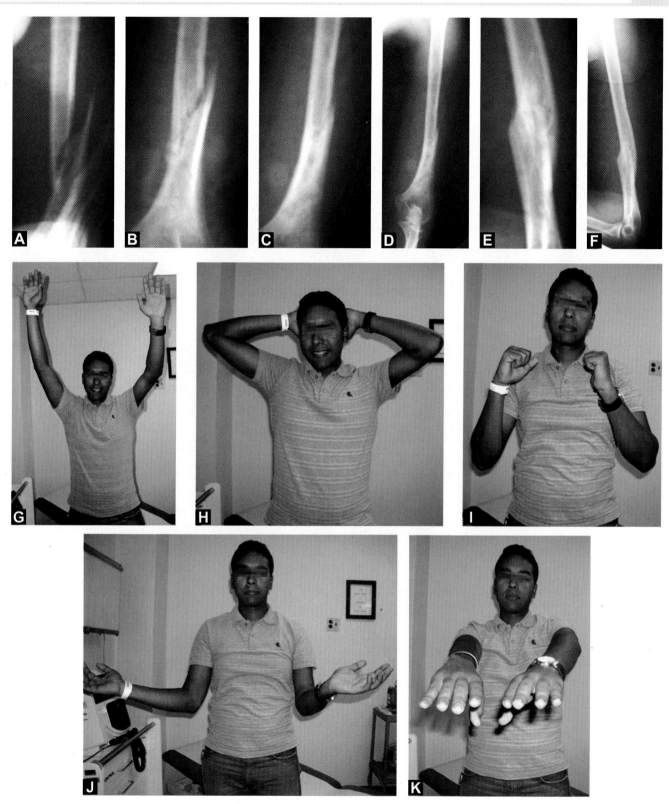

Figs 38.28A to K: (A) Radiograph of oblique, comminuted fracture at the junction of the middle and distal thirds of the humerus. (B and C) Radiographs taken 4 weeks after the accident. (D to F) Radiographs obtained 3 months after the initial injury. (G to K) Clinical photographs obtained 8 weeks after the initial insult, at the time of removal of the brace. Notice the residual limitation of external rotation, which probably disappeared with continued use of the extremity.

39

The Distal-third Fracture

A few examples of case studies for fractures in the distal-third of the humerus are illustrated in Figures 39.1 to 39.15.

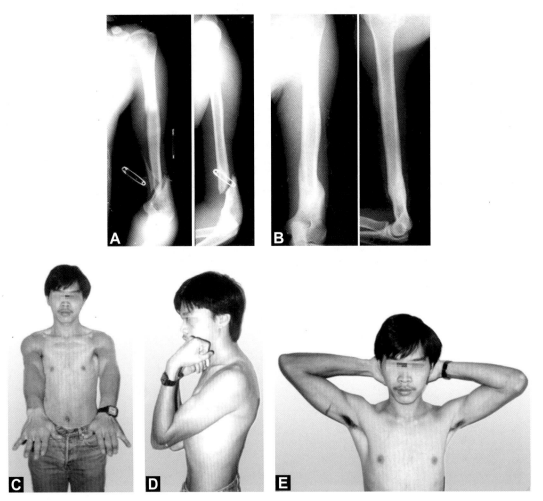

Figs 39.1A to E: (A) Radiograph of supracondylar fracture in a 23-year-old man. The fracture was treated with a functional brace that was applied 14 days after the injury. (B) Radiographs obtained after healing of the fracture. Notice the mild varus angular deformity. (C to E) Patient demonstrates the mild varus angulation of his humerus and very good range of motion of his shoulders and elbows.

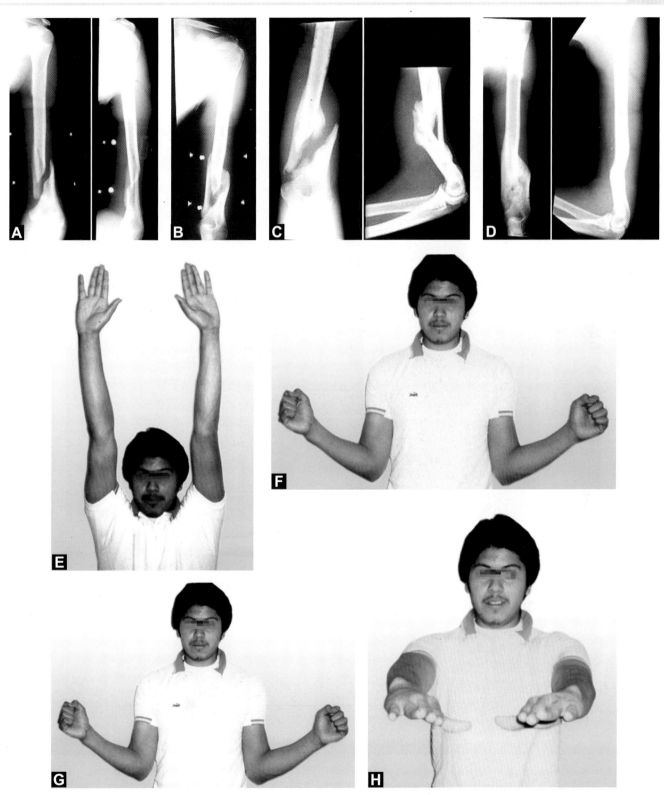

Figs 39.2A to H: (A) Radiograph of oblique fracture of the distal humerus obtained through a brace applied 7 days after the initial injury. (B) Radiograph taken 2 months after the injury showing a healed fracture. The brace was discontinued at this time. (C) Radiograph demonstrating a new fracture following the hitting of a ball with a bat a few days after removal of the brace. (D) A brace was reapplied and the fracture healed solidly. (E to H) Patient demonstrates the function of his elbows and shoulders.

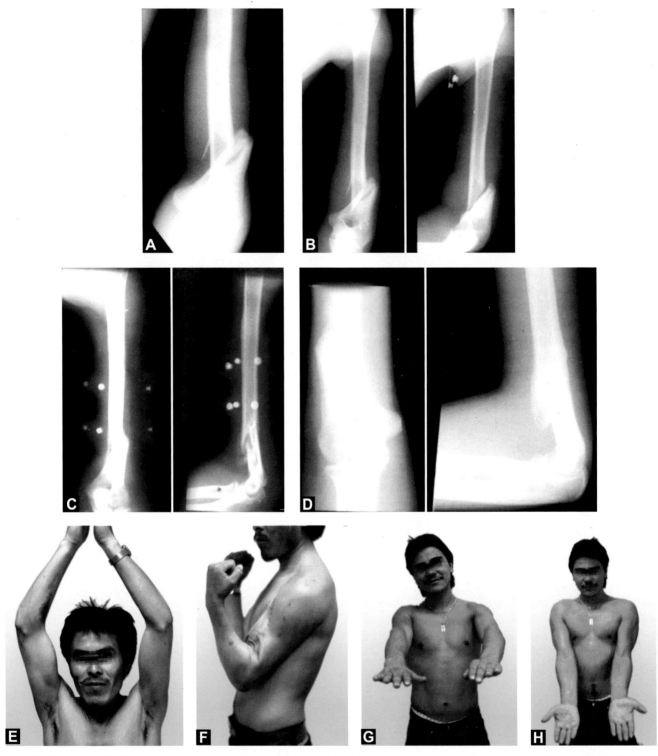

Figs 39.3A to H: (A) Radiograph of open displaced fracture in the distal-third of the humerus treated with a functional brace. (B) Radiograph showing the original deformity in both planes. (C) Radiograph obtained through the brace showing some spontaneous improvement in the alignment of the fragments. (D) Last radiograph showing the healed fracture but with a residual angular deformity. (E to H) Patient demonstrates the function of his shoulders and overall alignment of the injured extremity.

NOTE: Transverse fractures located in the distal third of the humerus are among the most difficult to manage by nonsurgical means. Angular deformities do not always improve with gravity and compression of soft tissues; surgical management has therefore become the treatment of choice.

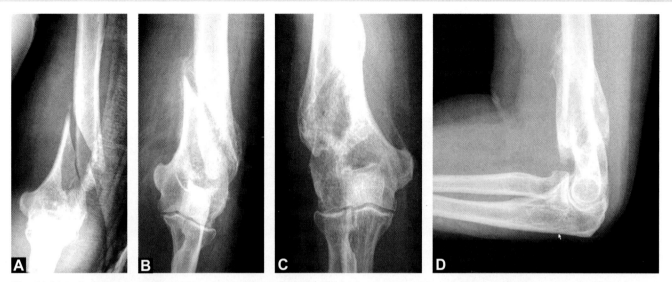

Figs 39.4A to D: (A) Radiograph of oblique fracture in the distal-third of the humerus in a 68-year-old man treated with a brace. (B) Radiograph illustrating the spontaneous alignment of the fragments and early callus 7 weeks after the initial injury. (C and D) Radiographs showing solid union of the fracture 4 months after the initial insult.

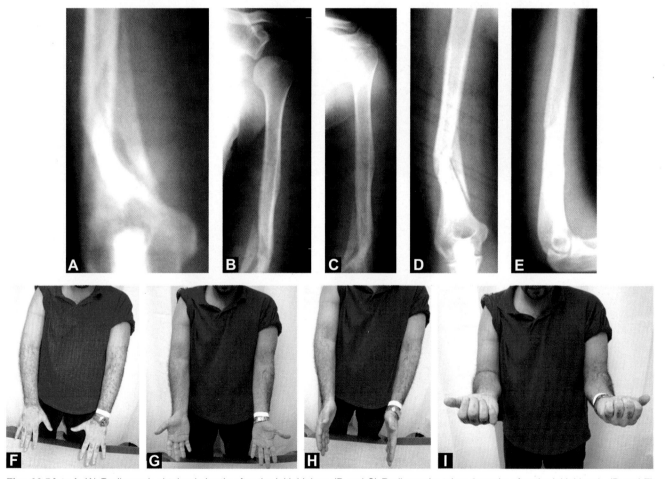

Figs 39.5A to I: (A) Radiograph obtained shortly after the initial injury. (B and C) Radiographs taken 6 weeks after the initial insult. (D and E) Final radiographs taken after completion of healing. Notice the acceptable alignment of the healed fragments. (F to I) Patient demonstrates the residual varus deformity and range of motion of his elbows.

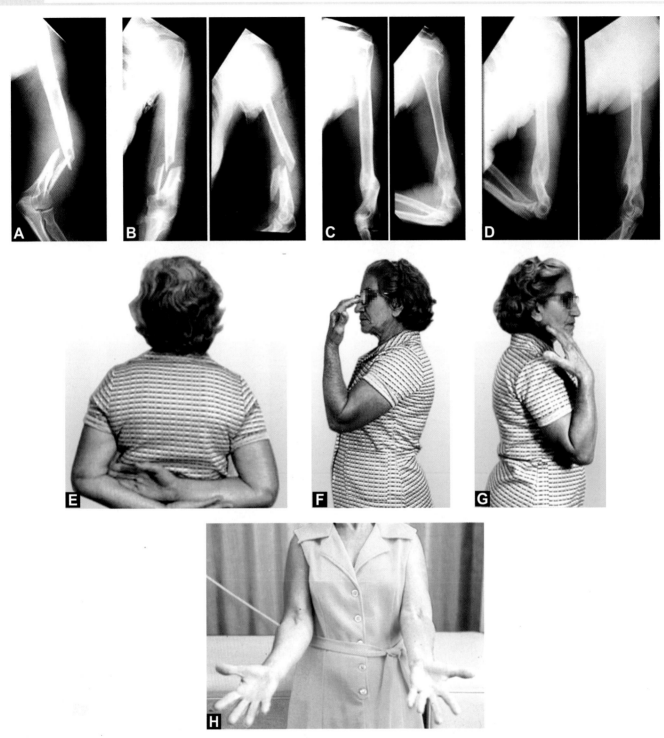

Figs 39.6A to H: (A) Radiograph of comminuted fracture of the distal-third of the humerus. (B) Radiograph obtained shortly after application of the brace 2 weeks after the initial injury. (C and D) Radiographs showing solid union of the fracture with a residual varus deformity. Notice the radiologically demonstrated range of motion of the elbow. (E to G) Patient demonstrates range of motion of the elbows 4 months after the initial injury. (H) Photo taken 9 months after the fracture occurred showing the residual loss of near-normal carrying angle.

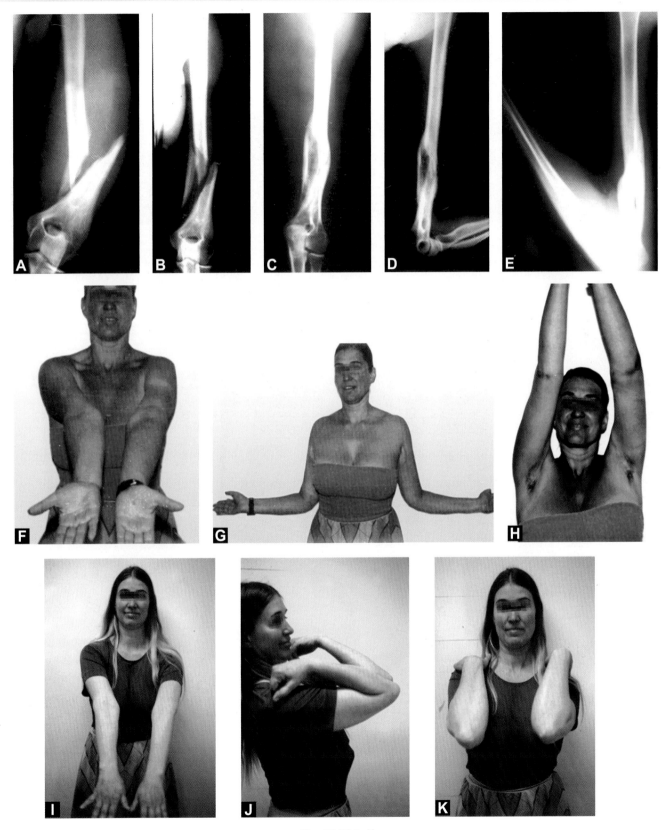

Figs 39.7A to K

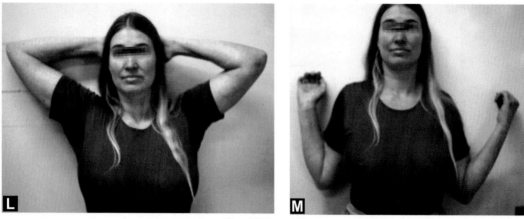

Figs 39.7L and M

Figs 39.7A to M: (A) Radiograph of comminuted fracture of the distal-third of the humerus. (B) Radiograph obtained following application of the brace 12 days after the original fracture. (C to E) Radiographs illustrating the healed fracture and the range of motion of the elbow. (F to H) Patient demonstrates the loss of carrying angle and the overall range of motion of her elbows and shoulders. (I to M) Photos taken 9 months after the initial insult.

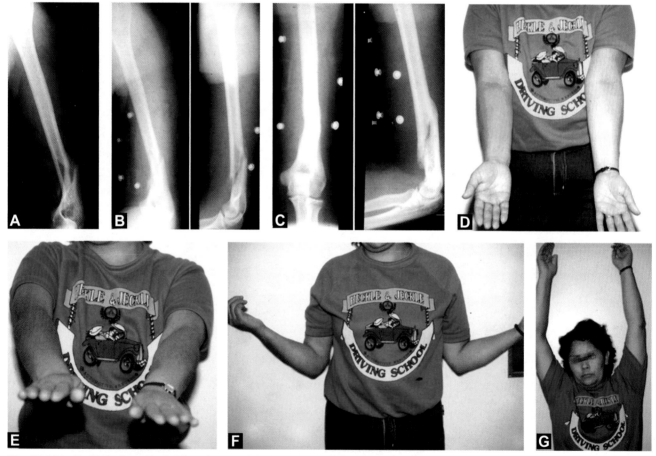

Figs 39.8A to G: (A) Radiograph of oblique fracture of the distal end of the humerus. (B) Radiographs obtained 10 days after the injury following application of the brace. (C) Radiographs showing solid union of the fracture 3 months after the injury. (D to G) Patient demonstrates the motion and appearance of her arms.

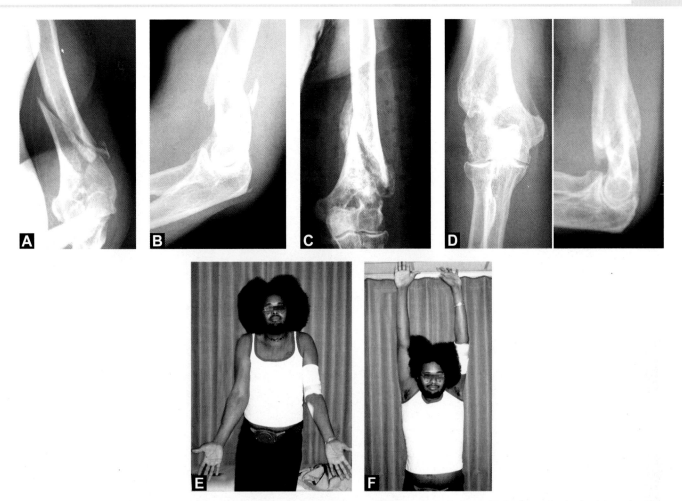

Figs 39.9A to F: (A and B) Radiographs of fracture of the distal humerus showing an oblique fracture. (B) Radiograph obtained 8 weeks after the injury showing early callus formation. (D) Final radiographs showing acceptable alignment of the healed fragments. (E and F) Patient demonstrates the function of his arms prior to the discontinuation of the brace.

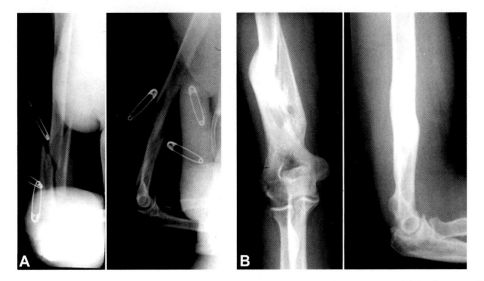

Figs 39.10A and B: (A) Radiographs illustrating a comminuted fracture in the distal-third of the humerus. (B) Radiograph obtained 4 months after the initial injury showing solid union of the fracture with mild varus angular deformity.

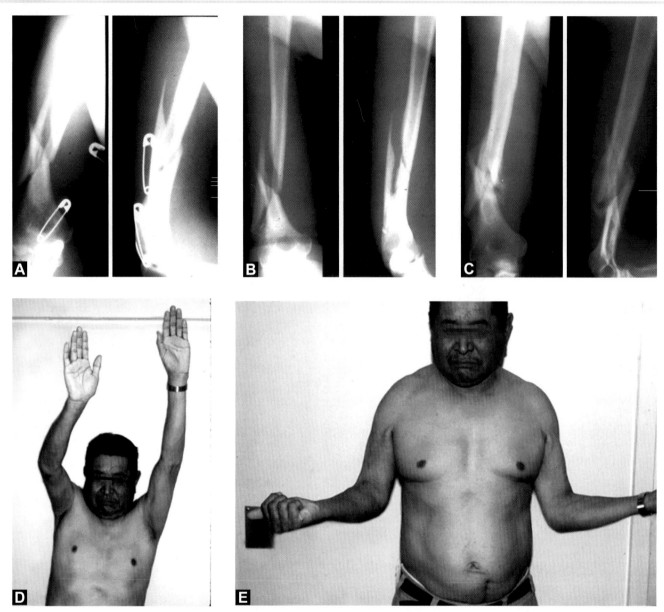

Figs 39.11A to E: (A) Radiograph of comminuted fracture of the humerus with a free fragment on the lateral side. This pattern of fracture is not very common. (B) Radiograph obtained 2 weeks after the injury following application of the brace. (C) Radiograph showing early callus but also an angular deformity that probably was the result of leaning on the elbow. The patient was lost to follow-up following this visit. (D and E) Photos of the patient obtained the day the last x-rays were taken. Notice the limitation of motion of the elbow and that of external rotation.

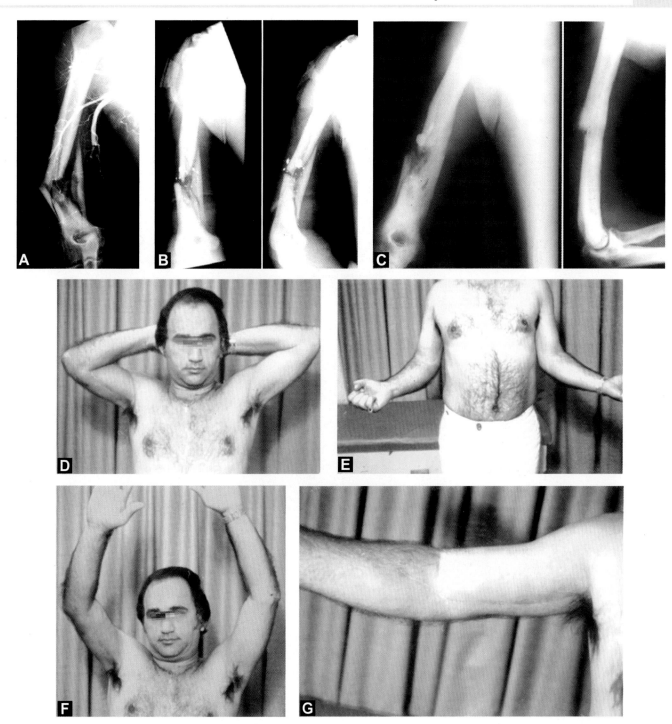

Figs 39.12A to G: Radiograph of a fracture produced by a low-velocity bullet. Notice the associated vascular injury. (B) After surgical treatment of vascular injury, a brace was applied. (C) Radiograph showing solid healing of the fracture. (D to G) Patient demonstrates the function of his injured arm.

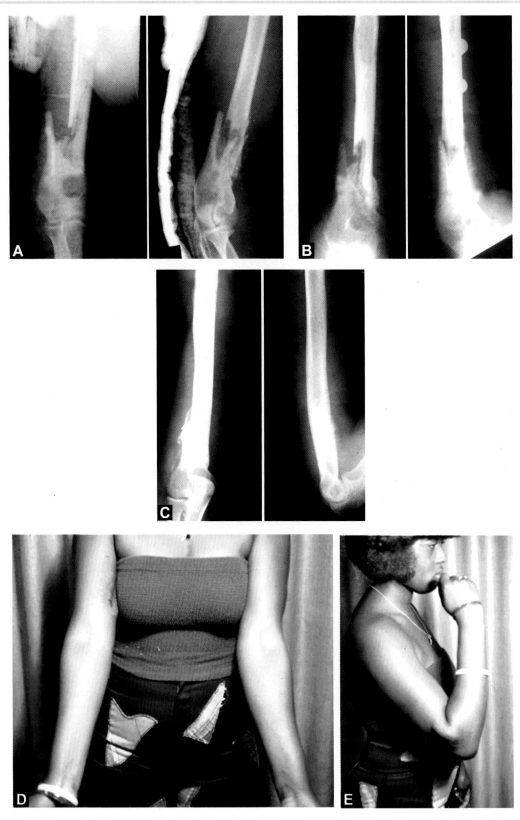

Figs 39.13A to E: (A) Radiograph of fracture produced by a low-velocity bullet. (B) Radiograph taken after application of the brace 3 weeks post-injury. (C) Radiograph illustrating solid union of the fracture. (D and E) Patient demonstrates the range of motion of her elbows and shoulders.

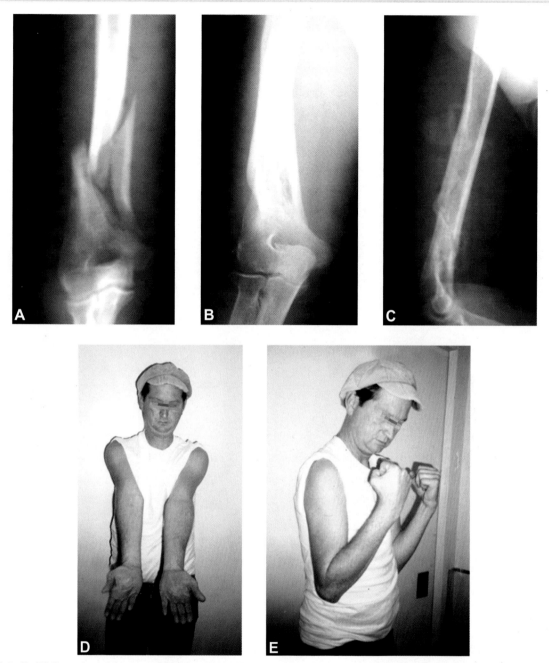

Figs 39.14A to E: (A) Comminuted fracture of the distal-third of the humerus. Notice the typical medial free fragment. (B and C) Radiographs obtained after completion of healing. (D and E) Patient demonstrates the cosmetic appearance of his arms and the range of motion of his elbows.

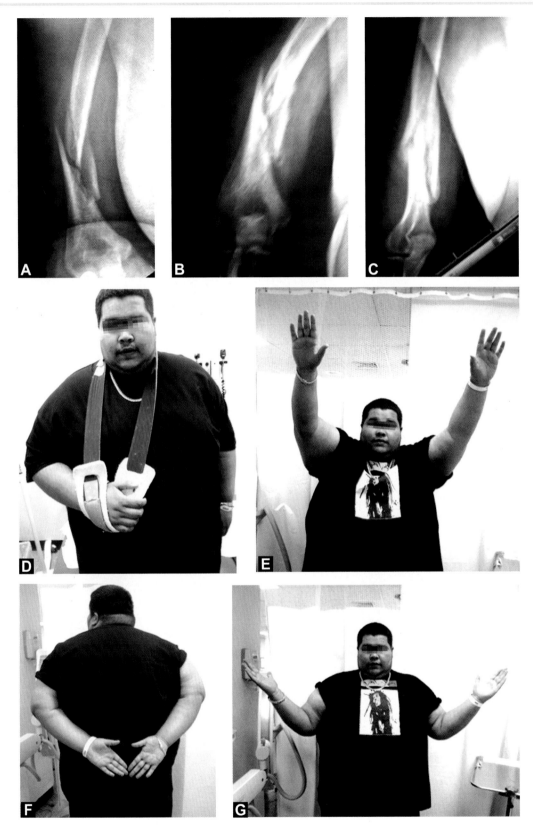

Figs 39.15A to G: (A) Radiograph of comminuted fracture in the distal-third of the humerus. (B) Radiograph obtained 2½ weeks after the initial injury. (C) Radiograph after completion of healing 3 months after the initial insult. (D to G) The patient, a severely obese person, demonstrates the range of motion of his shoulders on the day the brace was discontinued.

40

The Segmental Fracture and Representative Examples

There appears to be no difference in the management and final outcome between simple and segmental humeral fractures. The same principles apply to both types. The compression of the soft tissues by the humeral sleeve, the early introduction of function, and the extension of the elbow at an early date result in adequate restoration of alignment in most instances.

Some of the representative examples illustrating segmental fractures are shown in Figures 40.1 to 40.6.

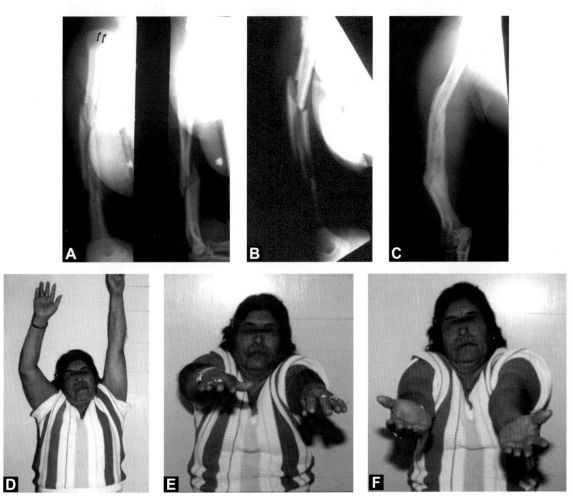

Figs 40.1A to F

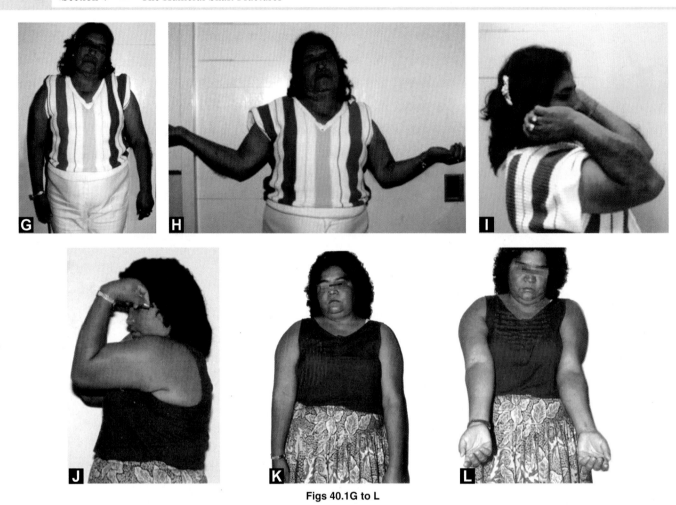

Figs 40.1G to L

Figs 40.1A to L: (A) Radiograph of double segmental fracture of the humerus sustained in an automobile accident by an obese woman. Notice the subluxation of the shoulder. (B) Radiograph obtained after application of the brace 10 days after the initial injury. An angular deformity is already apparent. Her large adipose tissues created a fulcrum leading to the angulation. (C) Radiograph obtained approximately 1 year after the initial injury. The subluxation had corrected after the initiation of active elbow exercises. The angular deformity remained unchanged. (D to I) Patient demonstrates the overall appearance of her fractured arm and the function of the shoulder and elbow. These photos were taken 3 months after the initial insult. (J to L) Photos of patient showing the cosmetic appearance of her arms and the degree of flexion of her elbow.

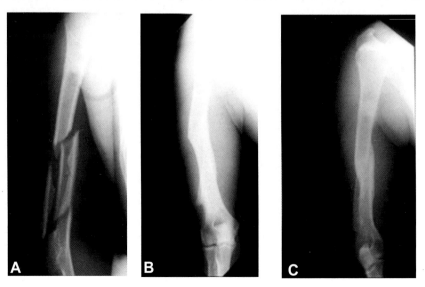

Figs 40.2A to C:

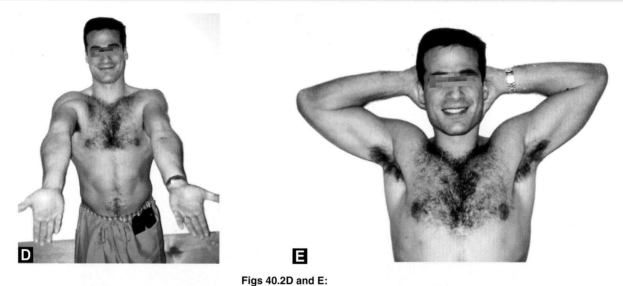

Figs 40.2D and E:

Figs 40.2A to E: (A) Radiograph of segmental fracture of the humerus. The fracture had been treated at another institution some years before we had an opportunity to know the patient. (B and C) Radiographs obtained 5 years after the initial fracture. (D and E) Patient demonstrates the esthetic appearance of the broken arm and the function of his elbows and shoulder. The patient indulges in sports and experiences no problems of any kind.

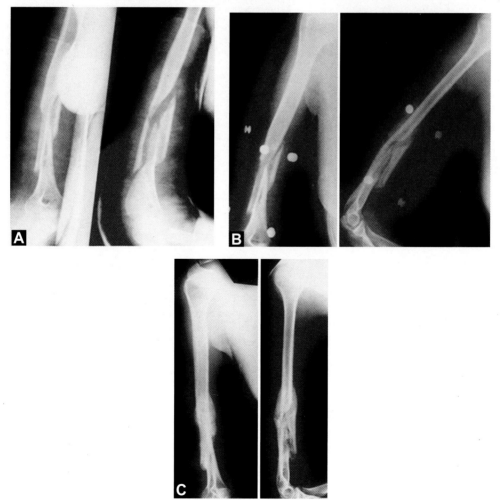

Figs 40.3A to C: Sequential radiographs of segmental fracture illustrating the progression of healing and maintenance of adequate alignment.

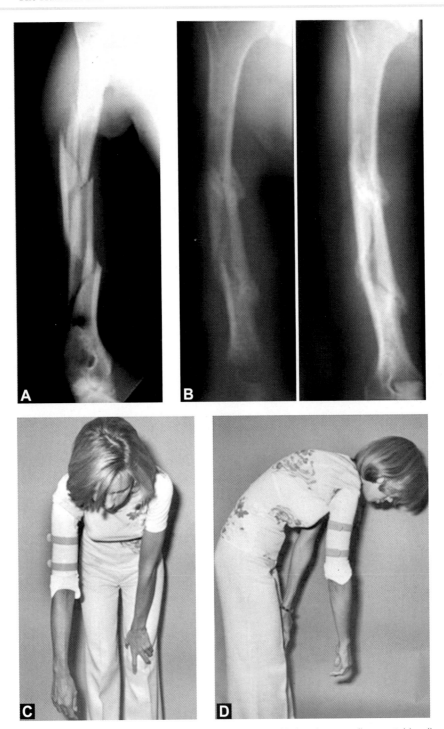

Figs 40.4A to D: (A) Radiograph of double segmental fracture of the humerus. Notice the overall acceptable alignment of the fragments. (B) Radiographs obtained after healing of the fracture, which had been treated with a functional brace. (C and D) Patient demonstrates the performance of pendulum exercises initiated shortly after the application of the brace.

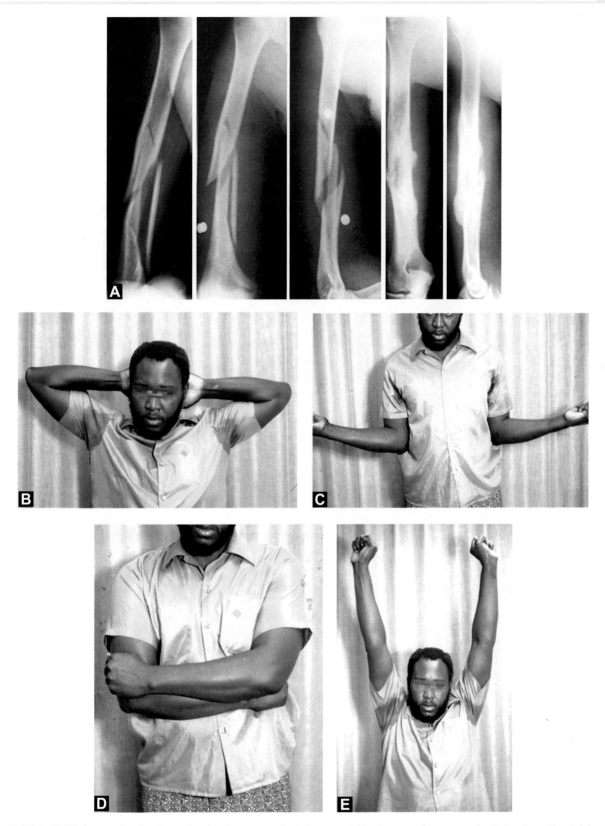

Figs 40.5A to E: (A) Composite of radiographs showing a comminuted-segmental fracture and the progression to healing without deformity. (B to E) Patient demonstrates the range of motion of his injured extremity.

Figs 40.6A to G

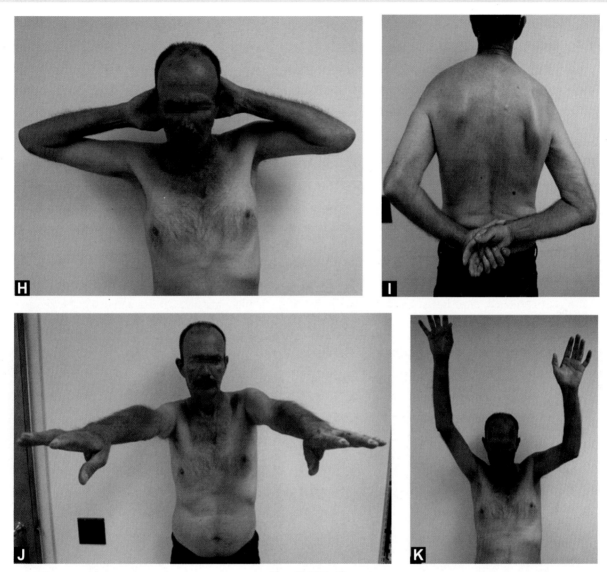

Figs 40.6H to K

Figs 40.6A to K: (A and B) Radiographs of a segmental fracture that occurred from a pedestrian-automobile collision. The patient was allegedly taken to a Nursing Home where orthopedic care was not sought until 1 month later. (C to E) Radiographs obtained in various positions 6 months post-injury. (F to K) Patient demonstrates the range of motion of his asymptomatic extremity.

41

Bilateral Shaft Fractures

Our experience with bilateral humeral fractures treated with functional braces is limited, most likely due to the fact that these special situations were managed by surgical means in an effort to avoid the initial period of shoulder immobilization that is required with closed functional methods (Figures 41.1A to K). In other instances, it was avoided due to the associated multiple organ compromise.

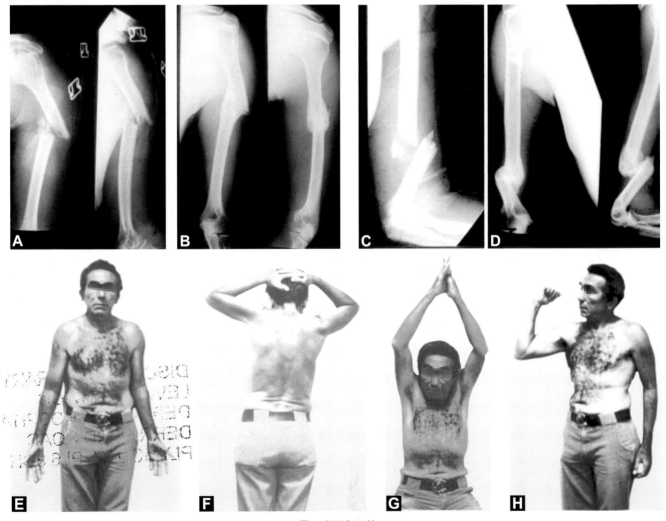

Figs 41.1A to H

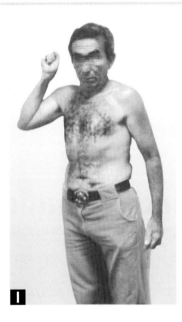 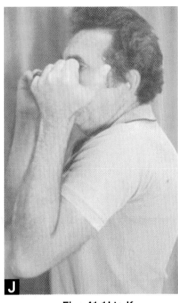 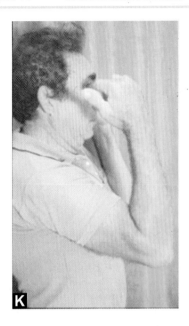

Figs 41.1I to K

Figs 41.1A to K: (A to D) Radiographs of bilateral humeral fractures sustained in an automobile accident. The patient had associated chest injury. When first seen by us, 3 weeks had already elapsed. The fractures healed with marked angular deformities. (E to I) Patient demonstrates the range of motion of his shoulders and elbows 6 months after the initial insult. (J and K) Photographs taken a year later. Notice the acceptable cosmetic appearance of his arms and further improved function.

42

Delayed Unions and Nonunions

Nonunion of humeral fractures, particularly in open ones, continues to challenge the orthopedic surgeon despite advances made in the management of the acute fracture. It is widely acknowledged that plating has failed to render the anticipated results. Radial nerve injury taking place at the time of surgery is a rather common complication with either plating or intramedullary fixation.[1-14] It is not always easy to determine with precision when a fracture is likely to develop nonunion. In other long bones, it is not uncommon to see fractures demonstrate no evidence of clinical or radiological union for long periods of time, and still observe eventual healing. The humerus seems to behave differently. A humeral diaphyseal fracture that demonstrates frank motion at the fracture site 2 or 2½ months after the injury is not likely to unite spontaneously. Such motion is of a greater diagnostic significance than the absence of peripheral callus. We have observed fractures with no radiologically demonstrable callus 2 months after the initial injury, but without gross motion at the fracture site, eventually heal solidly (Figures 42.1A to 42.2C).

Fractures associated with peripheral nerve injury are the ones most likely to develop nonunion, particularly if the injured nerve affects the function of the flexor and extensor of the elbow. These fractures, as a rule, demonstrate initial axial separation between the fragments (Figures 42.3A 42.4D). Axial distraction between fragments can also indicate major

soft tissue damage that requires earlier active use of the surrounding musculature. Failure to see a rapid correction of the distraction often calls for surgical intervention (Figures 42.5A to D).

Despite the fact the humerus is less likely to show eventual union of a fracture that a few months after the injury still fails to demonstrate clinical and radiological stability, we have observed in a few instances of subsequent union (Figures 42.6A and B). Most often, these people had had intensive, early physical therapy exercises, and union did not take place until such activities were discontinued. Rest and continued passive pendulum exercises were the only additional therapy. The next patient is a good example (Figures 42.1A to G). He was a physician who had sustained a closed oblique fracture without associated peripheral nerve injury. Active abduction and elevation of the arm was encouraged and monitored by professional occupational therapists.

The following radiographs illustrate an instance when spontaneous union of a mid-diaphyseal fracture of the humerus eventually show union, despite the fact that several months after the initial injury, there was no evidence of callus formation. The patient was an obese, elderly diabetic woman who rejected surgery to overcome what appeared to be a nonunion. She continued to wear the brace. It took one year before the fracture healed.

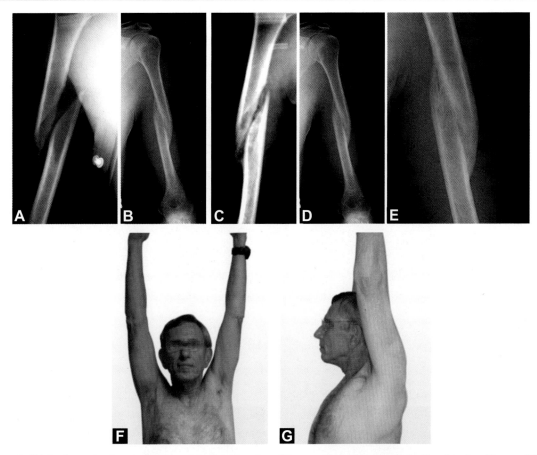

Figs 42.1A to G: (A) Radiograph of acute fracture of the humerus in a 55-year-old physician treated with a functional brace. (B) Radiograph obtained 4 weeks after the initial injury. Allegedly, the patient had been instructed to carry-out active elevation and abduction from the very outset. (C) Four months later, there was no clinical or radiological evidence of healing. Patient was then encouraged to discontinue all active exercises of the shoulder, and to limit the activities to pendulum exercises and active flexion and extension of the elbow. (D and E) The fracture healed spontaneously. These radiographs were obtained 22 months after the initial injury. (F and G) Painless full range of motion of all joints returned. Patient demonstrates the elevation of the shoulders.

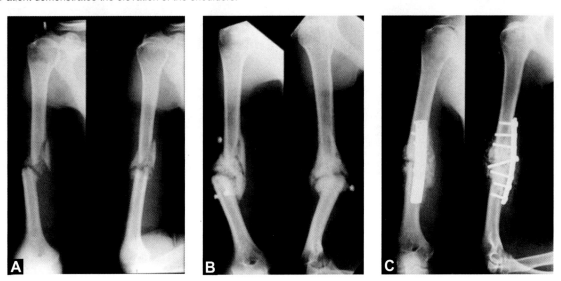

Figs 42.2A to C: (A) Radiograph of fracture of the humeral diaphysis obtained 2 months after the initial injury. Notice the distal distraction between the major fragment and the absence of peripheral callus. (B) Radiograph taken 4 months later showing an angular deformity and no evidence of healing. (C) Radiograph obtained following plating of the nonunion, reinforced with an autologous bone graft.

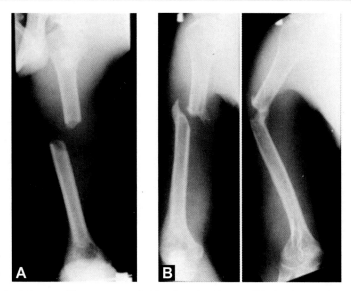

Figs 42.3A and B: (A) Radiograph of distracted fracture treated with a functional brace. (B) The fracture failed to unite as illustrated in this film.

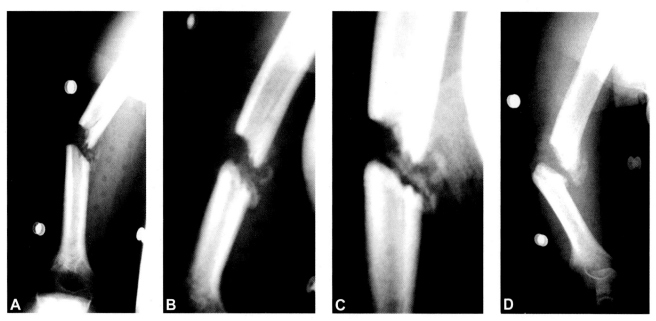

Figs 42.4A to D: Radiograph of established nonunion of an open fracture treated with a functional brace.

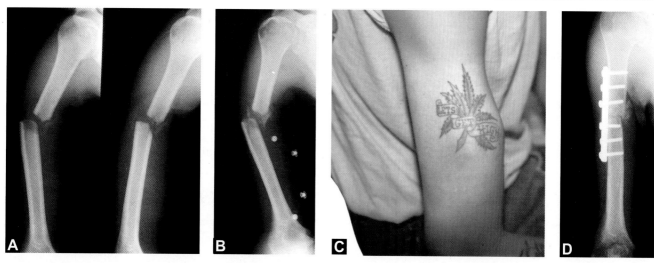

Figs 42.5A to D: (A) Radiograph of transverse fracture in the middle-third of the humerus taken 2 months after the initial insult, showing axial distraction between the fragments. The patient had suffered a radial palsy initially. (B) Radiograph obtained 1 month later showing some peripheral callus. There was however, frank motion at the fracture site. Early return of nerve function was detected at this time. (C) Appearance of the tattooed arm of the 24-year-old "gang" member. (D) Radiograph taken after plating and grafting of the nonunited bone. Patient was lost to follow-up.

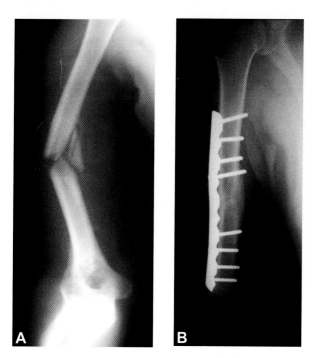

Figs 42.6A and B: (A) Radiograph of a nonunited open fracture that had been treated with a functional brace. (B) Radiograph showing solid union following plating.

REFERENCES

1. Aiken GK, Rorabeck CH. Distal humeral fractures in the adult. Clin Orthop Relat Res. 1986; 207:191-7.

2. Bleeker WA, Nijsten MW, ten Duis HJ. Treatment of humeral shaft fractures related to associated injuries: A retrospective study of 237 patients. Acta Orthop Scand. 1991; 62(2):148-53.

3. Foulk DA, Szabo RM. Diaphyseal humeral fractures: Natural history and occurrence of nonunion. Orthop 1995; 18(4):333-5.

4. Flinkkila T, Hyvonen P, Lakovaara M, Linden T, Ristiniemi J, Hamalainen M. Intramedullary nailing of humeral shaft fractures: A retrospective study of 126 cases. Acta Orthop Scand. 1999; 70(2):133-6.

5. Foulk DA, Szabo RM. Diaphyseal humerus fractures: Natural history and occurrence of nonunion. Orthopedics. 1995; 18(4):333-5.

6. Jawa A, McCarthy P, Doornberg J, Harris M, Ring D. Extra-articular distal-third diaphyseal fractures of the humerus. J Bone and Joint. 2006; 88A(11):2343-7.

7. Joshi A, Labbe M, Lindsey RW. Humeral fracture secondary to civilian gunshot injury. Injury. 1998; 29 Suppl 1:SA13-17.

8. Liebergall M, Jaber S, Laster M, Aub-Snieneh K, Mattan Y, Segal D. Ender nailing of acute humeral shaft fractures in multiple injuries. Injury. 1997; 28(9-10):577-80.

9. Lin J, Hou SM. Antegrade locking nailing for humeral shaft fractures. Clin Orthop. 1999; 365:201-10.

10. Lin J. Treatment of humeral shaft fractures with humeral locked nail and comparison with plate fixation. J Trauma. 1998; 44(5):859-64.

11. Moran MC. Distal interlocking during intramedullary nailing of the humerus. Clin Orthop. 1995; 317:215-8.

12. Ring D, Perey BH, Jupiter JB. The functional outcome of operative treatment of ununited fractures of the humeral diaphysis in older patients. J Bone Joint Surg. 1999; 81A(2):177-90.

13. Sarmiento A, Waddell JP, Latta LL. Diaphyseal Humeral Fractures: Treatment Options. An Instructional Course. AAOS J Bone and Joint Surg. 1999; 83A(10):1566-79.

14. Svend-Hansen H, Skettrup M, Rathcke MW. Complications using the Seidel intramedullary humeral nail: outcome in 31 patients. Acta Orthop Belgica. 1998; 64(3):291-5.

43

Clinical and Radiological Results

The orthopedic literature dealing with functional bracing of humeral diaphyseal fractures has indicated a high degree of success, as depicted by the high union rate, and the obvious absence of infections and nerve injury.[1-25]

We have reported several times on the results obtained with functional bracing of humeral shaft fractures. The following data is based on a published review of 922 fractures treated in that manner, from which 620 (67%) were available to follow-up.[19] Four hundred and sixty five (75%) of the fractures were closed, and 155 (25%) were open. Nine patients (6%) who had an open fracture and seven (less than 2%) who had a closed fracture had a nonunion after bracing. In 87% of the 565 patients for whom antero-posterior radiographs were available, the fractures healed with less than 16° of varus angulation, and in 81% of the 546 for whom lateral radiographs were available, it healed with less than 16° of anterior angulation. At the time of brace removal, 98% of the patients had limitation of shoulder motion of 25° or less.

The average age of the patients was 36 years (range, 16 to 83 years) at the time of injury. There were 391 male patients (63%) and 229 female patients (37%). Three hundred and three (49%) of the fractures were in the right humerus, and 317 (51%) were in the left humerus; 465 (75%) were closed, and 155 (25%) were open. One hundred and eighteen (76%) of the open fractures were gunshot injuries, and the remaining 37 (24%) resulted from motor-vehicle accidents. One hundred and ninety-two patients (32%) sustained the fracture in a fall to the ground; 118 (19%) from a gunshot; 211 (34%) in a motor-vehicle accident; and 99 (16%) from various causes, such as a bicycle accident, a direct blow to the arm, or a twisting force.

Ninety-two fractures (15%) were in the proximal-third of the humeral diaphysis, 303 (49%) were in the middle third, 219 (35%) were in the distal-third, and six (1%) were segmental. One hundred and one fractures (16%) were transverse, 149 (24%) were oblique, 364 (59%) were comminuted, and six

(1%) were segmental. Twelve (2%) had an associated inferior glenohumeral subluxation.

Sixty-seven patients (11%) had an associated radial nerve palsy. Fifty-two (78%) of the palsies were associated with a closed fracture and 15 (22%) with an open fracture. Twenty-eight (42%) of the 67 fractures were transverse, 14 (21%) were oblique, and 25 (37%) were comminuted. The mechanism of injury was a fall for 16 patients (24%), a motor-vehicle accident for 24 (36%), a low-velocity gunshot for 23 (34%), and unknown for four (6%).

In the instances in which a nerve injury was due to a penetrating injury or a high-velocity gunshot wound, operative exploration was performed and, if necessary, the nerve was repaired. We were unable to determine the exact number of patients in this category. The fractures in these patients were stabilized by other orthopedists within the department, and we were unable to follow them. Only patients who had an open fracture or an associated injury were admitted to the hospital. The humeral fractures of an unknown number of patients who had multiple injuries were treated by operative or nonoperative methods, and these patients were not included in our series.

Initially, the injured extremity was stabilized in an above-the-elbow cast or coaptation splint that held the elbow in 90° of flexion, for an average of 9 days (range, 0 to 35 days). None of the fractures were manipulated. Patients were evaluated in the outpatient department approximately 1 week (range, 3 days to 5 weeks) after the initial injury. If the acute symptoms had subsided and the injured extremity was not swollen, a brace was applied and the patient was given a collar-and-cuff sling to wear. The brace consisted of two plastic shells that encircled the arm with two adjustable Velcro straps to hold the shells together. The brace extended from approximately 2 inches (5 cm) distal to the axilla to 2 inches proximal to the olecranon. Patients were shown how to adjust the brace and tighten the Velcro straps several times a day to accommodate the changes in the girth of the extremity that occurred as the swelling subsided and muscle atrophy developed. The brace was worn at all times, except during bathing.

Patients were instructed on the performance of pendulum exercises immediately after the application of the initial cast or splint, and the exercises were continued after the application of the brace. The collar-and-cuff sling was taken off for a few minutes several times a day to permit active and passive exercises of the elbow and to regain full extension of the elbow as soon as possible. Active elevation and abduction were not allowed, since such exercises could lead to angular deformity. The patients were also instructed not to lean on the elbow, on the arm of a chair, a table, or their lap, as leaning on the elbow of a fractured extremity during the early stages of healing may cause varus angulation. Such angulation is more likely to occur in association with transverse fractures, particularly when the bone fragments contact each other; it is less likely to occur in association with oblique fractures, where elastic pistoning of the fragments takes place.

At the time of application of the original sling that is applied after the completion of the above-the-elbow cast or coaptation splint, if the elbow is flexed to 90° and then held in the sling, the angular deformity occurs. This is also more likely to happen if the patient had held the shoulder in a shrugged position during the sling application, and then relaxes (Figure 43.1). The accompanying force creates or aggravates the deformity.

Patients were seen 1 week after the application of the brace, and radiographs were made to evaluate the position of the fragments. Once extension of the elbow was achieved, use of the collar-and-cuff was continued until clinical signs of intrinsic stability were confirmed. Once this stability is confirmed by the patients' own feelings and the appearance of early callus in recent radiographs, patients were allowed to discontinue the sling during ambulation but encouraged its use during decumbency. During the next 4 weeks, patients increased the frequency and intensity of exercises involving passive rotation of the shoulder and active flexion and extension of the elbow.

Fracture treatment was the same for the 67 patients (11%) who had an associated radial nerve palsy at the time of the injury. A cock-up wrist splint was not used in anticipation that once the elbow reached full extension, the wrist spontaneously extends to neutral, precluding the development of a permanent flexion contracture of the fingers and wrist. Patients were instructed to perform active and passive extension of the fingers and wrist several times a day.

RESULTS

We were able to follow 620 (67%) of the 992 patients who had a fracture of the humeral diaphysis to the point of complete healing. The result have been summarised in Figures 43.2A to 43.3. A large number of patients discontinued their visits to the outpatient clinic as soon as the injured extremity became painless and functional.

The functional brace was removed upon confirmation of clinical and radiological union of the fracture. Which occurred at an average of 11.5 weeks (range, 5 to 22 weeks). Union was arbitrarily defined as being present when osseous bridging between the main fragments was observed on at least one radiograph and there was no pain at the fracture site.

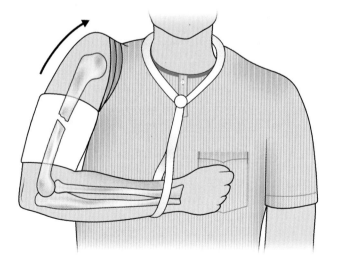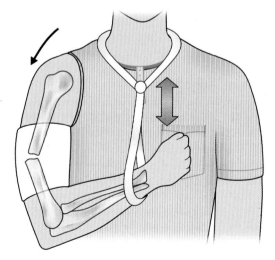

Fig. 43.1: The natural apprehension the patient experiences at the time of application of the original sling prompts him/her to shrug the shoulder. When the shoulder relaxes, a varus angular deformity may occur. It is therefore important to ascertain that the sling is applied after the shoulder is no longer in a shrugged position.

The 465 closed fractures healed with a median of 9.5 weeks (range, 5 to 19 weeks) and the 155 open fractures, at a median of 14 weeks (range, 8 to 22 week). The median healing time was 12 weeks (range, 8 to 22 weeks) for the 101 transverse fractures, 10 weeks (range, 5 to 17 weeks) for the 149 oblique fractures, 11 weeks (range, 5 to 18 weeks) for the 149 oblique fractures, 10 weeks (range, 5 to 17 weeks) for the 364 comminuted fractures, and 12 weeks (range, 8 to 21 weeks) for the 6 segmental fractures. The median healing time was 10 weeks (range, 4 to 14 weeks) for the 92 fractures located in the proximal third of the humeral diaphysis, 10 weeks (range, 6 to 22 weeks) for the 303 fractures located in the middle-third, 9 weeks (range, 6 to 22 weeks) for the 219 fractures located in the distal-third, and 12 weeks (range, 8 to 21 weeks) for the 6 segmental fractures.

Sixteen patients (3%) required operative intervention because of nonunion. The mechanism of injury was a fall to the ground for four of these patients, a motor-vehicle accident for nine, and a low-velocity gunshot for three. Nine open fractures and seven closed fractures failed to unite. Of the nine nonunions of open fractures, four (two transverse and two comminuted) were in the middle-third of the humerus and five (two transverse and three comminuted) were in the distal-third of the humerus. Of the seven nonunions of closed fractures, four (three transverse and one comminuted) were in the middle-third of the humerus and three (two transverse and one comminuted) were in the distal-third. Distal distraction between the fragments in the nonunions was observed in seven patients on radiographs made with the patients standing.

Four (less than 1%) of the patients had a refracture between the 2nd and the 8th week after removal of the brace. Two of the refractures occurred after a fall; one during sports activities; and one, from an unknown mechanism. The four refractures healed following reapplication of the brace.

Five hundred and sixty five patients (91%) were available for measurements of antero-posterior angulation. The most recent lateral radiographs were available for measurement of angulation in 546 patients (88%).

The 101 transverse fractures healed at an average of 9° of varus angulation; the 149 oblique fractures, in an average of 4°; and the 364 comminuted fractures, in an average of 8°.

Nerve function did not return in one of the 67 patients who had a radial nerve palsy. Because of the relatively short duration of follow-up of many of the patients, we are not in a position to state the ultimate degree of recovery that might have taken place. As we stated, in unknown number of patients a repair of the lacerated nerve were followed at another service and were not seen in our clinic.

The 12 patients who had an inferior subluxation of the shoulder demonstrated spontaneous correction of the subluxation, but no accurate data was kept concerning the speed of recovery. We believe, however, that the early

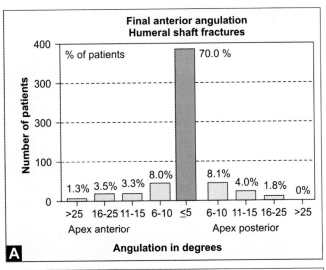

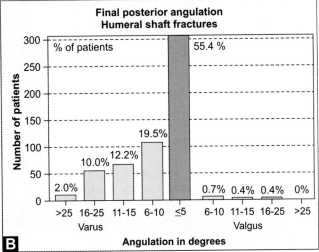

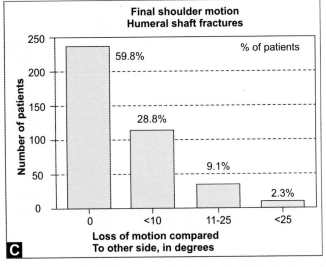

Figs 43.2A to C: (A) Barograph illustrating the final anterior and posterior angular deformities. (B) Barograph illustrating the final varus-valgus at the fracture site. (C) Barograph illustrating the loss of motion of the shoulder at the time of removal of the functional brace.

introduction of active contractions of the biceps and triceps expedites the recovery.

Once the fracture was clinically stable and there were radiographic signs of healing, the patients were asked by the examining residents to flex, abduct, and rotate the shoulders. The range of motion was recorded on specially designed forms, and the final recording of the motion measured at the time of the last contact with the patient.

Elbow motion was recorded for 301 (48 %) of the patients.

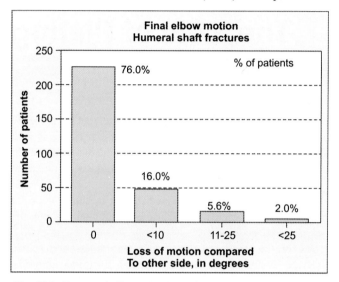

Fig. 43.3: Barograph illustrating loss of motion of the elbow at the time of removal of the brace.

REFERENCES

1. Balfour GW, Mooney V, Ashby ME. Diaphyseal Fractures of the Humerus Treated with a Ready-Made Fracture Brace. J Bone Joint Surg. 1982; 64A:11.
2. Bruggemann H, Kujat R, Tscherne H. Funkionelle Frakturebehandlung nach. Sarmiento an Unterschenkel, Unterarm und Oberarm. Orthopaede. 1983; 12:143.
3. Ekholm R, Tidemark J, Tornkvist H, Adami J, Ponzer S. Outcome after closed treatment of humeral shaft fractures. J Orthop Trauma. 2006 Oct; 20(9):591-6.
4. Ekkernkamp A, Kayser M, Althoff M. Knozept der Funktionellen Therapie am Beispiel des Frischen Geschlossenen Oberarmschaftbruches. Zentralbl Chir. 1989; 114:788.
5. Klestil T, Rangger C, Kathrein B, Huber B, Waldegger M. Sarmiento Bracing of Humeral Shaft Fractures: A comparative study. SOT (Finnish Orthop Journal). 1997; 2.
6. Latta LL, Sarmiento A, Tarr R. The Rationale of Functional Bracing of Fractures. Clin Orthop. 1980; 146:28-36.
7. Latta LL. Sarmiento A. Fracture Casting and Bracing. ASOP Publishing Inc. 2008.
8. Latta LL, Sarmiento A. Functional Bracing of selected Upper Extremity Fractures. AAOS Atlas of Orthoses and Assistive Devices. Mosby Saunders: Philadelphia. 2008: 261-9.
9. McMaster WC, Tivnon MC, Waugh TR. Cast Brace for the Upper Extremity. Clin Orthop. 1975; 109:126.
10. Naver L, Aalberg JR. Humeral Shaft Fractures Treated with a Ready-Made Fracture Brace. Arch Orthop Trauma Surg. 1986; 106:20-2.
11. Osterman PAW, Ekkerkamp A, Muhr G. Functional Bracing of Fractures of the Humerus: An analysis of 195 cases. Proc 60th Amer Acad Orthop Surg. 1993; 69.
12. Sarmiento A, Kinman PB, Galvin EG, Schmitt RH, Phillips JG: Functional Bracing of Fractures of the Shaft of the Humerus. J. Bone Joint Surg. 1977; 59A:596.
13. Sarmiento A, Latta LL. Closed Functional Treatment of fractures. Springer-Verlag, Berlin, GFR. 1981.
14. Sarmiento A, Zych GA, Zagorski JB, Latta LL. Functional Bracing of Diaphyseal Humeral Fractures. J Bone Joint Surg, 1999
15. Sarmiento A, Horowitch A, Aboulafia A, Vangsness CT Jr. Functional Bracing of comminuted extra-articular fractures of the Distal-Third of the Humerus. J. Bone Joint Surg. 1990; 72B-2:283-7.
16. Sarmiento A, Latta LL. Functional Fracture Bracing. J Amer Acad Orthop Surg. 1999; 7-1:66-75.
17. Sarmiento A, Zagorski JB, Zych GA, Latta LL, Capps CA. Functional Bracing of Humeral Shaft Fractures. J. Bone Joint Surg. 2000; 82A4:478-86
18. Sarmiento A, Latta LL. Functional Fracture Bracing. A review Article Journal AAOS. 1999; 7(1):66-78.
19. Sarmiento A, Ross SDK, Racette WL. Functional Fracture Bracing. Atlas of Orthotics. The CV Mosby & Company. 1985; 358-70.
20. Sarmiento A, Waddell JP, Latta LL. Diaphyseal Humeral Fractures: Treatment Options. An Instructional Course. AAOS J Bone and Joint Surg. 1999; 83A(10):1566-79.
21. Sarmiento A, Latta LL. The Evolution of Fracture Bracing J. Bone Joint Surg (B). 2006; 88-8(2):141-8.
22. Sarmiento A, Latta LL. Conservative treatment of humeral shaft fractures. Unfallchirurg. German Trauma Assoc. 2007.
23. Sharma VK, Jain AK, Gupta RK, Tyagi AK, Sethi PK. Non-operative treatment of Humeral Shaft Fracture: A comparative study. J Indian Med Assoc. 1991; 89:157.
24. Wasmer G, Worsdorfer O. Functional Management of Humeral Shaft Fractures with Sarmiento Cast Bracing. Unfallheilkunde. 1984; 87:309.
25. Zagorski JB, Latta LL, Zych G, Finnieston AR. Diaphyseal Fractures of the Humerus. Treatment with pre-fabricated Braces. J Bone Joint Surg. 1988; 70A:607.

44

Other Treatment Modalities: The Role of Plating

Of the various modalities currently available for the care of humeral fractures, plating is a popular one. However, even the most enthusiastic surgeons favoring internal osteosynthesis, recognize the high complication rate following plate fixation, such as radial nerve injury, nonunion and infection.[1-17]

Closed diaphyseal humeral fractures that show an initial axial distraction between fragments is a rather common situation that often requires surgical stabilization. It has been our experience that such gap may lead to nonunion, particularly if there is an associated nerve injury. The large gap between the fragments is often overcome if the associated nerve injury is limited to the radial nerve providing that early active flexion exercises to the elbow (and extensors if the triceps had retained its innervation) are carried out. If the nerve injury involves additional nerves – e.g. brachial palsy— the prognosis regarding improvement in the length of the gap is poor. Under this circumstance it is best to approach the fracture in a surgical manner.[6,8] If the accompanying soft tissue damage is significant the use of external fixators is usually the safest method of treatment. In the absence of major soft tissue damage, plating is usually recommended. Intramedullary nailing under this circumstance is probably not the best and safest approach (Figures 44.1 to 44.5).

Plating is usually chosen when there is additional systemic pathology, such as chest injury or other associated pathology, hoping that in this manner the patient can be mobilized earlier.

Many surgeons use plating with some frequency in fractures with angular deformities because of the fear that deformities, even of a few degrees, are accompanied with impaired function. We have, through the course of this manuscript, proven that most deformities identified through radiographs are clinically inconsequential, since the humerus tolerates angular deformities better than virtually any other long bone in the body. In addition, another reason for the performance of surgery is the mistaken belief that the presence of a radial palsy requires exploration. Our experience as well as the experience of many other investigators has documented that such palsies have a very good prognosis if managed conservatively.

Since patient cooperation and ability to stand erect are necessary requirements for the use of functional bracing, the polytraumatized patient is usually managed surgically. However, the presence of another fracture does not preclude the use of functional bracing of the fractured humerus. Numerous times we have treated patients who had humeral fractures amenable to closed functional care, who had either a tibial or femoral fracture or an isolated ulnar fracture. Several examples have been described in the text. The femoral fractures had been stabilized with interlocking nails and the tibias either with functional braces or intramedullary fixation.

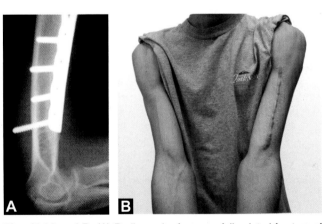

Figs 44.1A and B: (A) Radiograph of successfully plated fracture of the humerus. The most distal screw was left protruding into the soft tissues creating discomfort. It was subsequently removed. (B) The ultimate function was very good, but the surgical scar was a source of unhappiness to the young patient.

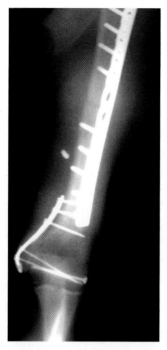

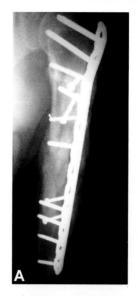

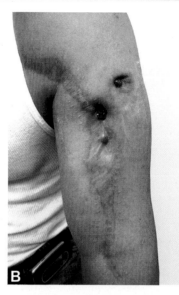

Figs 44.4A and B: Radiograph of a fracture produced by a low-velocity projectile, treated with a plate and multiple screws. It became infected. B) Photograph of the infected arm 2 years after the initial injury.

Figs 44.2: Radiograph of an appropriately treated open fracture of the humeral diaphysis using a plate. An associated nerve injury and an intra-articular fracture justified the procedure.

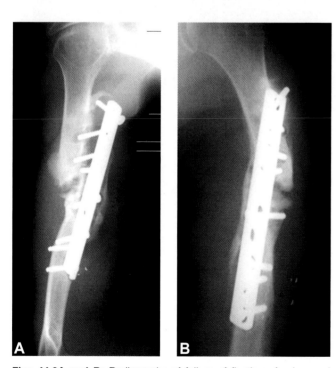

Figs 44.3A and B: Radiographs of failure of fixation of a humeral fracture treated with a plate. An appropriate number of screws had been used. It is likely that the presence of nonunion placed unsupportable stresses on the screws, leading to their eventual separation from the plate.

EXTERNAL FIXATORS

One of us (A.S.) described years ago external fixators as "nonunion making machines and instruments of the devil." They are, however, a most effective means to handle major open fractures of the humerus, particularly when associated with peripheral nerve or vascular injuries.[1,10,14,16,18,19] With their use, inspection of the skin is possible and further debridements can be carried out without difficulty.

The rigid immobilization of the fragments creates an unphysiological environment that might lead to nonunion.[16,20-27] Pin-track infection is common, which may contaminate the fracture site. The appropriate time for their discontinuance is not easy to determine. Most people remove them when the condition of the wound is satisfactory. Others prefer to keep the fixator in place until the fracture is united.

The following representative example illustrates a proper use of the system, which allowed for the care of the wound and the subsequent performance of the bone graft (Figures 44.6A to E).

INTRAMEDULLARY NAILING

The success with intramedullary nailing in the care of femoral and tibial fractures prompted interest in the possibility of using a comparable method in the care for diaphyseal humeral fractures. Results were less than satisfactory in the hands of many surgeons, due to the frequent development of damage to the rotator cuff and the associated pain and disability, as well

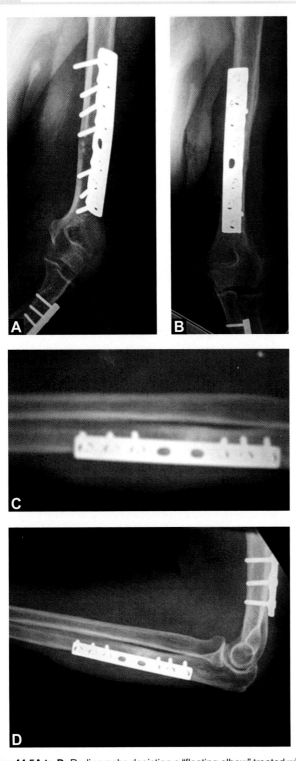

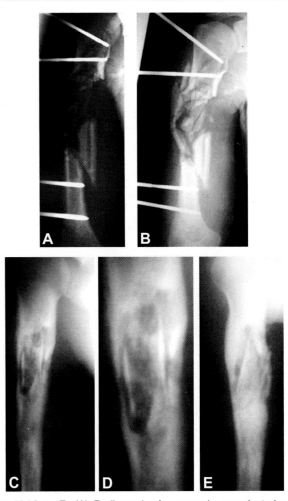

Figs 44.6A to E: (A) Radiograph of a severely comminuted open fracture of the humerus, the result of a high-velocity projectile. (B) Radiograph taken after deliberate shortening of the humerus and evidence of early healing of the grafted bone. (C) Radiograph taken a year later showing an infection with a possible sequestrum. (D and E) Fifteen months after the initial injury, the wound was still draining but the fracture appeared to be solidly united. The sequestrum has not as yet incorporated.

Figs 44.5A to D: Radiographs depicting a "floating elbow" treated with plate fixation of the humerus and ulna. Notice the cortical atrophy of the humerus underneath the plate. This atrophy may result in a new fracture if the plate is eventually removed. If the humeral fracture is an appropriate one for bracing management and the isolated ulnar fracture is not open and displaced significantly, functional bracing of both fractures usually render good results.

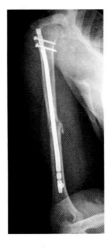

Fig. 44.7: Radiograph of a fracture of the humerus treated with an intramedullary nail. Healing seems to be taking place.

as radial nerve injury and nonunion. Reports indicating good clinical results have also been published. In order to avoid damage to the rotator cuff, inserting of the nail in a retrograde fashion, by entering the bone at the supracondylar level, has been advocated (Figure 44.7). This effort has not been as rewarding as it was initially anticipated, since iatrogenically induced fractures at the site of entrance of the nail, as well as nerve injuries have been frequently reported.[5,11,14,17,28-38]

It appears at this time that intramedullary nailing of humeral diaphyseal fractures is not recommended. If surgery is necessary, plating is the preferred method of treatment.

REFERENCES

1. Bleeker WA, Nijsten MW, ten Duis HJ. Treatment of humeral shaft fractures related to associated injuries: A retrospective study of 237 patients. Acta Orthop Scand. 1991; 62(2):148-53.
2. Foulk DA, Szabo RM. Diaphyseal humeral fractures: Natural history and occurrence of nonunion. Orthop 1995; 18(4):333-5.
3. Gill DR, Torchia ME. The spiral compression plate for proximal humeral shaft nonunion: A case report and description of a new technique. J Orthop Trauma. 1999; 13(2):141-4.
4. Ekholm R, Adami J, Tidemark K, Hansson K, Tornkvist H, Ponzer S. Fractures of the shaft of the humerus: An epidemiological study of 401 fractures. J Bone Joint Surg Br. 2006 Nov; 88(11)-1469-73.
5. Flinkkila T, Hyvonen P, Lakovaara M, Linden T, Ristiniemi J, Hamalainen M. Intramedullary nailing of humeral shaft fractures: A retrospective study of 126 cases. Acta Orthop Scand. 1999; 70(2):133-6.
6. Foulk DA, Szabo RM. Diaphyseal humerus fractures: Natural history and occurrence of nonunion. Orthopedics. 1995; 18(4):333-5.
7. Gardner MJ, Voos JE, Wanich T, Helfet DL, Lorich DG. Vascular complications of minimally invasive plating of proximal humeral fractures. J Orthop Trauma. 2006 Oct; 20(9):602.
8. Heim D, Herkert F, Hess P, Regazzoni P. Surgical treatment of humeral shaft fractures - the Basel experience. J Trauma. 1993; 35(2):226-32.
9. Jawa A, McCarthy P, Doornberg J, Harris M, Ring D. Extra-articular distal-third diaphyseal fractures of the humerus. J Bone and Joint. 2006; 88A(11):2343-7.
10. Joshi A, Labbe M, Lindsey RW. Humeral fracture secondary to civilian gunshot injury. Injury. 1998; 29 Suppl 1:SA13-17.
11. Lin J. Treatment of humeral shaft fractures with humeral locked nail and comparison with plate fixation. J Trauma. 1998; 44(5):859-64.
12. Olerud S, Dankwardt-Lilliestrom G. Fracture healing in compression osteosynthesis. Acta Orthop Scand Suppl. 1971; 137:1-44.
13. Ring D, Perey BH, Jupiter JB. The functional outcome of operative treatment of ununited fractures of the humeral diaphysis in older patients. J. Bone Joint Surg. 1999; 81A(2):177-19.
14. Sarmiento A, Waddell JP, Latta LL. Diaphyseal Humeral Fractures: Treatment Options. An Instructional Course. AAOS J Bone and Joint Surg. 1999; 83A(10):1566-79.
15. Uhthoff HK, Dubuc FL. Bone structure changes in the dog under rigid internal fixation. Clin Orthop. 1970; 81:40-7.
16. Ward EF, Savoie FH, Hughes JL. Fractures of the diaphyseal humerus. In: Browner, Jupiter, Levine, Trafton (Eds). Skeletal Trauma. WB Saunders. 1992; 2:1177-200.
17. Wu CC, Shih CH. Treatment of nonunion of the shaft of the humerus: Comparison of plates and Seidel interlocking nails. Comments. Canadian J. Surg. 1992; 35(6):576.
18. Emmerson KP, Sher JL. A method of treatment of nonunion of humeral shaft fractures following treatment by locked intramedullary nail: A report of three cases. Injury. 1998; 29(7):550-2.
19. Wisniewski TF, Radziejowski MJ. Gunshot fractures of the humeral shaft treated with external fixation. J Orthop Trauma. 1996; 10(4):273-87.
20. Latta LL, Sarmiento A, Tarr R. The Rationale of Functional Bracing of Fractures. Clin Orthop. 1980; 146:28-36
21. Perren SM. Physical and biological aspects of fracture healing with special reference to internal fixation. Clin Orthop Relat Res. 1979; 138:175.
22. Perren SM, Rahn B. Biomechanics of fracture healing I: Historical review and mechanical aspects of internal fixation. Orthop Surg. 1978; 2:108.
23. Sarmiento A, Latta LL, Tarr R. The effects of Function on Fracture Healing and Stability. AAOS Instructional Course. Mosby Saunders: Philadelphia. 1994; XXXIII.
24. Sarmiento A, Mullis DL, Latta LL, Tarr R, Alvarez R. A quantitative comparative analysis of Fracture Healing under the influence of compression plating vs. closed weight bearing Treatment. Clin Orthop. 1980; 149-232.
25. Sarmiento A, Latta L, Tarr R. Principles of fracture healing Part II: The effects of function on fracture healing and stability. Amer Acad Orthop Sur Instr Course Lectures. Mosby Saunders: Philadelphia. 1984; XXXIII.
26. Sarmiento A, Latta LL. The Evolution of Fracture Bracing J. Bone Joint Surg (B). 2006; 88-8(2):141-8.
27. Sarmiento A. The functional bracing of fractures. JBJS (A). Classics Techniques. 2007; 89 Suppl 2(2):157-69.
28. Crates J, Whittle AP. Antegrade interlocking nailing of acute humeral shaft fractures. Clin Orthop. 1998; 350:40-50.
29. Hems TE, Bhuller TP. Interlocking nailing of humeral shaft fractures: The Oxford experience 1991 to 1994. Injury. 1996; 27(7):485-9.
30. Liebergall M, Jaber S, Laster M, Aub-Snieneh K, Mattan Y, Segal D. Ender nailing of acute humeral shaft fractures in multiple injuries. Injury. 1997; 28(9-10):577-80.
31. Lin J, Hou SM: Antegrade locking nailing for humeral shaft fractures. Clin Orthop. 1999; 365:201-10.
32. Lin J, Inoue N, Valdevit A, Hang YS, Hou SM, Chao EY. Biomechanical comparison of antegrade and retrograde nailing of humeral shaft fracture. Clin Orthop. 1998; 351:203-13.
33. Moran MC. Distal interlocking during intramedullary nailing of the humerus. Clin Orthop. 1995; 317:215-8.
34. Rommens PM, Blum J, Runkel M. Retrograde nailing of humeral shaft fractures. Clin Orthop. 1998; 350:26-39.
35. Rodriguez-Merchan EC. Hackethal nailing in closed transverse humeral shaft fractures after failed manipulation. Int. Orthop. 1996; 20(3):134-6.
36. Rupp RE, Chrissos MG, Ebraheim NA. The risk of neurovascular injury with distal locking screws of humeral intramedullary nails. Orthopedics. 1996; 19(7):593-5.
37. Svend-Hansen H, Skettrup M, Rathcke MW. Complications using the Seidel intramedullary humeral nail: outcome in 31 patients. Acta Orthop Belgica. 1998; 64(3):291-5.
38. Thomsen NOB, Mikkelsen JB, Svendsen RN, Skovgaard N, Jensen CH, Jorgensen U. Interlocking nailing of humeral shaft fractures. J Orthop Sci. 1998; 3(4):199-203.

The Isolated Ulnar Fracture

45

Rationale of Functional Treatment

Plating of isolated ulnar fractures is a popular method of treatment and the overall reported results are mixed.[1-10] Postoperative infection is low, and nonunion and implant failure do not occur with great frequency. However, refracture following plate removal is not uncommon and the cost of surgical treatment remains higher.[10,11]

The popularity of surgical plating came as a result of observing that nonunion was not infrequently encountered when the limb was immobilized in a cast that extended from the head of the metacarpals to above the elbow. Such a cast had been used in accommodation to the long-held premise that joints above and below a fracture require immobilization. Today, the theory of rigid immobilization and interfragmentary fixation has been proven flawed, and replaced with evidence-supported data that freedom of motion of joints and physiologically induced motion at the fracture site are conducive to fracture healing.[4-10,12-27] The high rate of success with functional bracing of isolated ulnar fractures makes it difficult to justify the routine plating of these fractures. There are, however, instances when open surgery is the treatment of choice. There is no doubt that the period of relative disability that follows an isolated ulnar fracture is much shorter when the fracture is treated nonsurgically.

Since isolated ulnar fractures are usually the result of direct blows over the forearm, the most common displacement of the fragments is in a radial deviation. Since the damage that such an injury does to the stabilizing interosseous membrane is minimal, the displacement of the fragments is usually mild.[16,23-26] Shortening is not possible, since the intact radius prevents such a development. When the forearm is placed in a relaxed attitude of supination, the angular deformity usually improves. In any event, the common residual angulation does not result in a noticeable loss of prono-supination. As a matter of fact, it is our view that the surgical trauma produced at the time of plate fixation is more likely to create a greater degree of limitation of motion. A synostosis between the two

bones is a complication we have not observed with the use of functional braces.

Initial angular deformity in a volar direction is usually of a mild degree and the clinical consequences are rarely of any significance. Major angular deformity may be seen in severe open fractures associated with significant amount of soft tissue damage. These fractures may require stabilization with external fixators or plates. Their functional prognosis is guarded.

REFERENCES

1. Altner PC, Hartman JT. Isolated fractures of the ulnar shaft in adults. Surg Clin North Am. 1992; 52:1.
2. Burwell HN, Charnley AD. Treatment of forearm fractures in adults with particular reference to plate fixation. J Bone and Joint Surg. 1964; 46B:405-25.
3. Brakenbury PH, Corea JR, Blakenmore ME. Nonunion of Isolated Fractures of the Ulnar Shaft in Adults. Injury. 1981; 12:371.
4. Bruggemann H, Kujat R, Tscherne H. Funkionelle Frakturebehandlung nach Sarmiento an Unterschenkel, Unterarm und Oberarm. Orthopaede, 1983: 12:143.
5. Ekkernkamp A, Muhr G, Indikation and Technik der Funktionellen Knochenbruchbehandlung Oper- und Unterarm. Unfallmed. Landesver. Gewerblich, GEW. BG. 1985.
6. Gefuhr P, Holmich P, Orsness T, Soelberg M, Drasheninnikoff M, Kjersgaard AG. Isolated Ulnar Shaft Fractures: Comparison of Treatment by a Functional Brace and Long-Arm Cast. J Bone and Joint Surg. 1992; 74B:757.
7. Grace TG, Witmer BJ. Isolated Fractures of the Ulnar Shaft. Orthop. Trans. 1980; 4:299.
8. Hackstock H, Helmreich M. Isolierte Bruche des Ellenschaftes -Behandlung mit Sarmiento Brace, Verbandtechnik. 1989; 2:6.
9. Hackstock H. Funktionelle Schienenbehhandlung von Frakturen. Isolated Ulnar Fractures. Orthopade 1988; 17:41-51.
10. Pollock FH, Pankovich AM, Prieto JJ, Lorenz M. The Isolated Fracture of the Ulnar Shaft - Treatment without Immobilization. J. Bone Joint Surg. 1983; 65A:339.

11. Hidaka S, Gustilo RB. Refracture of Bones of the Forearm after Plate Removal. J. Bone and Joint Surg. 1984; 66A:1241.

12. Goodship A, Kenwright J. The influence of induced micromovement upon the healing of experimental tibial fractures. J. Bone Joint Surg Br. 1985; 67:650-5.

13. Latta LL, Sarmiento A, Tarr RR. The Rationale of Functional Bracing of Fractures. Clin Orthop & Rel Res. 1980; 146:28-36.

14. Latta LL, Sarmiento A. Principles of non-operative Fracture Treatment. Skeletal Trauma. Browner B et al. (Eds). Mosby Saunders Publishing. 1997.

15. Park SH, O'Connor K, McKellop H, Sarmiento A. The Influence of active Shear or Compressive Motion on Fracture Healing. Jour. Bone and Joint Surg. 1998 June; 80A(6):868-78.

16. Sarmiento A, Latta LL, Zych G, McKeever P, Zagorski J. Isolated Ulnar Shaft Fractures Treated with Functional Braces. Journ. Of Orthopaedic Trauma. 1998; 12(6):420-4.

17. Sarmiento A, Kinman P, Murphy R, Phillips J. Treatment of Ulnar Fractures by Functional Bracing. Jour Bone and Joint Surg. 1976; 58A(8):1104-7.

18. Sarmiento A, Cooper JS, Sinclair WF. Forearm Fractures - Early Functional Bracing - A Preliminary Report. J. Bone & Joint Surg. 1975; 57A:297-304.

19. Sarmiento A, Ebramzadeh E, Brys D, Tarr R. Angular Deformities and forearm Function. Ortho. Res. 1992; 10-1:121-33.

20. Sarmiento A, Latta LL, Tarr RR, Alvarez R. A Quantitative Comparative Analysis of Fracture Bracing Under the Influence of Compression Plating versus Closed Weight Bearing Treatment. Clin. Orthop. 1980; 149:232-9.

21. Sarmiento A, Latta LL. Closed Functional Treatment of Fractures. Springer-Verlag. 1981 Feb.

22. Sarmiento A, The functional bracing of fractures. JBJS (A). Classics techniques. 2007; 89 Suppl 2(2):157-69.

23. Latta LL, Sarmiento A. Casting and Bracing of Fractures. A.S.O.P. 2008.

24. Moore TM, Lester DK, Sarmiento A. The Stabilizing Effect of Soft Tissue Constraints in Artificial Galeazzi Fractures. Clin. Orthop. & Rel. Res. 1985; 194:189-94.

25. Schneiderman G, Meldrum RD, Bloebaum RD, Tarr R, Sarmiento A. The Interosseous Membrane of the Forearm Structure and Its Role in Galeazzi Fractures. Trauma. 1993; 35(6).

26. Tarr RR, Garfinkel AI, Sarmiento A. The Effects of Angular and Rotational Deformities of Both Bones of the Forearm: An in vitro Study. J. Bone and Joint Surg. 1984; 66A(1):65-70.

46

Indications and Contraindications

Most isolated ulnar fractures are the result of a direct blow over the forearm and in most instances, the fracture is of a closed type. When a fracture of the ulnar diaphysis occurs following a fall on the outstretched hand, an associated dislocation of the radial head is almost always present. This condition, known as a Monteggia fracture, is a clear indication for surgical intervention due to the difficulties encountered in maintaining a manually achieved reduction.

The above observations suggest that the majority of isolated ulnar fractures can be successfully treated with functional braces that permit early use of the extremity without the need for the prevention of prono-supination of the forearm, and flexion and extension of the elbow and wrist.

We recognize that the functional brace does not immobilize the fractured fragments. This is a desirable feature, since immobilization retards healing. This is true for all other types of braces used in the care of tibial or humeral fractures. In the case of the ulna, simply the brace provides comfort and holds the forearm in the desirable relaxed attitude of supination, which assists in maintaining the two bones as far apart as possible.

Pankovich and his associates reported successful results in treating isolated ulnar fractures simply with the use of an elastic bandage.[1] Their work further supports the concept that immobilization is not necessary. However, the brace provides a degree of comfort the bandage does not accomplish.

Low-grade open fractures can also be treated in this manner following appropriate debridement of the injured soft tissues. More severe open fractures associated with major soft tissue damage may require stabilization with external fixators until the condition of the area is satisfactory and free of infection. At that point, internal fixation and bone grafting may be indicated.

REFERENCE

1. Pollock FH, Pankovich AM, Prieto JJ, Lorenz M. The Isolated Fracture of the Ulnar Shaft - Treatment without Immobilization. J. Bone Joint Surg. 1983; 65A:339.

47

Acute Management: Closed Fractures

In order to provide relief from the acute pain that accompanies any fracture, we prefer to stabilize the arm in an above-the-elbow cast that holds the elbow in a position of 90° of flexion and the forearm in a relaxed attitude of supination. The position of relaxed supination is more likely to place the fragments in the most anatomical alignment. In addition, it helps in restoring earlier prono-supination of the forearm, because that routine daily activities call for the use of pronation more frequently than supination. In other words patients, by necessity, pronate their forearm and regain the initially lost motion. Furthermore, in the event that a permanent loss of motion of the forearm would take place, it is best to lose the last few degrees of pronation rather than supination. The shoulder girdle, through an inconspicuous motion of flexion, abduction and rotation compensates for that loss. A comparable inconspicuous mechanism for the loss of supination does not exist.

The initial long-arm cast is not always necessary. If the energy that produced the fracture was moderate and the accompanying pain and swelling are not significant, a below-the-elbow cast or splint may suffice. In some instances, the functional brace can be applied initially.

When a cast or splint is used initially, it does not need to be held in place for more than 1 week. Most patients, at that time, experience only from minimal to moderate discomfort. Those who use their fingers from the very outset, are more likely to get rid of pain sooner. This is something important to keep in mind when dealing with bilateral fractures.

48

Open Fractures

Low-energy produced open fractures rarely demonstrate significant displacement between the fractured fragments. The intact radius and interosseous membrane prevent major displacement. In open fractures resulting from high-energy injuries and associated with major soft tissue damage, the displacement between the fragments may be significant due to damage to the stabilizing interosseous membrane.[1,2] These fractures require appropriate debridement of the wound, and not infrequently, stabilization with plates or external fixators. Less severe fractures can be managed with functional braces as soon as the wounds begin to show healthy signs of healing.

The presence of an open wound does not preclude the use of braces since they are removable and permit cleansing of the wound and frequent dressings change.

In most instances, the initial above-the-elbow cast is more comfortable than the below-the-elbow cast. It can be removed at the end of the first week. The brace is then applied. A sling or collar- and-cuff is also applied in order to eliminate the pain that the dependent arm is likely to produce.

The brace ("sleeve") permits unencumbered use of the arm since it does not extend over the elbow or wrist. It simply limits prono-supination. The brace must be adjustable in order to effectively compress the soft tissues and, in that manner, provide comfort.

REFERENCES

1. Sarmiento A, Cooper JS, Sinclair WF. Forearm Fractures - Early Functional Bracing - A Preliminary Report. J Bone & Joint Surg. 1975; 57A:297-304.
2. Sarmiento A, The functional bracing of fractures. JBJS (A). Classics techniques. 2007; 89 Suppl 2(2):157-69.

49

The Pre-fabricated Brace:
Instructions and Expectations

CLINICAL EXPERIENCE

The orthopedic literature is relatively rich in reports indicating a high degree of success with closed functional bracing of isolated ulnar fractures.[1-13]

The following is an abbreviated version on an article published in 1998 reporting in 444 isolated ulnar fractures with pre-fabricated functional braces.[8] All patients had their fractures initially stabilized in above-elbow Plaster of Paris casts holding the forearm in relaxed attitude of supination. The brace was applied on the average of 18 days (range 1-66 days). Delays in seeking initial Emergency Room care or in obtaining appointment at the outpatient clinic explained the delay in brace application. The orthopedic team would have preferred the application of the brace to have taken place no later than 7 days after the initial insult.

Hospitalization was not required for closed fractures. Patient with open fractures were admitted to the hospital for debridement and intravenous antibiotic therapy for 3 days. Patients were instructed to report to a special Fracture Brace Clinic 1 week later and then at monthly intervals.

The degree of activity of the injured arm was left at the discretion of the patient and to be determined by the degree of symptoms. No restrictions on the use of the fractured extremity were imposed.

The prefabricated brace is removable and adjustable with Velcro straps. It comes in three different sizes and extended from below the elbow to above the wrist without interfering with elbow or wrist motion. The brace is applied with the forearm still held in a relaxed attitude of supination in order to separate the radius and the ulna as much as possible. Its snugness over the soft tissues limits prono-supination to approximately 50% of its normal range. Patients are encouraged to maintain the snugness of the brace at all times and to remove it daily for

hygienic purposes. As symptoms begin to subside, patients are encouraged to carry out gentle prono-supination of the forearm for short periods of time without the brace.

Of the 444 patients, 278 patients with 287 (65%) fractures were available to follow-up out of which 186 (67%) were males and 92 (33%) were females. The mean age was 35 years (range 21-82). Nine patients (3%) had bilateral ulnar fractures. One hundred and twenty (42%) occurred in the right forearm and 167 (58%) in the left forearm.

One hundred and sixty-one fractures (56%) were located in the distal-third of the ulnar diaphysis; 111 (39%) in the middle-third and 15 (5%) in the proximal-third.

One hundred and sixteen (40%) fractures were oblique, 96 (33%) were transverse, 68 (24% were comminuted and seven (3%) were segmental.

Closed fractures were diagnosed in 258 (90%) patients and open fractures in 29 (10%) patients.

RESULTS

Braces were removed when clinical and radiological union of the fracture was diagnosed based on absence of pain at the fracture site and early bony bridging of the fragments. The average length of brace usage was 64 days (range 23-206 days). Union took place in 99% of patients. Three fractures (1%) developed nonunion and five (1.3%) had delayed union. Shortening of the ulna averaged 1.1 mm (range 0-10 mm).

Final radial angulation averaged 5° (range 0-18°). Dorsal angulation averaged 5° (range 0-20°).

The range of motion of the elbow, wrist and forearm, as recorded at the time the brace was discontinued, indicated a loss of elbow extension that averaged 5° (0-30); and that of flexion of 3° (range 0-30).

Proximal-third fractures had an average loss of pronation of 12° (range 0-60) and that of supination of 1° (range 0-10) Middle-third fractures had a loss of pronation of 10° (range 0-45) and that of supination of 2° (range 0-25).

Distal-third fractures had an average loss of pronation of 5° (range 0-35); and that of supination of 7° (range 0-40).

Three (1%) patients with open fractures developed synostosis between the radius and ulna eliminating all pronation and supination. These patients had concomitant head injuries.

Using the criteria outlined by Altner and Hartman,[14] the clinical results recorded at the time of brace removal, as far as range motion is concerned, 247 patients (89%) had an excellent result; 21 (7.5%) patients had a good result and 10 patients (3.5%) had a poor result. It is assumed that the limitation of motion recorded at the time of brace removal decreased with continued use of the extremity. It is very likely, therefore, that the percentage of patients in the good and excellent categories was ultimately higher had we had the opportunity to evaluate them several months later.

DISCUSSION

The popularity of plate fixation of ulnar fracture is probably strongly influenced by the long accepted belief that rigid immobilization of fracture fragments and interfragmentary fixation create the ideal environment for diaphyseal fracture healing. In fact, there is currently ample evidence to indicate that rigid immobilization of diaphyseal fractures delays healing and that motion at the fracture site is a most important factor in osteogenesis[6,15-17] The incidence of 1% nonunion reported in this large group of patients testifies to the value of the hypothesis that motion at the fracture is desirable for fracture repair. The peripheral callus that forms in the presence of motion at the fracture site has superior mechanical properties than the callus seen when fracture immobilization is carried out.[6,16-18] Contributing to the wide use of osteosynthesis in the management of this fracture is also the perception that loss of anatomical alignment results in impairment of function. Though malalignment of a significant degree results in loss of prono-supination, clinical and laboratory studies have indicated that mild angular deformities produce minimal impairment of function.[4,6,8-13,19-21] Severe degree of angulation of ulnar fragments is very unlikely in isolated fractures of the ulna. For it to occur, either an associated fracture of the radius or a dislocation of the ulna at either end of the forearm is necessary. The presence of a strong interosseous membrane further prevents angulation from reaching high degrees especially when the mechanism of injury is a direct blow or a projectile striking the bone. Functional bracing treatment is contraindicated in the care of isolated ulnar fractures when there is an associated dislocation of the radial head. The

clinical and radiographic results in this large series support the premise that minor angular deformities are associated with minimal residual limitation of motion. Other investigators have reported comparable clinical results (Figures 49.1 and 49.3).[1-15,13,19]

From the radiological point of view, anatomical restoration of alignment of fractures is more readily achievable with surgical techniques producing a more esthetic appearance of the fractured bone. The esthetic alignment shown on the x-ray does not necessarily show parallel function. Even 10° of malalignment of fractures of both bones of the forearm leave a functional extremity with minimal, if any, discernible cosmetically detectable deviation.[8-10,19,21] It is likely that the cosmetic appearance of a fractured forearm healed with a few degrees of malalignment is more acceptable than that produced by the scars left by the surgical intervention.

The economic implications of fracture care in the current fiscal/political atmosphere is an important factor, which in earlier years did not play an important role. Surgical treatment of ulnar fractures is more expensive than the non-surgical one, see Tables 49.1 to 49.3. The fact that surgical removal of the implant is necessary or desirable, in many instances, further increases the cost of surgical care. The need to protect the plated bone from major stresses, particularly after the removal of the implant, precludes those labor or athletic activities that might place the bone in jeopardy, for an additional period of time.[22] According to a report by Gefuhr,[3] a group of patients treated with functional braces returned to work at a median time of 33 days. This study suggests that closed functional bracing of isolated ulnar fractures produces good functional and cosmetic results without the possible complications associated with surgery and anesthesia. The residual limitation of motion of the forearm is minimal and the overall cost of care significantly lower, see Tables 49.1 to 49.3.

Table 49.1: Cost of surgical plating of Isolated ulnar fractures	
Emergency Room Charges:	$ 144.00
X-Rays	$ 125.00
E.R. Physician	$ 90.00
Supplies	$ 150.00
$ 479.00	
Hospitalization	
Operating Room	
Fixation device	
Laboratory	
Hospital Room	$ 5492.00
Anesthesiologist	$ 900.00
Orthopedic Surgeon's global fee	$ 1650.00
Three F.U. X-Rays	
$ 50.00 each.	$ 150.00
TOTAL:	**$ 8671.00**

Table 49.2: Loss of motion (degrees) with angulation of the ulna								
			Proximal fracture		Middle fracture		Distal Fracture	
Degrees of angulation	Direction of angulation	n	Loss of pronation	Loss of supination	Loss of pronation	Loss of supination	Loss of pronation	Loss of supination
5	Dorsal	3	− 2 (1)	3 (1)	9 (3)	1 (3)	3 (3)	6 (6)
5	Volar	3	− 1 (1)	4 (3)	11 (4)	2 (6)	2 (4)	2 (3)
5	Radial	3	− 3 (2)	1 (1)	13 (2)	3 (6)	5 (6)	1 (4)
5	Ulnar	3	—	—	11 (5)	− 1 (5)	1 (3)	0 (1)
10	Dorsal	3	2 (2)	4 (1)	10 (2)	4 (8)	7 (4)	13 (7)
10	Volar	3	0 (1)	9 (7)	14 (6)	8 (13)	16 (16)	3 (3)
10	Radial	3	5 (2)	1 (2)	17 (4)	17 (2)	12 (13)	12 (11)
10	Ulner	3	—	—	—	—	—	—
15	Dorsal	3	8 (1)	4 (1)	—	—	9 (6)	23 (3)
15	Volar	3	—	—	15 (5)	24 (10)	15 (16)	9 (3)
15	Radial	3	11 (2)	6 (1)	33 (1)	31 (1)	24 (1)	20 (1)
15	Ulnar	3	—	—	—	—	—	—

Table 49.3: Cost of closed functional bracing of isolated ulnar fractures		
Emergency Room Charges:	$114.00	
X- Rays	125.00	
E.R. Physician	90.00	
Supplies	150.00	$ 379.00
Hospitalization NONE		
Anesthesiologist. NONE		
Orthopedic Surgeon? global fee.	$900. 00	$ 900.00
3 F.U. X-Rays		
$50.00 each	$ 150.00	$ 150.00
Functional Brace.	$100.00	$ 100.00
TOTAL:		**$1529.00**

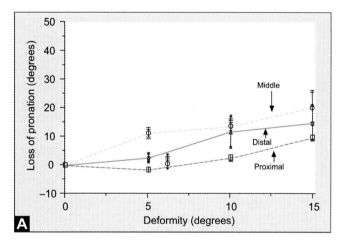

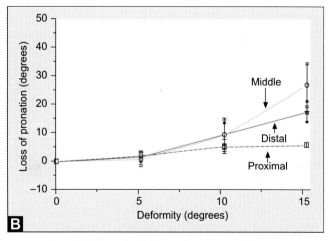

Figs 49.1A and B: Relationship between deformity and loss of motion.

The ulna fracture brace, or "sleeve," must be adjustable in order to make possible its frequent removal and re-application for hygienic purposes and to ensure the maintenance of its desirable snugness against the soft tissues. Velcro straps are best for this purpose. Circular casts that cannot be adjusted slip distally as swelling subsides and atrophy of the musculature takes place. The brace should be short enough to make possible free motion of the wrist and elbow, regardless of the location of the fracture (Figures 49.2A to H). Obviously, rigid immobilization of fragments is not necessary. All the brace accomplishes is probably nothing more than provision of comfort and protection to the arm from inadvertent forceful contact with hard objects.

Patients are encouraged to use the extremity to the maximum degree allowed by pain. In most instances, the pain present at the time of application of the brace is only moderate. It is our opinion that the early introduction of function results in a more rapid disappearance of acute symptoms and faster healing.

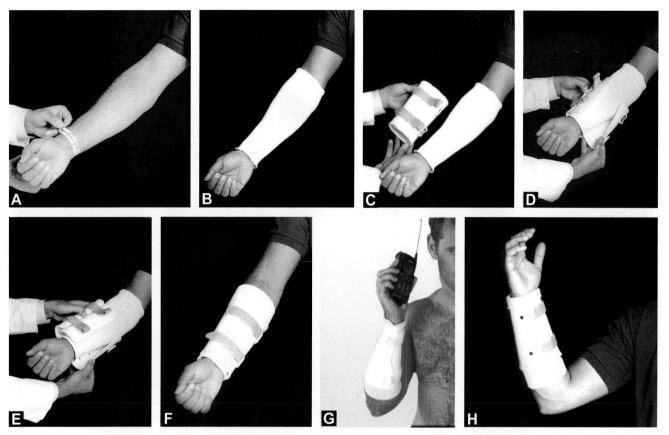

Figs 49.2A to H: Photographs of the sequential steps taken during the application of the ulnar brace; the adjustable Velcro straps; and the range of motion of the elbow and wrist.

The brace should be adjusted on a frequent basis during the first few days in order to maintain the desirable compression of the soft tissues and to prevent the distal displacement of the sleeve over the wrist. The brace may be removed for hygienic purposes as often as necessary and the collar-and-cuff permanently discontinued as soon as the systems subside.

Flexion and extension of the elbow are rapidly regained. Pronation and supination required a longer period of time because such motions are more painful. In a few instances, we have treated patients with functional braces who had sustained bilateral isolated ulnar fractures. Their recovery was rapid and uneventful.

BRACE REMOVAL AND FOLLOW-UP

The brace is permanently discontinued as soon as radiographs show evidence of early callus formation, the symptoms have completely subsided and unencumbered motion has been achieved. We do not believe the brace is necessary after that time, even if the amount of osseous callus is not abundant according to the radiographs.

EXPECTED OUTCOMES

At the time of completion of healing, there is usually full range of motion of the elbow. The motion of the wrist may be slightly limited for an additional few weeks, particularly when the fracture was located close to the wrist joint. Permanent loss of pronation and supination is found in a small percentage of patients, particularly in those with fractures located in the proximal-third of the bone (Figures 49.2 and 49.3). The overall functional results are most gratifying. (See RESULTS)

MANAGING COMPLICATIONS

We are not aware of any complications that can be directly traced to the brace other than possible allergic reaction to the stockinet or to the plastic material of the appliance. Increase of angulation at the fracture site is known to take place in situations when major initial displacement was corrected at the time of application of the brace. Usually, the intrinsic stability of the fracture provided by the interosseous membrane ensures that the original displacement will remain unchanged.

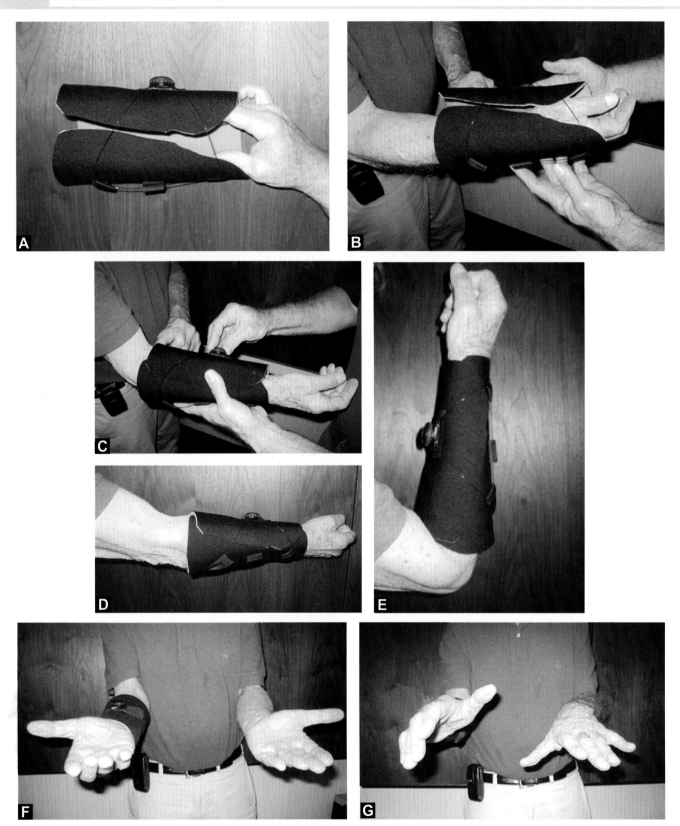

Figs 49.3A to G: The brace allows unrestricted elbow and wrist motion, but prevents complete pronation.

SYNOSTOSIS

Synostosis is extremely rare when forearm fractures are treated with functional braces. We found out this to be true even in the relatively small number of fractures of both bones of the forearm treated with functional braces. Perhaps the early introduction of function prevents the building of a bridge between the two bones.

Synostosis is more common following plate fixation. Fractures associated with head injuries are known to develop heterotopic bone. We had the opportunity to observe one instance of synostosis following an isolated ulnar fracture. This complication requires surgical excision of the bony bridge. The prognosis is not always good since a residual limitation of motion is usually identified.

DELAYED UNIONS AND NONUNIONS

Most isolated ulnar fractures demonstrate radiological union within 2 to 2½ months. Most demonstrate large peripheral callus. There are instances, however, when a gap between the fragments remains present for a longer period of time, suggesting a delayed union or a nonunion. If the associated symptoms are minimal or non-existent, skillful neglect is the most appropriate approach. In most instances, radiological healing eventually becomes apparent (Figures 49.4A and B). Failure to achieve bony union calls for surgery and possibly grafting if the nonunion has remained painful.

Nonunion has been reported to be less than 3%. In our series, the nonunion rate was 1%. Infection may occur in open fractures, but this complication is unrelated to the bracing method (See RESULTS).

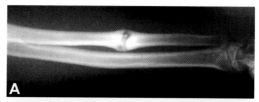
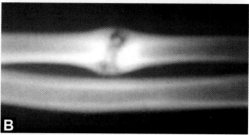

Figs 49.4: Radiographs of healed ulnar fracture demonstrating a lack of bony trabeculae at the center of the bone. This not uncommon finding is inconsequential, since virtually the defect eventually disappears.

SKIN PROBLEMS

Allergic reactions to the stockinette of plastic material are rare. Poor hygiene is the most likely cause of skin irritation. The frequent removal of the brace and washing of the arm and hand, which is possible and recommended from the very outset, prevents skin problems. If present, it is probably due to excessive perspiration and a reaction to heat.

REPRESENTATIVE EXAMPLES

Some of the representative examples illustrating closed functional bracing of ulnar fractures are shown from Figures 49.5 to 49.10.

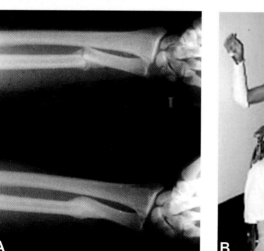
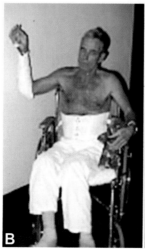
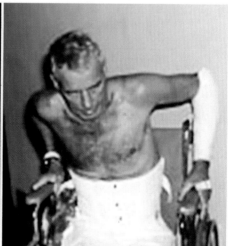

Figs 49.5A and B: (A) Radiograph of an ulnar fracture showing early callus, and the patient, a paraplegic, illustrating the ulnar brace, which we originally constructed as a Munster-like prosthesis. Shortly afterwards we realized that the supracondylar extension was unnecessary. (B) The freedom of motion of the elbow and wrist made it possible for the patient to engage in transfer activities less than 3 weeks after the initial insult.

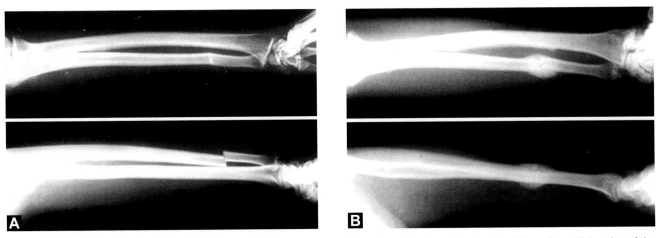

Figs 49.6A and B: (A) Transverse fracture in the distal-third of the ulna. Since the radius is not fractured and there is no dislocation of the proximal or distal radio-ulnar joints, shortening of the fragments is impossible. (B) Radiograph of the fracture solidly united with abundant peripheral callus. The fracture was treated with an ulnar brace that allowed full range of motion of the elbow and wrist, and only limited prono-supination of the forearm.

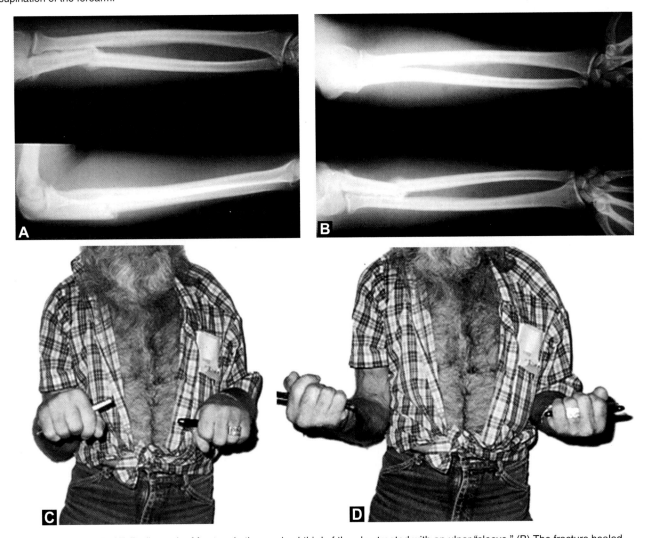

Figs 49.7A to D: (A) Radiograph of fracture in the proximal-third of the ulna treated with an ulnar "sleeve." (B) The fracture healed uneventfully. (C and D) Patient illustrates the mild and inconsequential limitation of pronation.

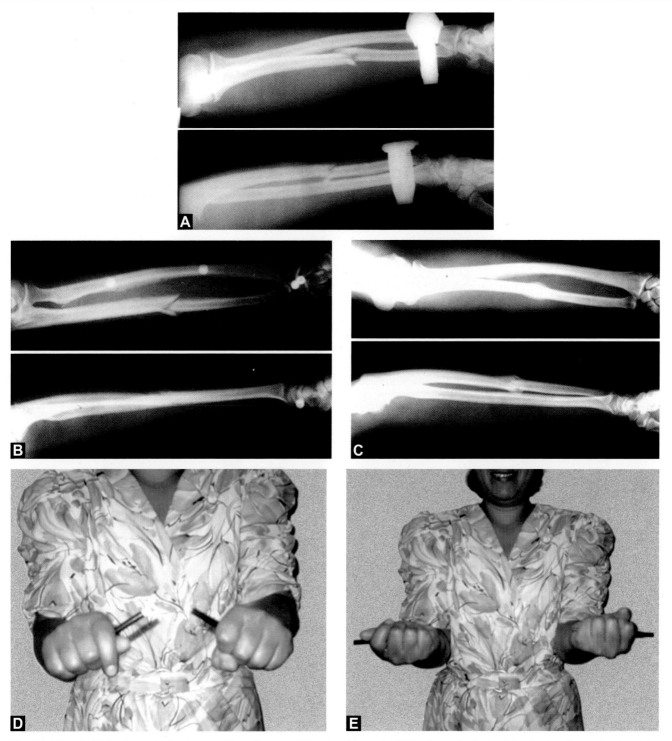

Figs 49.8A to E: (A) Radiograph showing an oblique fracture of the ulnar diaphysis. (B) Radiograph obtained shortly after the application of the ulnar brace. (C) The fracture healed with abundant peripheral callus. (D and E) Patient demonstrates normal pronation and supination of her forearms.

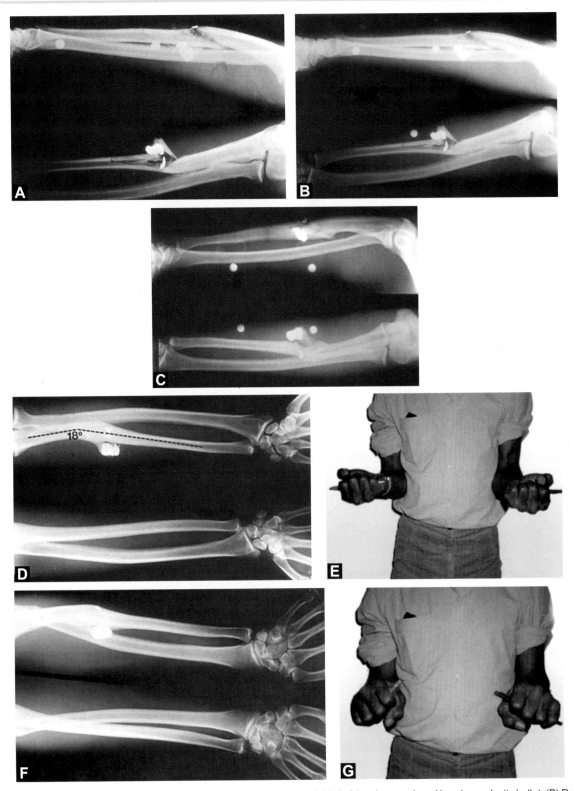

Figs 49.9A to G: (A) Radiograph of slightly comminuted fracture in the proximal-third of the ulna, produced by a low-velocity bullet. (B) Radiograph of the forearm in supination shortly after the application of the ulnar brace. (C) Radiograph obtained approximately 2 months after the initial injury showing evidence of progressive union. (D and E) Radiograph and clinical photograph of the forearms demonstrating normal supination of the injured forearms. (F and G) Radiograph and clinical photograph of the forearms demonstrating a residual limitation of pronation, which the patient readily and inconspicuously compensates with shoulder rotation.

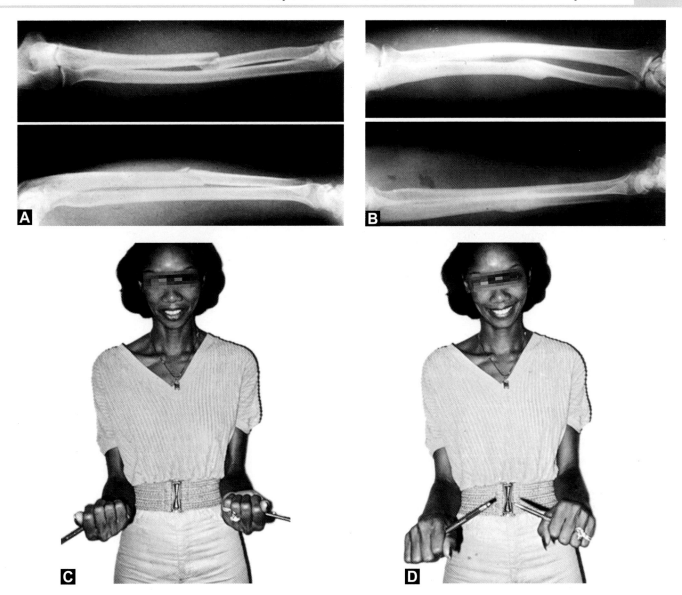

Figs 49.10A to D: (A and B) Radiograph of the initial diaphyseal fracture of the ulna and after completion of healing demonstrating solid union with abundant peripheral callus. (C and D) Patient shows a minimal, inconsequential limitation of pronation of the forearm.

REFRACTURE

Diaphyseal fractures that are treated with functional braces usually heal with peripheral callus. Under those circumstances, the likelihood of refracture is minimal. If a new fracture were to occur, it would be either above or below the old fracture, since the bone at the level of the old fracture is stronger than the rest of the diaphysis. When an ulnar fracture is plated, the cortices under the plate experience thinning. If a new injury to the forearm were to produce a fracture, the changes are that it will occur either at the level of a defect left by a removed screw or at the level of the old fracture. Its management

would be functional braces if the fracture meets the criteria for nonsurgical care.

RANGE OF MOTION

It is logical to expect a temporary weakness of grip in all patients who sustain diaphyseal ulnar fractures. However, since the period of inactivity is relatively short, the resulting muscular weakness is mild and the recovery thereof is rapid. The same applies to the residual limitation of motion. Some patients demonstrate a mild loss of pronation of the forearm, but inconspicuous compensation occurs with mild flexion, abduction and internal rotation of the shoulder. This mechanism is similar to that used by below-the-elbow amputees who pronate the terminal device in the same manner. The limitation of pronation detected at the time the brace is permanently discontinued, tends to improve with the return to normal activities without the hindrance that the brace posed.

POST-BRACING MANAGEMENT

Patients should avoid early, prolonged dependency of the injured extremity because of the likely possibility of distal edema developing. Frequent tightening of the fist and wrist active exercises assist in the prevention and correction of this problem.

The patient can temporarily remove the brace in order to carry out active prono-supination of the forearm when the degree of discomfort permits it. Most patients seem to be able to do so after one week of wearing the brace. Washing of the forearm can be done as often as desired.

DATA

The following tables depict the initial results obtained with the first 142 patients with isolated ulnar fractures treated with a functional brace. Subsequently, a report was made on over 400 similar fractures. The results did not differ significantly with the original ones except for a greater loss of pronosupination in fractures located in the proximal third (Table 49.4 to 49.10).

Table 49.4: Results of open treatment of isolated fr of the ulna[a]

	Method	No of Fractures
Smith and Sage (1957)[b]	Medullary	79
Smith (1959)[c]	Medullary	73
DeBuren (1962)[d]	Planting	77

Table 49.5: Isolated fractures of tl

Age distribution	
Range	16–75
Average	34
Mode	31
Median	35
Nature	
Closed	130
Open	12
Total	142
Location	
Proximal 1/3	4
Middle 1/3	55
Distal 1/3	82
Segmental	1
Total	142

Table 49.6: Healing time distributed by location of isolated ulnar fracture

	Healing time (weeks)		
	Range	Average	Median
Proximal 1/3	7.0–15.9	10.3	
Middle 1/3	6.3–22.3	8.9	8.4
Distal 1/3	6.0–15.9	7.9	8.1

Table 49.7: Average loss of function in treatment of isolated ulnar fractures

	No of cases	Loss of motion (degrees)		
		Pronation	Supination	Total
Proximal 1/3	4	2	4	6
Middle 1/3	55	5	3	8
Distal 1/3	82	5	7	12
Segmental	1	5	3	8
Total	142			

Table 49.8: Criteria for results of treatment of isolated fractures of the ulna

	Forearm rotation	Joint motion
Excellent	90%	90%
Good	70-89%	70-89%
Poor	< 70%	< 70%

REFERENCES

1. Bruggemann H, Kujat R, Tscherne H. Funkionelle Frakturebehandlung nach Sarmiento an Unterschenkel, Unterarm und Oberarm. Orthopaede, 1983: 12:143.
2. Ekkernkamp A, Muhr G, Indikation and Technik der Funktionellen Knochenbruchbehandlung Oper- und Unterarm. Unfallmed. Landesver. Gewerblich, GEW. BG. 1985.
3. Gefuhr P, Holmich P, Orsness T, Soelberg M, Drasheninnikoff M, Kjersgaard AG. Isolated Ulnar Shaft Fractures: Comparison of Treatment by a Functional Brace and Long-Arm Cast. J Bone and Joint Surg. 1992; 74B:757.
4. Hackstock H, Helmreich M. Isolierte Bruche des Ellenschaftes -Behandlung mit Sarmiento Brace, Verbandtechnik. 1989; 2:6.
5. Hackstock H. Funktionelle Schienenbehandlung von Frakturen. Isolated Ulnar Fractures. Orthopade 1988; 17:41-51.
6. Latta LL, Sarmiento A, Tarr RR. The Rationale of Functional Bracing of Fractures. Clin Orthop & Rel Res. 1980; 146:28-36.
7. Latta LL, Sarmiento A. Casting and Bracing of Fractures. A.S.O.P. 2008.
8. Sarmiento A, Latta LL, Zych G, McKeever P, Zagorski J. Isolated Ulnar Shaft Fractures Treated with Functional Braces. Journ. Of Orthopaedic Trauma. 1998; 12(6):420-4.
9. Sarmiento A, Kinman P, Murphy R, Phillips J. Treatment of Ulnar Fractures by Functional Bracing. Jour Bone and Joint Surg. 1976; 58A(8):1104-7.

10. Sarmiento A, Cooper JS, Sinclair WF. Forearm Fractures - Early Functional Bracing - A Preliminary Report. J. Bone & Joint Surg. 1975; 57A:297-304.

11. Sarmiento A, Latta LL. Closed Functional Treatment of Fractures. Springer-Verlag. 1981 Feb.

12. Sarmiento A, The functional bracing of fractures. JBJS (A). Classics techniques. 2007; 89 Suppl 2(2):157-69.

13. Zych GA, Zagorski JB, Latta LL. Treatment of Isolated Ulnar Fractures with Prefabricated Fracture Braces. Clin Orthop. 1987; 219:194-200.

14. Altner PC, Hartman JT. Isolated fractures of the ulnar shaft in adults. Surg Clin North Am. 1992; 52:1.

15. Goodship A, Kenwright J. The influence of induced micromovement upon the healing of experimental tibial fractures. J. Bone Joint Surg Br. 1985; 67:650-5.

16. Latta LL, Sarmiento A. Principles of non-operative Fracture Treatment. Skeletal Trauma. Browner B et al. (Eds). Mosby Saunders Publishing. 1997.

17. Park SH, O'Connor K, McKellop H, Sarmiento A. The Influence of active Shear or Compressive Motion on Fracture Healing. Jour. Bone and Joint Surg. 1998 June; 80A(6):868-78.

18. Sarmiento A, Latta LL, Tarr RR, Alvarez R. A Quantitative Comparative Analysis of Fracture Bracing Under the Influence of Compression Plating versus Closed Weight Bearing Treatment. Clin. Orthop. 1980; 149:232-9.

19. Pollock FH, Pankovich AM, Prieto JJ, Lorenz M. The Isolated Fracture of the Ulnar Shaft - Treatment without Immobilization. J. Bone Joint Surg. 1983; 65A:339.

20. Sarmiento A, Ebramzadeh E, Brys D, Tarr R. Angular Deformities and forearm Function. Ortho. Res. 1992; 10-1:121-33.

21. Tarr RR, Garfinkel AI, Sarmiento A. The Effects of Angular and Rotational Deformities of Both Bones of the Forearm: An in vitro Study. J. Bone and Joint Surg. 1984; 66A(1):65-70.

22. Hidaka S, Gustilo RB. Refracture of Bones of the Forearm after Plate Removal. J. Bone and Joint Surg. 1984; 66A:1241.

The Colles' Fracture

50

Rationale of Functional Treatment

The orthopedic community has witnessed, in recent years, interest in the surgical treatment of fractures of the distal radius. A number of comparative studies between internal osteosynthesis and external fixation have been published. Conspicuous for their absence are analyses of clinical results with non-surgical methods of treatment, as if such a traditional method had been rendered obsolete.

Improved metallurgical and imaging techniques have documented the worth of many surgical methods used in fracture care, such as closed intramedullary nailing of long bone fractures. As far as we are concerned, the same cannot be said about the surgical treatment of distal radius fractures. In general, the literature has not convincingly supported the current enthusiasm with the surgical approach and there is no evidence that long-term results are superior, except in the case of intra-articular, comminuted, displaced fractures. Several reports have indicated significantly improved results with the use of volar plating in the case of these fractures.[1-4]

A final verdict regarding the true indications for surgery has not yet been rendered and the genesis of the trend is not completely clear. However, there should be no doubt that the volar approach to the distal radius and the use of a plate has been a major and most important contribution to the treatment of Colles' fractures. The pioneer work of J. Orbay in Miami in the year 2000 started a revolution of great significance.

We can only suspect some of the subtle factors that underline the current preference for surgery: (1) The intuitive assumption that anatomical restoration of anatomy has to be superior to acceptance of deviations from the normal. (2) the emotional satisfaction that anatomical repositioning of the broken fragments brings to the surgeon. (3) The greater social prestige the surgeon gains from treating the pathological condition by surgical means. (4) The fact that surgical care is financially better recompensed. (5) The fear of litigation, since at this time it is wrongly perceived that a bad surgical result is easier to defend than one arising from conservative treatment. The surgeon can often claim in the face of complications that the surgical technique was appropriately implemented.

These skeptical views do not imply a failure to recognize the limitations of the non-surgical care of these fractures. Quite the contrary, certain distal radial fractures are best managed surgically. However, the vast majority of them may be treated successfully and inexpensively by closed means.[1,5-21]

Our discussion regarding the non-surgical treatment of wrist fractures is limited to the classical Colles' fracture. The Smith, chauffeur's and Barton's fractures have been discussed by others.

Distal radial fractures are usually lumped into the broad eponym of Colles' fractures, in recognition of the fact that it was Abraham Colles, of Scotland, who first described the fracture and proposed a treatment protocol.[9] The fact that his work was done long before the invention of radiography, enlarges the significance of his contribution. Obviously, he must have failed to recognize that among his patients, some had fractures that did not fit into his classical description. Two hundred years later, we have come to the conclusion that the Colles' fracture represents, however, over 90% of wrist fractures.

Colles, made the statement that his described distal radial fracture healed consistently, but some left a permanent "silver fork" deformity. This deformity, according to him, is not "associated with pain or disability."[5] It is generally agreed, that the vast majority of patients with Colles' fractures, with a residual deformity, become asymptomatic.[1,5-15,19-21]

REFERENCES

1. Downing N, Karantana A. A revolution in the management of Fractures of the distal radius? J Bone and Joint Surg Br. 2008; 90(10):1271-5.

2. Mudgal C et al. Plate fixation of Osteoporotic fractures of the distal radius. J. Orthop Trauma. 2008; 22(8 Suppl):S106-S15.

3. Orbay J. The treatment of unstable fractures of the distal radius with volar fixation. J Hand Surg. 2000; 5:103-12.

4. Orbay J, Fernandez D. Volar fixed-angle plate fixation for unstable distal radius fractures in the elderly patient. J Hand Surg. 2004; 29:96-102.

5. Abbaszadegan H, Conradi P, Jonsson U. Fixation not needed for undisplaced Colles' fractures. Acta Orthop Scand. 1990; 61:457-9.

6. Bacorn RW, Kurtzke JF. Colles' Fracture: A Study of two thousand cases from the New York Workmen's Compensation Bard. J Bone Joint Surg Am. 1953; 35A:643.

7. Bunger C, Solund K, Rasmussen P. Early Results After Colles' Fractures: Functional Bracing in Supination Versus Dorsal Plaster Immobilization. Arch Orthop Trauma Surg. 1984; 103:251-6.

8. Charnley J. The closed treatment of Common Fractures. London, E. and S. Livingstone Ltd. 1972; 128.

9. Colles A. On the fracture of the carpal extremity of the radius. Edinb Med Surg. J. 1814;10: 181. Clin Orthop Relat Res. 2006 Apr; 445:5-7.

10. Forward DP, Davis TR, Sithole JS. Do young patients with malunited fractures of the distal radius inevitably develop symptomatic post-traumatic osteoarthritis? J. Bone and Joint Surg Br. 2008; 90(5):629-37.

11. Gartland JJ, Werley CW. Evaluation of healed Colles' fractures. J. Bone and Joint Surg Am. 1951 Oct; 33A:895-907.

12. McQueen M, Caspers J. Colles' fractures. Does the anatomical result affect the final function? J Bone and Joint Surg Am. 1988; 70B:649-51.

13. Rosetzsky A. Colles' Fractures Treated by Plaster and Polyurethane Braces: A Controlled Clinical Study. J. Trauma. 1982; 22:910.

14. Sarmiento A, Pratt GW, Sinclair WF. Colles' fractures: Functional bracing in supination. J. Bone and Joint Surg Am. 1975; 57A:311.

15. Sarmiento A, Zagorski JB, Sinclair WF. Functional Bracing of Colles' Fractures: A Prospective Study of Immobilization in Supination versus Pronation. Clin Orthop Rel Res. 1980; 146:175-83.

16. Sarmiento A. Closed Treatment of Distal Radius Fractures. Techniques in orthopaedics. Philadelphia: Lippincott, Williams and Wilkins (Eds). 2000; 15(4):299-304.

17. Sarmiento A, Latta LL. Closed Functional Treatment of Fractures. Springer-Verlag. 1981 Feb.

18. Sarmiento A. The functional bracing of fractures. JBJS (A). Classics Techniques. 2007; 89 Suppl 2(Part 2):157-69.

19. Stewart HD, Innes AR, Burke FD. Functional Cast-Bracing for Colles' Fractures: A Comparison Between Cast-Bracing and Conventional Plaster Casts. J. Bone Joint Surg. 1984; 66(5):749.

20. Warwick D, Field J, Prothero D, Gibson A, Bannister GC. Function ten years after Colles' fractures. Clin Orthop Relat Res. 1993 Oct; 295:270-4.

21. Van der linden W, Ericson R. Colles' fracture: How should its displacement be measured and how should it be immobilized? J Bone Joint Surg Am. 1981; 63:1285-8.

51

Classification of Colles' Fracture

We have evaluated our results according to Gartland and Werley's criteria[9] as we considered their method sophisticated and practical. However, in an attempt to further improve their classification, we modified their criteria and classified the fractures into four types: Type I: Non-displaced extra-articular Type II: Displaced extra-articular. Type III: Non-displaced intra-articular. Type IV: Displaced intra-articular.[1] In retrospect, it appears that we did not emphasize with sufficient force the presence or absence of dislocation of the radio-ulnar joint. It was an error, because the stability of the radio-ulnar joint constitutes the single most important factor determining the behavior of these fractures. Frykman had included the distal-radial joint in his thorough classification, making his evaluation of results more appropriate.[8]

Following schematic drawings, from Figures 15.1 to 15.5 show various types of Colles fractures.

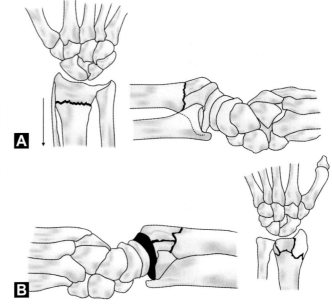

Figs 51.2A and B: (A) Schematic drawing of extra-articular non-displaced Colles' fracture. (B) Drawing of non-displaced intra-articular fracture.

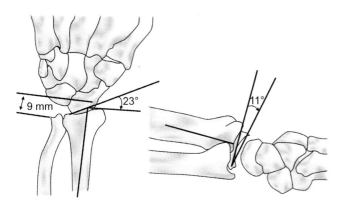

Fig. 51.1: Schematic drawings illustrating the average 23° ulnar tilt of the radial articulation and the average 11° of volar tilt.

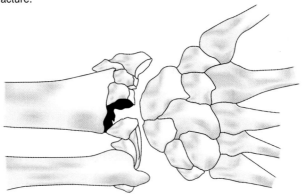

Fig. 51.3: Schematic drawing of comminuted intra-articular fracture of the distal radius.

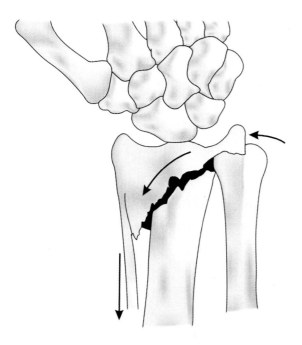

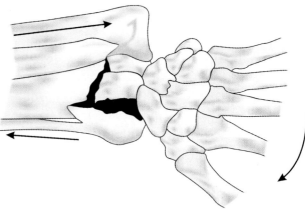

Fig. 51.5: Schematic drawing of comminuted, intra-articular fracture associated with a dislocated distal radio-ulnar joint. This situation represents the worse combination of unhealthy features that make this fracture a good candidate for internal fixation, preferably with a volar plate.

REFERENCES

1. Sarmiento A, Pratt GW, Sinclair WF. Colles' fractures: Functional bracing in supination. J. Bone and Joint Surg Am. 1975; 57A:311.
2. Frykman G. Fracture of the Distal radius including sequelae. Acta Orthop Scand. 1967; Suppl 108:3.

Fig. 51.4: Schematic drawing of long oblique fracture of the distal radius associated with a tear of the radio-ulnar ligament. This situation renders the fracture unstable with a tendency to shortening.

52

The Etiology of Recurrent Deformity

It has been repeatedly documented that many Colles' fractures, following reduction experience a recurrence of the deformity. This can only be explained on deforming muscular forces acting on the distal radial fragment, since weight bearing on the hand does not occur. We studied this phenomenon with electromyography and concluded that the recurrence of the deformity was more likely to be produced by the contraction of the brachioradialis muscle. The brachioradialis is the only muscle that inserts on the distal fragment and because of its location is capable of recreating the three typical features of the deformity: dorsal and radial tilt of the distal fragment and loss of the ulnar angulation of the radial articular surface.[1]

We demonstrated that on minimizing the function of the brachioradialis muscle, the recurrence of deformity was effectively reduced. Our studies further documented that stabilization of the forearm in pronation favor the function of the brachioradialis (Figures 51.1 to 51.3).

We concluded that the classical position of stabilization in pronation of the forearm and ulnar and volar deviation of the wrist was responsible for the frequent recurrence of deformity. We then undertook prospective clinical investigations that confirmed our thesis: the anatomical results obtained with fractures treated in forearm supination were superior to those treated in pronation.[1-3]

We conducted studies in patients under anesthesia, by electrically stimulating the brachioradialis and observing the recreation of the deformity (Figures 51.4A and B).

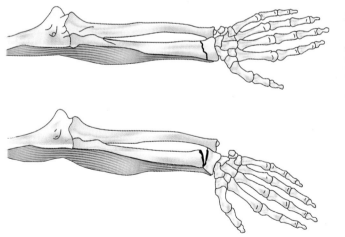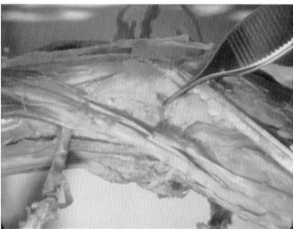

Figs 52.1: Schematic drawing of the likely role the brachioradialis muscle plays in the recreation of the typical deformity of radial deviation and dorsiflexion of the distal radial fragment. Since the muscle is a powerful flexor of the elbow in pronation, such a position favors the loss of fracture reduction.

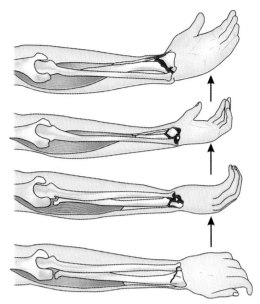

Figs 52.2: Schematic drawings illustrating the relationship of the brachioradialis muscle with the distal radius according to the rotation of the forearm.

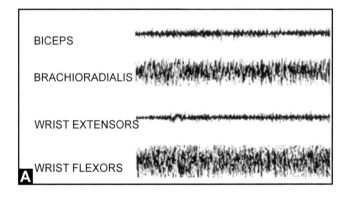

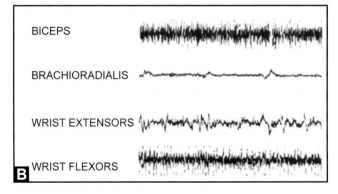

Figs 52.3A and B: (A) Electromyogram obtained during the lifting of an object with the forearm in pronation. Notice the weak tracing of the biceps and the strong tracing of the brachioradialis muscle. (B) When the forearm is in supination the activity of the brachioradialis is significantly reduced, while the contraction of the biceps increases.

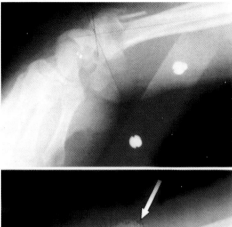

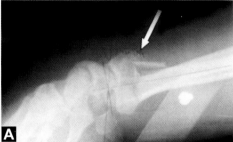

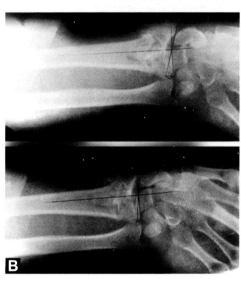

Figs 52.4: (A) (Top) Radiograph of reduced Colles' fracture prior to electrical stimulation of the brachioradialis muscle. (Bottom) Radiograph showing the dorsal displacement of the distal radial fracture following electrical stimulation of the brachioradialis muscle. (B) Antero-posterior radiograph demonstrating shortening of the radius under electrical stimulation.

REFERENCES

1. Sarmiento A. The Brachioradialis as a deforming force in Colles' fracture. Clin Orthop Relat Res. 1965; 38:86.
2. Sarmiento A, Pratt GW, Sinclair WF. Colles' fractures: Functional bracing in supination. J. Bone and Joint Surg Am. 1975; 57A:311.
3. Sarmiento A, Zagorski JB, Sinclair WF. Functional Bracing of Colles' Fractures: A Prospective Study of Immobilization in Supination versus Pronation. Clin Orthop Rel Res. 1980; 146:175-83.

53

The Distal Radio-ulnar Joint

It is our opinion that the single most important prognostic feature in Colles' fractures is the condition of the distal radio-ulnar joint; not necessarily the presence or absence of a fracture of the styloid process of the ulna but an initial subluxation or dislocation of the joint. The styloid process may be fractured in association with many intra-articular fractures, however, without an adverse effect in the ultimate prognosis. With or without a fracture of the styloid process, reduced, stable joint, muscular deforming forces cannot shorten the radius.

On the other hand, an extra- or intra-articular comminuted fracture may experience recurrence of the corrected deformity if the joint was initially dislocated. In the absence of the stabilizing tethering effect of the fibro-cartilage ligament, shortening of the radius is almost always inevitable (Figure 53.1). The deforming force of the surrounding muscles, particularly that of the brachioradialis makes the recurrence possible. This fracture requires either stabilization with external fixators or open reduction and internal fixation.

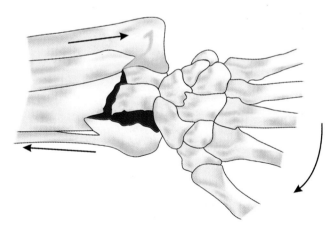

Fig. 53.1: Schematic drawing illustrating a dislocation of the distal radio-ulnar joint accompanying an intra-articular comminuted fracture. This comminution of factors make this fracture the worst case scenario, since recurrence of the dislocation is likely to occur once flexion of the elbow and function of the fingers are introduced.

54

The Long-oblique Fracture

The long oblique intra-articular fracture of the lateral aspect of the radius has a guarded prognosis when treated by nonsurgical means regardless of the accuracy of the closed reduction. The pull of the surrounding muscles recreates the deformity. The brachioradialis, being the only muscle attached to the distal fragment, easily shortens the radius upon its contraction (Figure 54.1). The position of pronation of the forearm does nothing but facilitate the creation of this complication. This fracture is best treated by surgical means. The fact that complications may result from surgery does not deny the value of the procedures and the need to use them in preference to non-surgical management under the described circumstances.

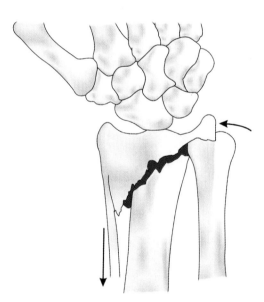

Fig. 54.1: Drawing depicting an oblique fracture of the distal radius, associated with a fracture of the ulnar styloid. The geometry of the fracture readily predisposes to proximal displacement of the fragment under muscle contractions, particularly that of the brachioradialis.

55

Late Arthritic Changes

Those who strongly propose surgical reduction of all displaced distal radial fractures seem to base their preference for the open method on the belief that anatomical repositioning of fragments, whether intra- or extra-articular, ensures better results by preventing late arthritic changes. We question unqualified support of that belief, since anatomical reduction of angulated fragments does not necessarily produce late joint degeneration. This is a rare complication, most likely to be secondary to articular damage that took place at the time of the injury. There is suggestive evidence in the literature indicating that impaction injury to articular cartilage may produce irreversible changes. Therefore, restoration of congruity does not necessarily prevent late arthritic changes under those circumstances. In weight-bearing bones, moderate residual angulation does not lead to joint disease. To suspect that moderate angular deformities in non-weight bearing extremities carry a worse prognosis is difficult to accept.

Mild intra-articular post-traumatic incongruity is easily tolerated as the cartilage undergoes remodeling. We demonstrated this fact in experimental animals. Re-approximation of intra-articular fragments does not necessarily preclude eventual joint degeneration. We found that instability is more important than incongruity by observing that intra-articular fractures, associated with incongruity, once made unstable, experience degenerative changes.[1,2]

Of equal importance is the fact that surgical repositioning of intra-articular fragments may cause additional damage by depriving osteo-cartilaginous fragments of blood supply. Even more important is the fact that most distal radial fractures are produced through an impaction mechanism, a mechanism known to be associated with irreparable damage to the articular cartilage. One can surmise that surgical reconstruction of damaged cartilage will not alter the permanent pathology that may have occurred at the time of the initial insult.

In a recent article, Forward et al "Do young patients with mal-united fractures of the distal radius inevitably develop symptomatic posttraumatic osteoarthritis?" concluded that "imperfect reduction of these fracture may not result in symptomatic arthritis in the long term."[3] They found out that patients who had their fractures treated with plates were more likely to experience long-term wrist pain. Others have demonstrated in various degrees that late symptoms following Colles' fractures that heal with mild deformities are usually asymptomatic.[4-18]

REFERENCES

1. Llinas A, McKellop HA, Marshall GJ, Sharpe F, Kirchen M, Sarmiento A. Healing and Remodeling of Articular Incongruities in a Rabbit Fracture Model. J Bone & Joint Surg. 1993; 75A(10):1508-23.
2. Lovasz G, Park SH, Ebramzadeh E, Benya PD, Llinas A, Bellyei A, Luck JV Jr, Sarmiento A. Characteristic of degeneration in an unstable knee with a coronal surface step-off. J Bone Joint Surg Br. 2001 Apr; 83(3):428-36.
3. Forward DP, Davis TR, Sithole JS. Do young patients with malunited fractures of the distal radius inevitably develop symptomatic post-traumatic osteoarthritis? J Bone and Joint Surg Br. 2008; 90(5):629-37.
4. Abbaszadegan H, Conradi P, Jonsson U. Fixation not needed for undisplaced Colles' fractures. Acta Orthop Scand. 1990; 61:457-9.
5. Bacorn RW, Kurtzke JF. Colles' Fracture: A Study of two thousand cases from the New York Workmen's Compensation Bard. J Bone Joint Surg Am. 1953; 35A:643.
6. Charnley J. The closed treatment of Common Fractures. London, E. and S. Livingstone Ltd. 1972; 128.
7. Colles A. On the fracture of the carpal extremity of the radius. Edinb Med Surg J. 1814;10: 181. Clin Orthop Relat Res. 2006 Apr; 445:5-7.
8. Downing N, Karantana A. A revolution in the management of Fractures of the distal radius? J Bone and Joint Surg Br. 2008; 90(10):1271-5.

9. Forward DP, Davis TR, Sithole JS. Do young patients with malunited fractures of the distal radius inevitably develop symptomatic post-traumatic osteoarthritis? J Bone and Joint Surg Br. 2008; 90(5): 629-37.

10. Gartland JJ, Werley CW. Evaluation of healed Colles' fractures. J. Bone and Joint Surg Am. 1951 Oct; 33A:895-907.

11. McQueen M, Caspers J. Colles' fractures. Does the anatomical result affect the final function? J Bone and Joint Surg Am. 1988; 70B:649-51.

12. Rosetzsky A. Colles' Fractures Treated by Plaster and Polyurethane Braces: A Controlled Clinical Study. J Trauma. 1982; 22:910.

13. Sarmiento A, Zagorski JB, Sinclair WF. Functional Bracing of Colles' Fractures: A Prospective Study of Immobilization in Supination versus Pronation. Clin Orthop Rel Res. 1980; 146:175-83.

14. Sarmiento A, Latta LL. Closed Functional Treatment of Fractures. Springer-Verlag. 1981 Feb.

15. Sarmiento A. The functional bracing of fractures. JBJS (A). Classics Techniques. 2007; 89 Suppl 2(Part 2):157-69.

16. Stewart HD, Innes AR, Burke FD. Functional Cast-Bracing for Colles' Fractures: A Comparison Between Cast-Bracing and Conventional Plaster Casts. J Bone Joint Surg. 1984; 66(5):749.

17. Warwick D, Field J, Prothero D, Gibson A, Bannister GC. Function ten years after Colles' fractures. Clin Orthop Relat Res. 1993 Oct; 295:270-4.

18. Van der linden W, Ericson R. Colles' fracture: How should its displacement be measured and how should it be immobilized? J Bone Joint Surg Am. 1981; 63:1285-8.

56

Immobilization: Pronation versus Supination

IMMOBILIZATION: PRONATION VERSUS SUPINATION

Not only does the position of supination diminishes the potentially harmful contractions of the brachioradialis but offers additional advantages: (1) Flexion of the fingers and wrist is carried out with greater ease when compared to pronation. This motion encourages maintenance of reduction since it tends to flex the distal radial fragment. (2) The radio-ulnar joint is most stable in that position. (3) Radiological evaluation of the condition of the fractured fragments is best conducted. Pronation of the forearm makes it more difficult. (4) Recognition of scaphoid-lunate dissociation is more easily observed with the wrist in supination. Pronation obscures the true relationship between the two bones. (5) Spontaneous improvement of lack of forearm motion takes place faster when the position of immobilization is that of supination since most activities of daily living require forearm pronation, therefore patients find themselves forcing the forearm into pronation. Since supination is required for fewer activities, a permanent limitation of supination is more likely to take place. If the forearm is immobilized in pronation, a permanent loss of the last few degrees of forearm pronation is inconspicuously compensated with a combined motion of shoulder flexion, abduction and internal rotation, a mechanism similar to the one used by upper extremity amputees who lack pronation of their forearm.

There is no universal agreement regarding the best position of immobilization and most people still use pronation on a regular basis.[1-4]

There is not a single, universal, non-surgical method of treatment for all Colles' fractures. Non-displaced or minimally displaced extra-articular fractures may be successfully treated with a below-the-elbow cast, followed by early use of the extremity. Displacement of the fragments is not likely to occur under those circumstances. Our data amply documented such prognosis.

Patients suffering with fractures that require manipulation and reduction do not require immediate reduction under all circumstances. Often, it is best to postpone forceful, traumatic manipulation in order to prevent or minimize the swelling produced by the injury. Measurement of pressure in the muscular compartments of the hand should be performed whenever clinical symptoms and findings suggestive of compartment syndromes in the making are suspected. Immediate reduction should be carried out in those fractures with major deformity since vascular and peripheral nerve complications are likely to occur. The reduction eliminates the compression and kinking of the nerve and vascular structures.

In order to facilitate the reduction and to minimize additional trauma to the tissues, finger skin traction using Chinese finger traps is most useful. In the elderly patient with thin and delicate skin, the fingers can be covered with adhesive tape over which the Chinese finger traps are placed. In that manner, the arm is suspended for a few minutes. A weight of no more than 10 pounds is placed over the distal arm. The traction should not be maintained longer than 5 minutes. This weight and time of traction are usually sufficient to disengage the fragments.

RESULTS

The following data was published by us a number of years ago, based on information from a prospective study comparing pronation versus supination (Table 56.1).[5,6]

Table 56.1: Loss of Length (at Least 2 mm)		
Type of Fracture	*Cost to Brace*	*Brace to Follow-up*
Type II		
Supination	23% (3/13)	8% (1/13)
	Range: 0–6 mm	Range: 0–5 mm
Pronation	33% (6/18)	39 (7/18)
	Range: 0–4 mm	Range: 0–8 mm
Type IV		
Supination	55% (11/20)	15% (3/20)
	Range: 0–3 mm	Range: 0–3 mm
Pronation	65% (13/20)	50 (10/20)
	Range: 0–5 mm	Range: 0–8 mm

TECHNIQUE

The technique of application of a functional Colles brace following immobilization of forearm has been illustrated in Figures 56.1 to 56.14.

The injured extremity is suspended with Chinese finger traps after appropriate sedation or anasthesia has been administered. After a few minutes, the fracture is then manipulated by applying additional manual traction, dorsiflexion of the wrist at the level of the fractures in order to further increase the dorsal deformity.

Once this has been accomplished, the distal fragment is brought into volar flexion in anticipation of obtaining the anatomical volar tilt of the distal radius. This manipulation is combined with pressure on the lateral aspect of the radial fragment. This is done in an attempt to correct the radial deviation created at the time of the injury.

However, upon completion of the reduction, the forearm should be supinated. The pronation and supination of the forearm should be tested at this time to ensure that there is no blockage in any direction. The forearm is then held in a relaxed attitude of supination with the wrist in ulnar deviation and mild volar flexion. In this position, the stabilizing cast is applied.[5-8]

It is best to begin the wrapping of the Plaster of Paris from distal to proximal, starting just above the wrist and extending to the distal upper arm. It is during this time that care should be exercised to ascertain that the position of relaxed supination is maintained and the supracondylar humeral region is molded appropriately.

The above-the-elbow cast may be replaced with Plaster of Paris cast or a plastic brace that resembles the shape of the Munster prosthesis used by below-the-elbow amputees with very short stumps. The brace permits flexion of the elbow and wrist. However, extension of the elbow is limited in approximately the last 30° and its flexion in the last 20°. Dorsiflexion of the wrist is completely prevented but flexion is possible.

A collar and cuff must be given to provide additional comfort, but may be discontinued when the distal swelling has disappeared and the painful symptoms have subsided. Active exercises of the elbow and hand are encouraged.

The Velcro straps of the brace must be adjusted frequently in order to maintain the desirable snugness of the brace and further enhance maintenance of the reduction.

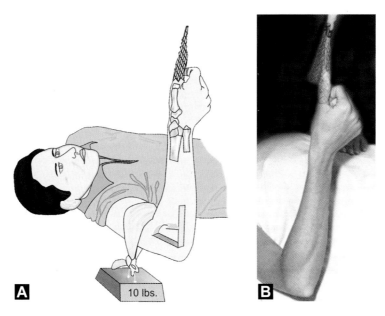

A   10 lbs.   **B**

Figs 56.1A and B: (A) Drawing and Photo depicting the arm suspended with Chinese finger traps, and counterweight over the distal arm.

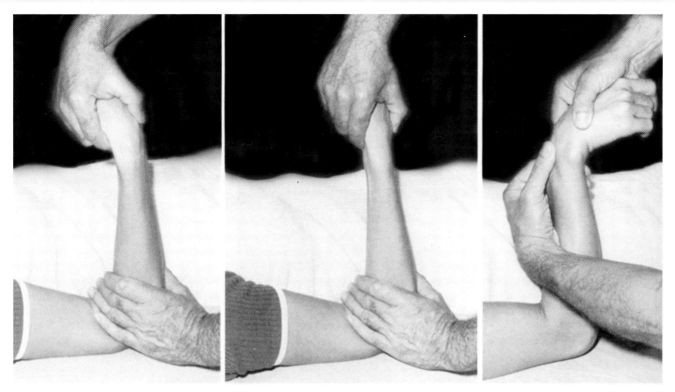

Fig. 56.2: The reduction requires manual traction, combined with localized pressure over the distal fragment. During this stage of the reduction, the forearm is held in pronation.

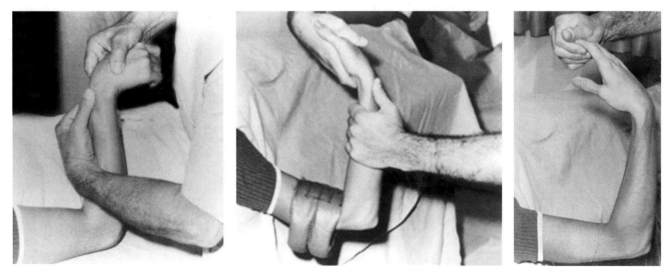

Fig. 56.3: After appropriate sedation and injection of the hematoma with an anesthetic, the fracture is manipulated by applying traction with the forearm in pronation. Pressure is applied over the distal radial fragment, both dorsally and laterally. Upon completion of the reduction in pronation, the forearm is supinated while maintaining slight pressure over the distal ulnar styloid, to ascertain that its relationship with the radius is normal.

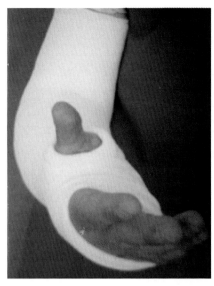

Fig. 56.4: Photographs of the completed above-the-elbow cast holding the elbow at 90° of flexion, the forearm in a relaxed attitude of supination, and the wrist in slight flexion and ulnar deviation.

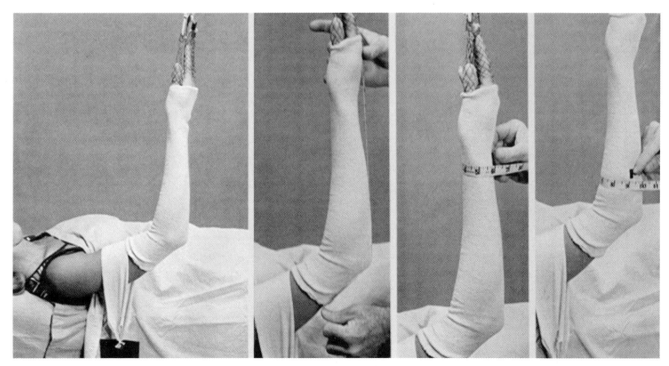

Fig. 56.5: Photos illustrating the application of a functional Colles' brace. The arm is suspended with Chinese finger traps with distal arm counterweight. The girth of the proximal and distal forearm is recorded in order to select the appropriate size of the Orthoplast sheet.

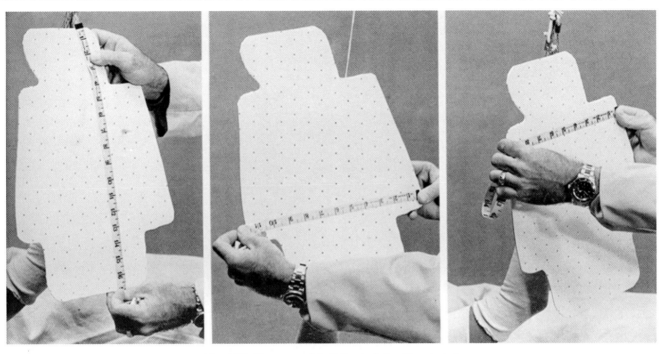

Fig. 56.6: The appropriate Orthoplast sheet is selected.

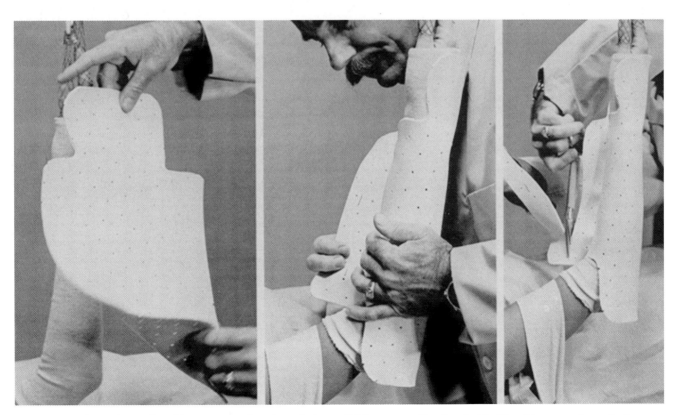

Fig. 56.7: The Orthoplast is dipped in warm water for a few minutes, until it becomes soft and malleable. Then it is wrapped over the forearm, (being held in supination) from below the elbow anteriorly, and to above the olecranon, posteriorly. Distally, it extends over the wrist to the base of the metacarpals.

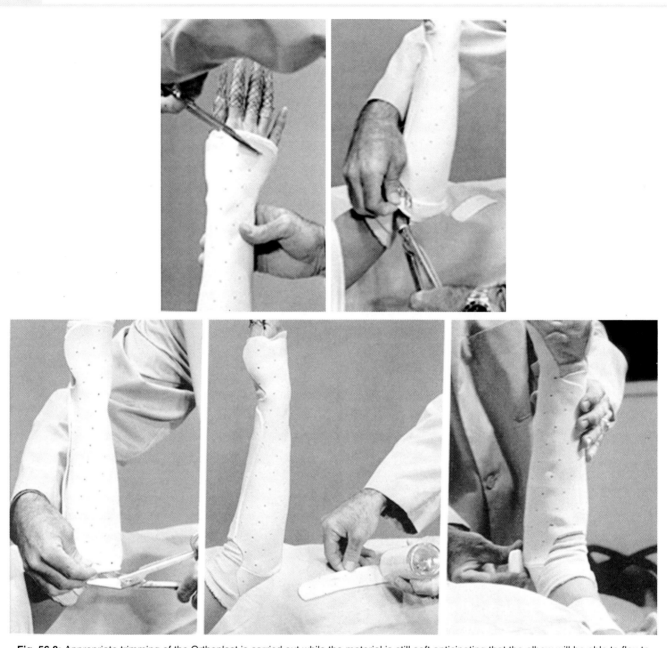

Fig. 56.8: Appropriate trimming of the Orthoplast is carried out while the material is still soft anticipating that the elbow will be able to flex to minus 20° and extend minus approximately 30°.

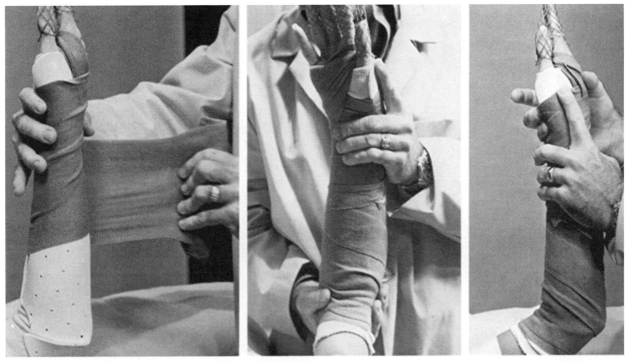

Fig. 56.9: While the Orthoplast is still soft, an elastic bandage, dipped in cold water, is firmly wrapped over the forearm. While ascertaining that the volar and dorsal surfaces of the forearm are flattened, and the wrist held in slight flexion and ulnar deviation. Proximately, the distal arm is firmly compressed in order to prevent prono-supination of the forearm.

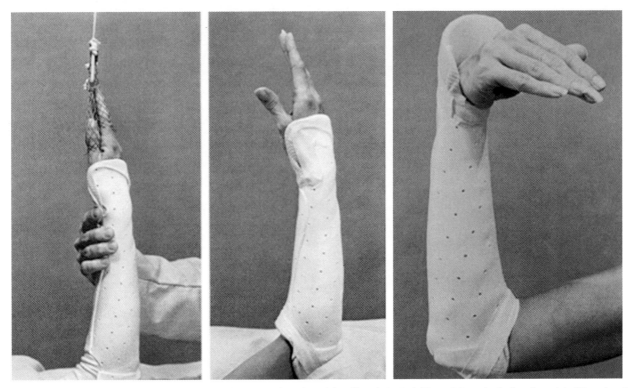

Fig. 56.10: Once the Orthoplast is chemically set, the range of motion of the elbow is tested. The wrist can be further flexed, but its extension is prevented by the dorsal extension of the plastic material. In flexion, the wrist cannot be actively forced into radial deviation.

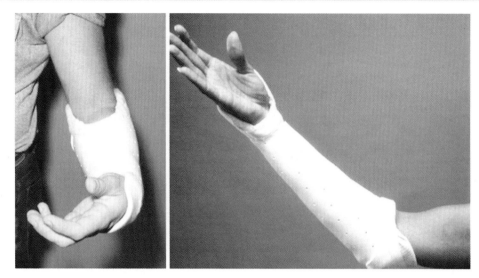

Fig. 56.11: Photos of the functional brace illustrating the supracondylar, Munster-like, extension over the distal humerus.

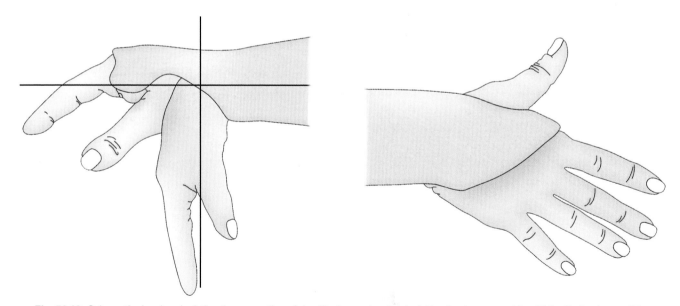

Fig. 56.12: Schematic drawing depicting the prevention of dorsiflexion and radial deviation the brace provides. Volar flexion is possible.

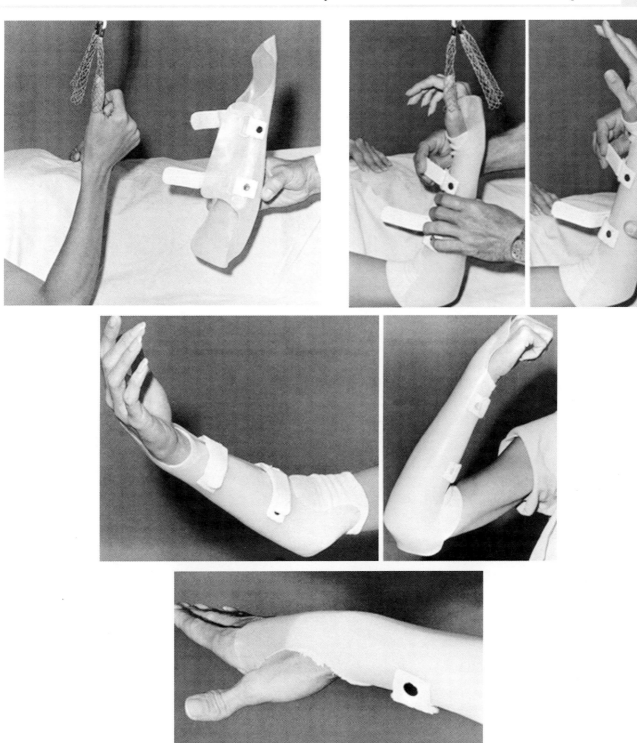

Fig. 56.13: Illustrations of a prefabricated brace with the characteristics described in the section describing the construction of the custom-made Orthoplast brace.

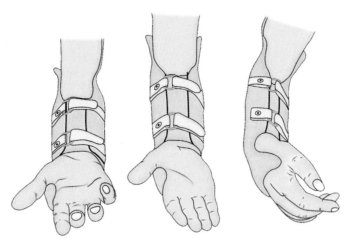

Fig. 56.14: Schematic drawing of the brace with adjustable Velcro straps. It illustrates the prevention of prono-supination by the firm molding of the distal humerus.

REPRESENTATIVE EXAMPLES

Some representative examples are shown in Figures 56.15 to 56.29.

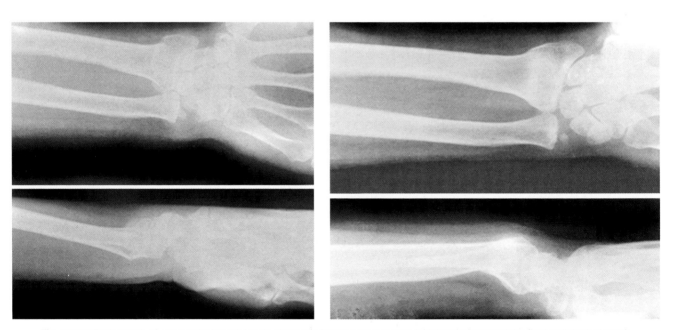

Fig. 56.15: Radiograph of extra-articular, minimally displaced fracture showing the initial pathology and the final radiological result.

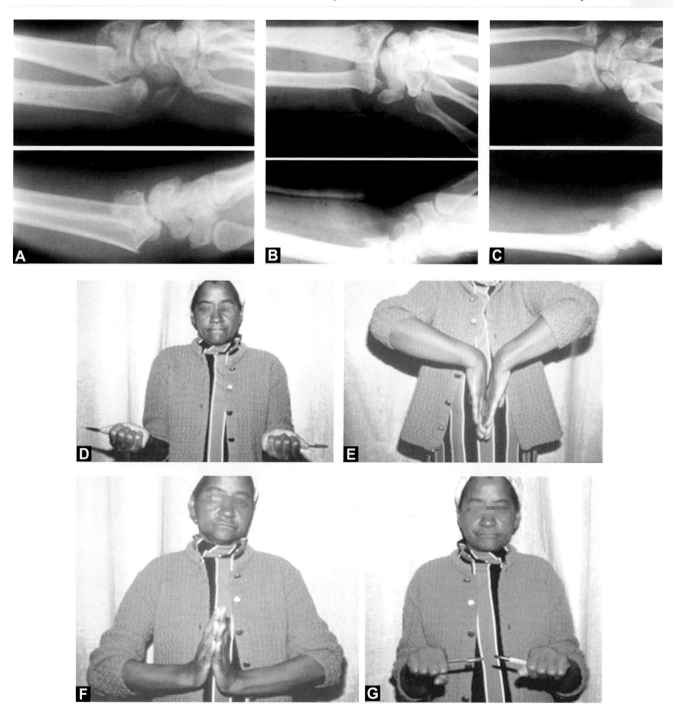

Figs 56.16A to G: (A) Radiograph of extra-articular, severely angulated fracture with what appeared to be an intact radio-ulnar joint. (B) Radiograph obtained after reduction of the fracture, which was stabilized in a brace in supination. Notice the volar displacement of the distal radial fragment. (C) The fracture healed uneventfully with a laterally displaced ulna, probably the result of a tear of the radio-ulnar ligament. (D to G) Patient demonstrates the mild residual loss of volar and dorsal motion, but normal prono-supination.

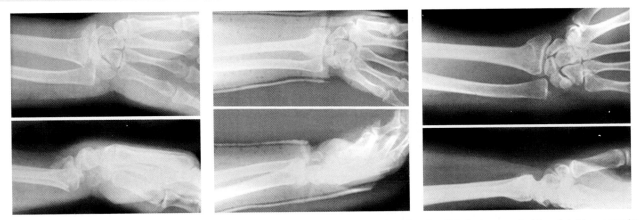

Fig. 56.17: Radiographs of a displaced extra-articular fracture illustrating the initial dorsal and radial displacement of the distal fragment; its reduction shown through the plastic brace; and the final radiological result.

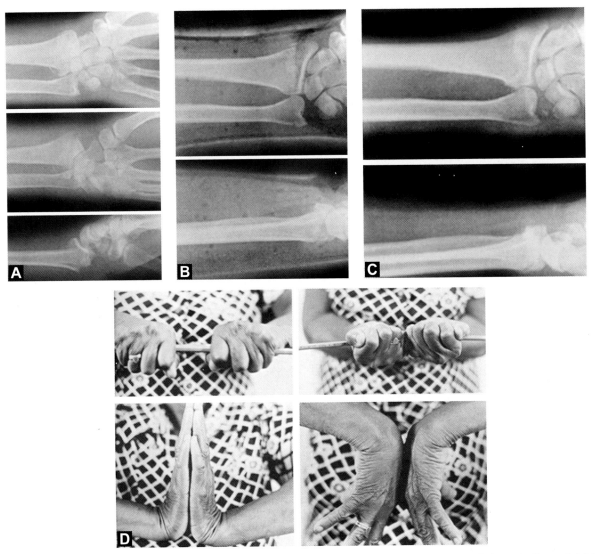

Figs 56.18A to D: (A) Radiographs of severely angulated extra-articular Colles' fracture. (B) Radiograph obtained after reduction and stabilization in an Orthoplast brace. (C) Radiograph showing the final radiological result. (D) Patient demonstrates the range of motion of her wrists. Notice the mild residual limitation of volar and dorsal motion.

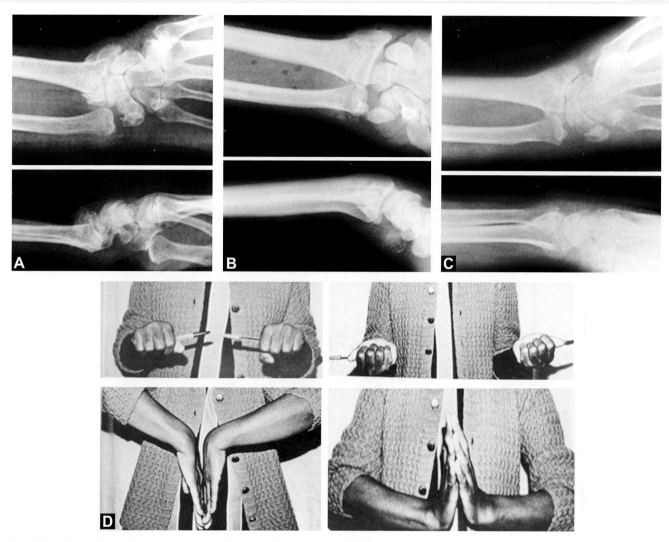

Figs 56.19A to D: (A) Radiograph of severely displaced Colles' fracture. (B) Radiographs taken through the brace after closed reduction of the fracture. (C) Radiographs after completion of healing. (D) Patient demonstrate a residual mild limitation of wrist flexion. It is very likely that the mild limitation will spontaneously subside.

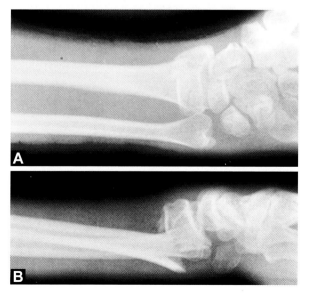

Figs 56.20A and B: (A) Radiograph of dorsally angulated Colles' fracture (B) radiograph showing the reduced fracture, stabilized in a cast in supination of the forearm.

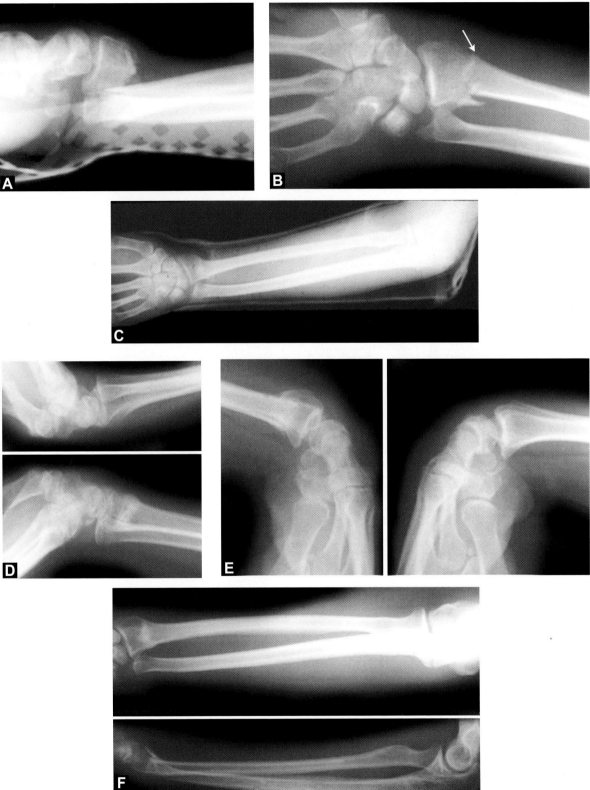

Figs 56.21A to F: (A) Radiographs of severely displaced extra-articular Colles' fracture. (B) Radiograph of the reduced fracture. (C) Radiograph obtained after application of the functional brace. (D and E) Radiographs obtained after completion of healing demonstrating the range of volar and dorsal motion. Notice the mild limitation of motion. (F) Radiograph taken 3 months after the initial insult.

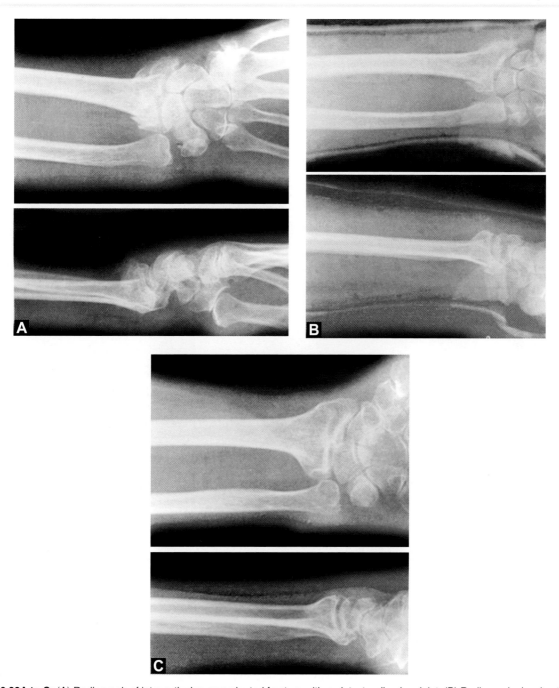

Figs 56.22A to C: (A) Radiograph of intra-articular, comminuted fracture with an intact radio-ulnar joint. (B) Radiograph showing the reduction of the fracture, but with increased radial tilt. (C) Radiograph obtained after completion of healing. Notice the loss of volar tilt.

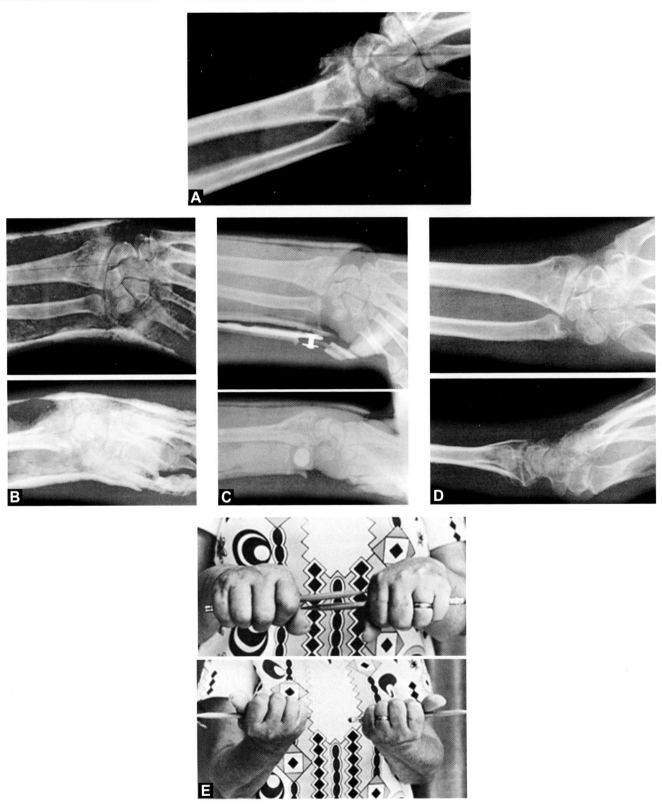

Figs 56.23A to E: (A) Radiograph of intra-articular fracture but with an intact radio-ulnar joint. (B) Radiographs obtained through the cast and brace. (C and D) Radiographs after completion of healing. Notice the residual mild loss of volar tilt and apparent remodeling of the joint. (E) Patient demonstrates a final mild limitation of supination.

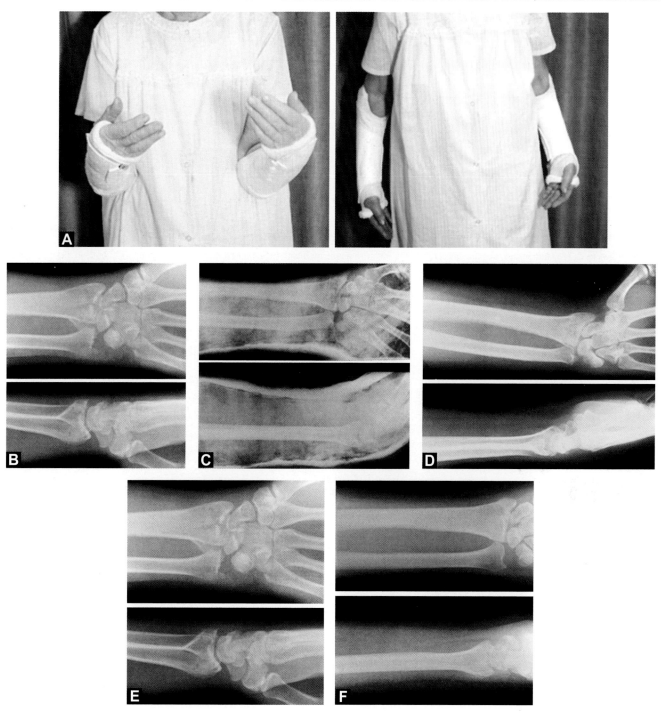

Figs 56.24A to F: (A) Photographs of patient with bilateral Colles' fractures illustrating the supination attitude of the forearms in the functional braces. (B to D) Sequential radiographs illustrating the initial fractures of the right wrist; the position in the brace and the final radiological result. (E and F) Radiographs of the left wrist illustrating the initial dorsal deviation of the distal radial fragment, and the final result. The fracture healed with an inconsequential residual dorsal tilt.

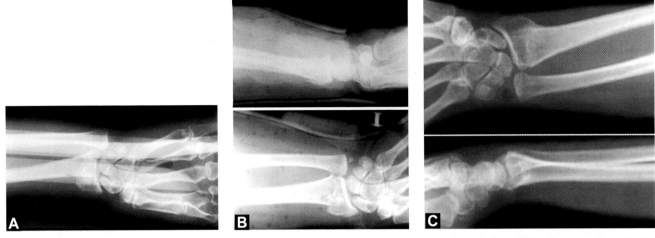

Figs 56.25A to C: (A) Radiograph of extra-articular Colles' fracture associated with a dislocated radio-ulnar joint. (B) Radiograph after reduction of the fracture and stabilization of the forearm in supination. (C) Radiograph showing the healed fracture. Notice the mild lateral subluxation of the radio-ulnar joint. The patient became totally asymptomatic.

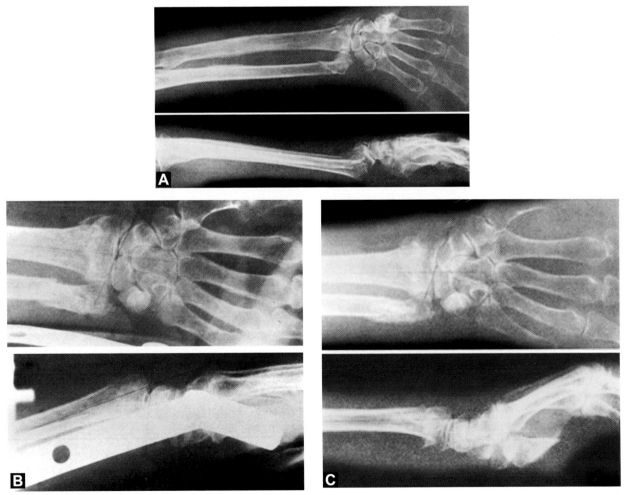

Figs 56.26A to C: (A) Radiograph of comminuted, intra-articular fracture associated with a fracture of the distal ulna. (B) Radiograph obtained after reduction and stabilization in a functional brace. (C) The fracture healed, but surgical resection of the distal ulna became necessary because of pain.

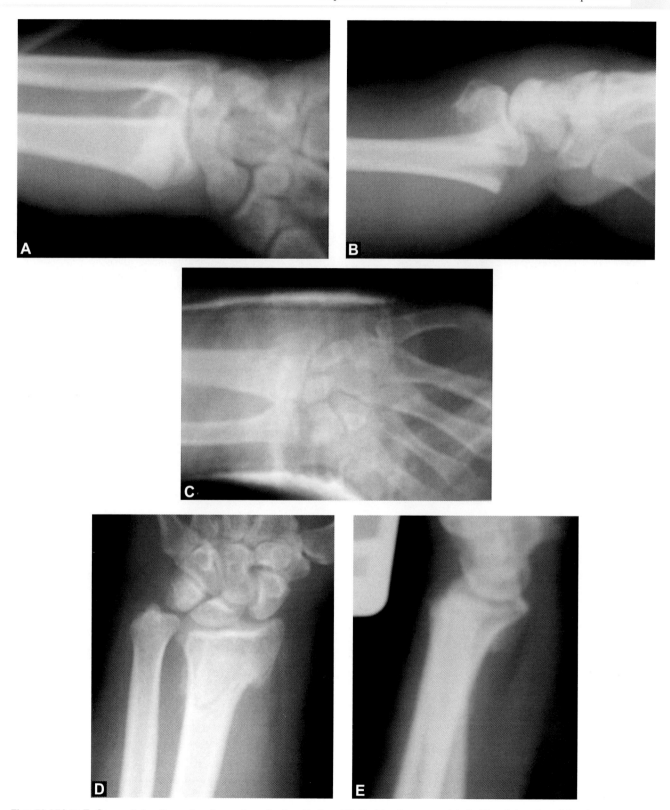

Figs 56.27A to E: Sequential radiographs of an extra-articular, displaced Colles' fracture, associated with a dislocation of the distal radio-ulnar joint. The fracture was reduced manually and held in a relaxed attitude of supination of the forearm. Notice the residual subluxation of the distal radio-ulnar joint.

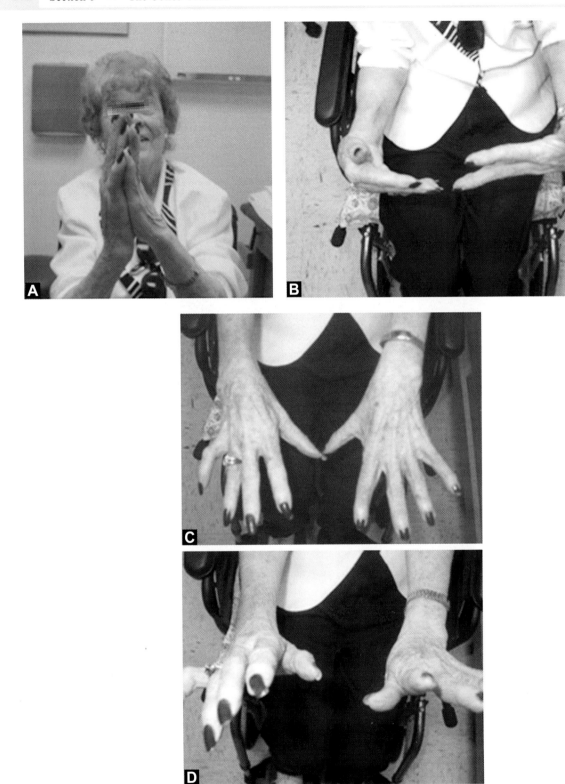

Figs 56.28A to D: Clinical photographs of the wrists of an elderly woman, who allegedly had sustained an intra-articular Colles' fracture with an associated dislocation of the radio-ulnar joint. Patient demonstrates a residual, but inconsequential loss of motion. The treating surgeons had chosen to accept the deformity in preference to a surgical intervention. It is likely that in a person of her age, surgery may have given her a similar degree of limitation of motion.

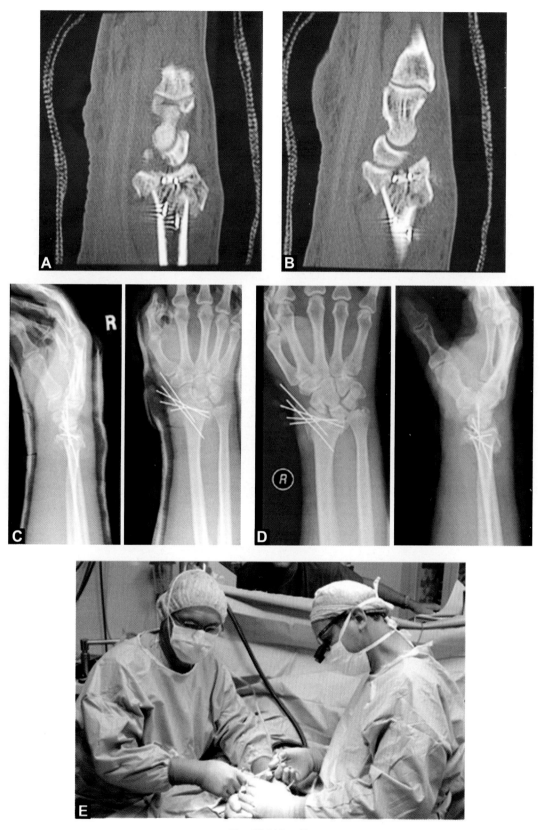

Figs 56.29A to E

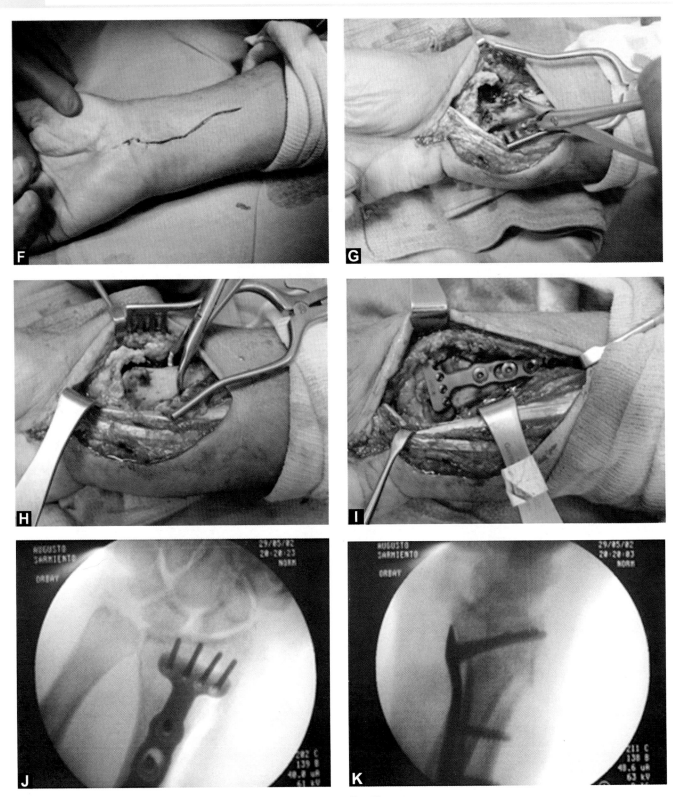

Figs 56.29F to K:

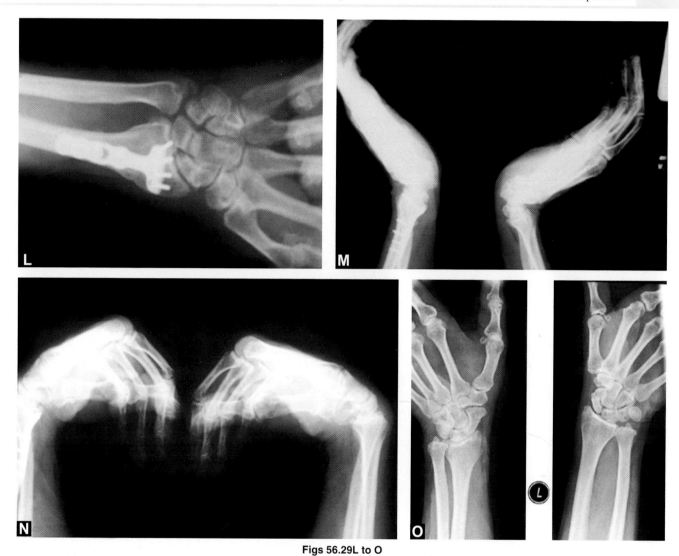

Figs 56.29L to O

Figs 56.29A to O: (A and B) CT can of the wrist of the senior author (AS) following a fall that produced an intra-articular, comminuted fracture of the right distal radius, associated with a dislocation of the radio-ulnar joint, and a nondisplaced fracture of the left navicular bone. (C) Radiograph following internal fixation with multiple pins. The dislocation and joint incongruity were corrected. (D) One week later, radiographs showed loss of reduction and a re-dislocation of the radio-ulnar joint. (E) Photograph of Jorge Orbay (Miami) and Diego Fernandez (Switzerland) performing the revision surgery, using a volar plate. (F to I) Sequential photographs of the steps taken in surgery to obtain reduction of the fracture and dislocation. (J to L) Intraoperative and post-operative radiographs illustrating the reduction of the fracture. (M and N) Radiographs obtained 5 years post operatively demonstrating the residual limitation of volar and dorsal motion. (O) Radiograph of the left wrist, showing no signs of complications from the nonsurgically treated fracture of the navicular bone. Both hands are asymptomatic 7 years post-surgery.

CONCLUSIONS

The place of surgery in the management of Colles' fractures should be limited to those fractures that when treated by non-surgical means are not likely to render satisfactory functional and cosmetic results. It is our opinion that the surgical approach to Colles' fractures has been greatly abused. To perform a surgical procedure in the treatment of a fracture that responds well to conservative means is difficult to justify. In the same manner, to deny the benefits of surgery when the surgical treatment has been shown to provide better results is also inexcusable. The fact remains that history and many years of experience have proven that the majority of Colles' fractures can be successfully and inexpensively without the need of a surgical intervention. Moderate angular deformity resulting from Colles' fractures does not lead to arthritic changes. There is nothing in the literature to refute that observation. Articular incongruity is well known to predispose to degenerative changes. However, mild incongruity is readily tolerated. This has been documented in animal investigations.[1,19] Instability, in the presence of incongruity, is the factor that leads to cartilage degeneration. It is likely that surgical attempts to reposition comminuted intra-articular fragments may create additional damage to the articular surface by devascularizing fragments already compromised.

Colles' fractures are almost always produced by an impaction injury. It has been proven that articular cartilage subjected to severe impaction forces experiences changes that may be of a permanent nature. Therefore, there is nothing to gain from routinely reapproximating permanently damaged structures in anticipation of late subsequent degenerative arthritis. Though all orthopedists agree that major incongruities should be corrected or improved, not all incongruities are unacceptable. Furthermore, it is not known at this time whether fractures that had the incongruity improved or corrected will do better in the long run.

We do not wish to dismiss the surgical treatment of Colles' fracture. We have acknowledged that surgery is the treatment of choice in the care of certain fractures. Those fractures, however, constitute the minority.

Surgery is necessarily associated with possible complications such as infection, adhesions, nerve or vessel injuries. For reasons we do not clearly understand, joint stiffness frequently follows the joint immobilization created by external fixators. Though, with time and therapy the stiffness improves in most instances, such a period of additional incapacitation is not only inconvenient but expensive.

Our work has demonstrated that stabilization of Colles fractures in a relaxed attitude of supination renders better results when dealing with fractures that required reduction by manipulation. The position of supination offers the following advantages:

1. Action of the brachioradialis muscle is reduced. This is important because this muscle is the only one attached to the distal radial fragment, and its activity is enhanced when the forearm is in pronation.
2. The tendency for dorsal and ulnar subluxation is reduced.

3. Excellent leverage on the radial collateral ligament can be obtained to avoid shortening of the radius.
4. Roentgenographic examination of the wrist is easier when the forearm bones are parallel. Identification of a scaphoid-lunate dislocation subluxation, which is difficult to recognize when the forearm is pronated becomes easier with supination.
5. Exercise of the fingers is also easier.
6. Recovery of pronation, after the immobilization is terminated, is automatic because use of the hand and gravity tend to pronate the forearm.
7. Any ultimate loss of pronation can be inconspicuously compensated for by humeral abduction and internal rotation. No such mechanism is possible for the loss of supination.

REFERENCES

1. Bunger C, Solund K, Rasmussen P. Early Results After Colles' Fractures: Functional Bracing in Supination Versus Dorsal Plaster Immobilization. Arch Orthop Trauma Surg. 1984; 103:251-6.
2. Gartland JJ, Werley CW. Evaluation of healed Colles' fractures. J Bone and Joint Surg Am. 1951 Oct; 33A:895-907.
3. Lovasz G, Park SH, Ebramzadeh E, Benya PD, Llinas A, Bellyei A, Luck JV Jr, Sarmiento A. Characteristic of degeneration in an unstable knee with a coronal surface step-off. J Bone Joint Surg Br. 2001 Apr; 83(3):428-36.
4. Van der linden W, Ericson R. Colles' fracture: How should its displacement be measured and how should it be immobilized? J Bone Joint Surg Am. 1981; 63:1285-8.
5. Sarmiento A, Pratt GW, Sinclair WF. Colles' fractures: Functional bracing in supination. J Bone and Joint Surg Am. 1975; 57A:311.
6. Sarmiento A, Zagorski JB, Sinclair WF. Functional Bracing of Colles' Fractures: A Prospective Study of Immobilization in Supination versus Pronation. Clin Orthop Rel Res. 1980; 146: 175-83.
7. Sarmiento A. Closed Treatment of Distal Radius Fractures. Techniques in orthopedics. Philadelphia: Lippincott, Williams and Wilkins. 2000; 15(4):299-304.
8. Sarmiento A, Latta LL. Closed Functional Treatment of Fractures. Springer-Verlag. 1981 Feb.

Fractures of Both Bones of the Forearm

57

Rationale and Indications

Plating is currently the most common method of treatment of fractures of both bones of the forearm. The technique of plating is simple, the incidence of complications is not high, and the final clinical outcome is satisfactory in most instances. However, the method may result in a higher incidence of nonunion with the development of synostosis and infection (Figure 57.1).

Plating gained popularity upon recognizing the difficulties encountered in reducing and maintaining the reduction in some instances. However, little attention has been given to the fact that the forearm tolerates well minor deviation from the normal. Ten degrees of angulation or 5 to 10° of malrotation are likely to go unnoticed from the cosmetic and functional points of view.[1-5]

Our experience with functional casting and bracing of fractures of both bones of the forearm have indicated that

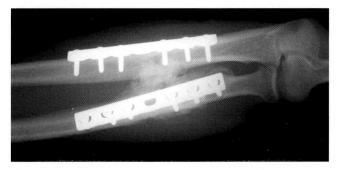

Fig. 57.1: Radiograph of synostosis following plating of both bones of the forearm. Although not a very common complication, its development results in loss of prono-supination of the forearm. Surgical removal of the bony bridge is usually accompanied with residual limitation of motion.

transverse fractures, once reduced and stabilized in a cast, are likely to suffer angulation, particularly if the initial injury produced major degrees of swelling. Upon the subsidence of swelling, the stabilizing cast loses its efficacy and the angular deformity develops. This complication is more likely to take place if one of the bones sustains a transverse fracture and the other bone sustains an oblique fracture. In this instance, the angulation is in the direction of the oblique fracture.

Forearm fractures experience at the time of the initial injury the total and final amount of shortening. This behavior is similar to that of tibial fractures. Closed fractures demonstrate in the vast majority of instances a degree of shortening that is minimal and inconsequential. That shortening, in the absence of major angular or rotary malalignment, produces none or minimal functional limitation of motion.[1,2,5]

The fracture of both bones of the forearm most amenable for closed functional casting or bracing is the one where the fractures are oblique or comminuted. The shortening remains essentially unchanged and the alignment of the fragments is usually maintained.

Functional casting or bracing is not indicated as the initial treatment. The swelling that results from the injury precludes the firm compression of the soft tissues that is necessary for success following bracing. The functional cast or brace can be applied only following a period of stabilization of the fracture in an above-the-elbow cast that holds the forearm in a relaxed position of supination. Once the brace is applied with the elbow in the same position of supination, the wrist is free to move in volar and dorsal directions, and the elbow can be flexed fully but its extension is limited in the last 20 to 25° (Figures 57.2 and 57.3, and Table 57.1 and 57.2).

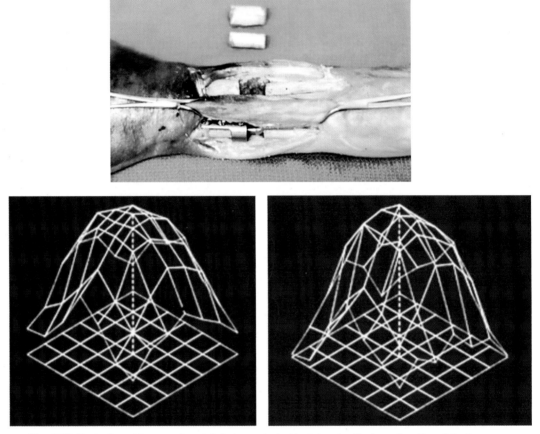

Fig. 57.2: Illustration of the experimental study conducted to determine the loss of motion of the forearm, according to the degree of angulation of the fracture.[5]

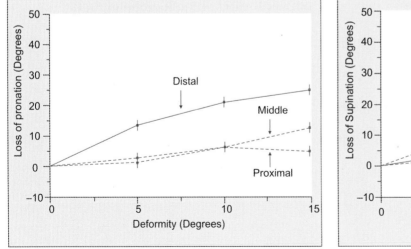
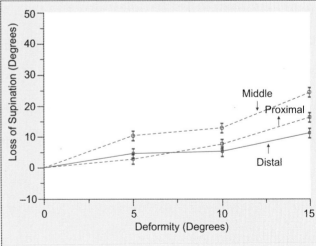

Fig. 57.3: Loss of motion depending on the degree of deformity

			Proximal fracture		Middle fracture		Distal Fracture	
Magnitude of angulation (Degrees)	Direction of angulation	n	Loss of pronation	Loss of supination	Loss of pronation	Loss of supination	Loss of pronation	Loss of supination
5	Dorsal	3	1 (6)	4 (5)	2 (3)	13 (3)	11 (3)	6 (1)
5	Volar	3	2 (6)	1 (4)	2 (3)	8 (7)	18 (3)	3 (3)
5	Radial	3	− 3 (6)	0 (2)	− 3 (3)	12 (6)	6 (4)	7 (2)
5	Ulnar	3	3 (5)	5 (6)	8 (7)	7 (5)	17 (3)	1 (2)
10	Dorsal	3	2 (4)	7 (8)	5 (2)	13 (2)	14 (5)	8 (3)
10	Volar	3	9 (7)	2 (5)	1 (2)	− 4 (4)	22 (2)	2 (4)
10	Radial	3	—	—	9 (4)	22 (3)	—	—
10	Ulnar	3	6 (3)	12 (6)	8 (8)	18 (7)	24 (3)	3 (2)
15	Dorsal	3	1 (1)	15 (11)	9 (3)	21 (1)	16 (2)	17 (2)
15	Volar	3	10 (8)	3 (3)	6 (2)	6 (6)	24 (5)	3 (3)
15	Radial	3	—	—	16 (3)	33 (8)	—	—
15	Ulnar	3	1 (5)	34 (30)	19 (1)	49 (1)	36 (1)	11 (1)

Table 57.1: Loss of motion (degrees) with angulation of the radius

Mean values of degrees loss of pronation and supination for each type of fracture in the radius are presented. Positive values indicate the mean loss of motion. Negative values indicate that on the average, the rotational motion actually increased with the deformity. Standard error in parentheses. Dash indicates deformity could not be produced in the cadaver forearm.

Table 57.2: Estimation errors

	Pronation	Supination	Average	n
Group I (n = 87)				
Radius	− 0.06	0.01	− 0.02	23
Ulna	0.06	0.05	0.06	43
Both	0.09	0.14	0.11	21
Group II (n = 18)				
Radius	− 0.17	0.04	− 0.06	5
Ulna	0.08	0.06	0.07	13

REFERENCES

1. Sarmiento A, Cooper JS, Sinclair WF. Forearm Fractures - Early Functional Bracing - A Preliminary Report. J Bone & Joint Surg. 1975; 57A:297-304.
2. Sarmiento A, Ebramzadeh E, Brys D, Tarr R. Angular Deformities and forearm Function. Ortho Res. 1992; 10-1:121-33.
3. Sarmiento A, Latta LL. The Closed Functional Treatment of Fractures. Springer-Verlag, Heidelberg, 1981.
4. Schneiderman G, Meldrum RD, Bloebaum RD, Tarr R, Sarmiento A. The Interosseous Membrane of the Forearm Structure and Its Role in Galeazzi Fractures. Trauma. 1993 Dec; 35:6.
5. Tarr RR, Garfinkel AI, Sarmiento A. The Effects of Angular and Rotational Deformities of Both Bones of the Forearm: An in vitro Study. J Bone and Joint Surg. 1984; 66A(1):65-70.

58

Technique and Representative Example

TECHNIQUE

There should be no doubt that at this time, the vast majority of fractures of both bones of the forearm are best treated with plate fixation, despite the unphysiological foundations of the technique. However, those biological disadvantages are often outweighed by the practical advantages.

The initial approach to an acute closed fracture of both bones encompasses the same basic principles that apply to all other fractures, i.e. determination of vascular or nerve injury and the possibility of a compartment syndrome. These factors must be observed for an adequate period of time. Though there are advantages to immediate reduction of the displaced fragments, it is best to simply and gingerly straighten out

the gross deformity without attempts being made to obtain the ideal reduction. This action, precipitously taken, might aggravate impending vascular complications. The application of a splint without manipulation should suffice. If by all indicators, the nature of the injury is thought to be benign, a permanent reduction can be carried out otherwise a period of observation is preferable.

We are under the positive impression that in all instances the initial stabilization of the fractured forearm is best in a position of relaxed supination, rather than the popular position of neutral. This position is based on the realization that it is in a relaxed position of supination that the two bones are as widely separate as possible. Obtaining good radiographs is better achieved (Figures 58.1 to 58.5).

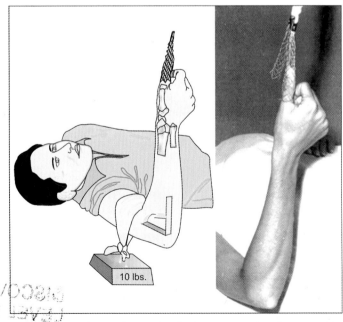

10 lbs.

Fig. 58.1: With the use of Chinese finger traps and a weight over the distal upper arm, the alignment of the fragments is best accomplished. The forearm should be held in a relaxed attitude of supination to best separate the two bones from each other.

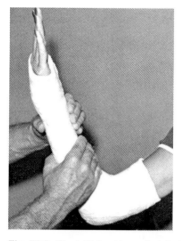
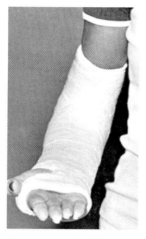
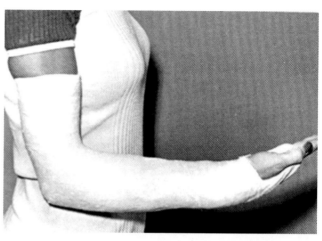

Fig. 58.2: The initial cast, applied during the acute stage of the condition, should be well padded in anticipation of increasing swelling. If clinical findings and symptoms indicate the possibility of significant additional swelling, it is best not to apply a circular cast but a splint that can be readily removed for further inspection of the extremity. These illustrations show the circular cast that holds the elbow at 90° of flexion, the forearm in a relaxed attitude of supination and the wrist in slight volar flexion.

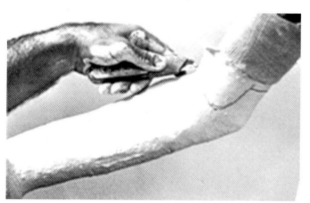
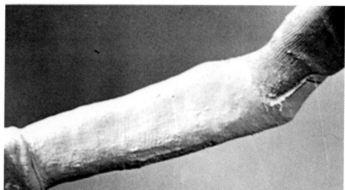
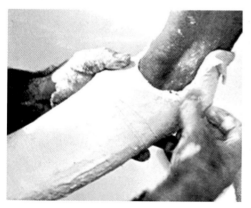
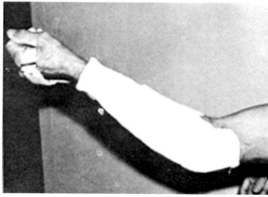
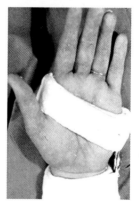

Fig. 58.3: The second cast, applied after the subsidence of acute swelling and pain, is similar to the original one but it has minimal padding and the proximal end is shaped to in a Munster-type fashion to allow flexion of the elbow (limited only in the last few degrees) and extension (limited in the last 30°). The wrist is freed and joined to the body of the cast with an artificial joint.

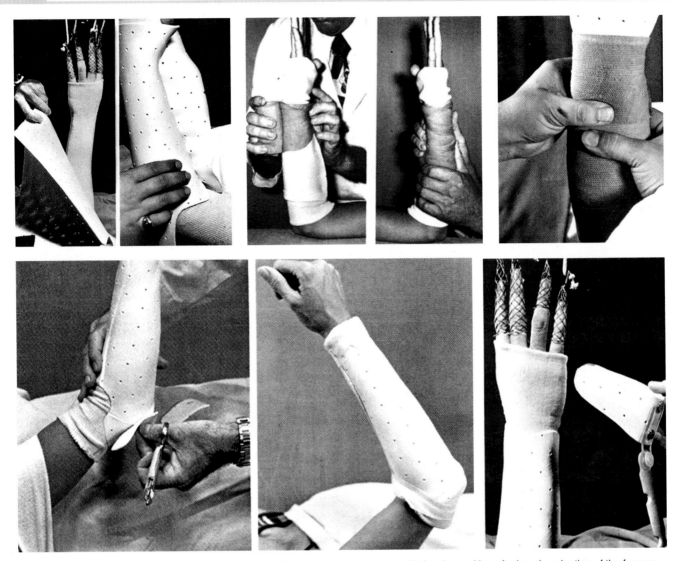

Fig. 58.4: Step-by-step illustrations of the application of the brace using Orthoplast. Notice the position of relaxed supination of the forearm and the firm compression of the material in the antero-posterior plane.

When the opportune time comes for a permanent reduction, it is best to suspend the extremity with Chinese finger traps with mild counter traction from the distal humerus. After a few minutes, the manipulation can be done.

Experience has indicated that obtaining anatomical reduction of transverse fractures in both bones is difficult to achieve and also difficult to maintain. This realization has given further credence to the advantages of plate fixation. The same is true for fractures where one bone has a transverse fracture and the other an oblique or comminuted fracture. In this instance, within a very short time, the reduced transverse fracture angulates towards the non-reducible bone.

It took us a great deal of laboratory work and extensive clinical observation regarding the effects of angulation in various directions and degrees to finally realize that a few degrees of malalignment is readily acceptable, since the resulting limitation of motion is inconsequential. Important is to recognize the fact that plate fixation does not always result in complete range of pronosupination. Much too often the final rotation of plated forearms is not different from that obtained with closed treatment. This is particularly true for fractures located close to the elbow joint where almost always, significant loss of forearm rotation is the norm. A bony synostosis between the radius and ulna readily develops.

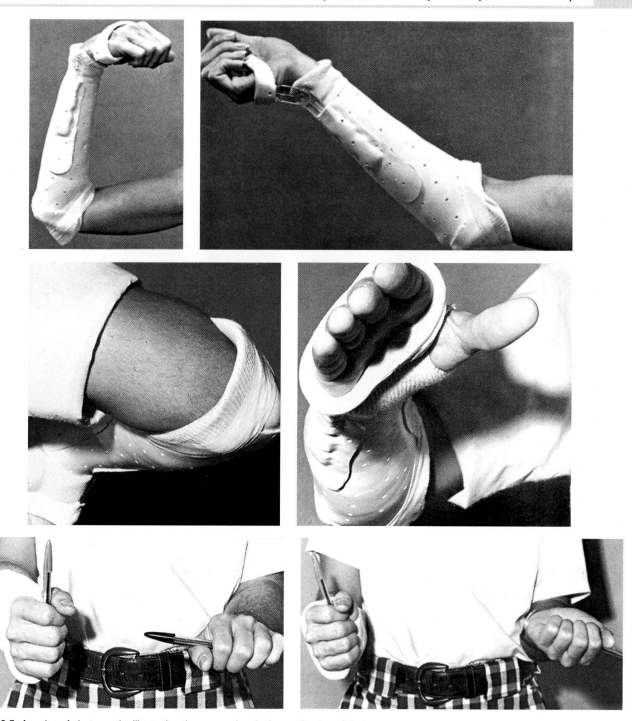

Fig. 58.5: A series of photographs illustrating the steps taken in the application of the brace and the ultimate range of motion the brace permits. Notice the flattening of the forearm being held in a relaxed attitude of supination. The flattening of the forearm separates the two bones as much as possible. The supracondylar extensions of the brace preclude full extension and limits flexion in the last few degrees. Upon completion of the procedure, prono-supination is not possible.

Of a major importance was the finding that the initial shortening of closed fractures of the forearm does not increase with the use of the extremity. This is the same mechanism that explains this phenomenon in axially unstable fractures of the tibia when associated with a fibular fracture. The tethering of the surrounding soft tissues, particularly the interosseus membrane prevents further shortening. We have obtained very good results when axially unstable fractures of both bones were treated without attempts to regain length or reduction, simply alignment of the fragments with the forearm in a relaxed position of supination.

Through the above-described studies, we found an explanation for the loss of reduction in some fractures. It appears that when the fracture in one of the bones is transverse and in the other bone oblique or comminuted, the reduction is difficult to maintain and the bones angulate toward the unstable fracture. The best clinical results were obtained in those instances when anatomical reduction was not attempted, as in the case of overriding comminuted or oblique fractures (Figure 58.6). In retrospect, we have concluded that our obsession with anatomical reduction of fractures of both bones of the forearm was a mistake. Had we accepted overriding of fragments, without panicking about a few degrees of angulation, we would have been able to say, with adequate data to prove the point, that transverse fractures of both bones of the forearm are best treated by internal fixation, but that oblique fractures do not always require it.

Once, we reviewed our experiences with surgical plating of fractures of both bones of the forearm and selected 20 patients who had healed their fractures uneventfully. Using a machine that recorded pronosupination only and eliminated any compensatory shoulder motion, we measured the pronosupination of the forearm. With only two exceptions, we discovered that all of the patients had a permanent loss of the last few degrees of pronosupination. The patients were not aware of the loss as they instinctively compensated with shoulder rotation.

I was discussing these experiences in front of a group of residents. One of them, who had recently joined the program, said to me, "Dr. Sarmiento, with all due respect I disagree with you. I broke my forearm a few years ago and had the fractures plated. Today, I have no limitation of motion at all." "Well," I responded, "you may be one of the rare exceptions. Let me examine your arms. Take off your shirt and stand here." I placed his elbows against his chest and asked him to maintain them in that position. I then put pencils in his clenched fists. He then pronated and supinated his forearms. Lo and behold he lacked the last 8° of pronation and was unaware of the loss.

Achievement of anatomical reduction and maintenance of reduction in a cast is extremely difficult in many instances. The experiences of other surzions with the use of thin Kirschner wires have reinforced my long-held belief that the reported failure rate of intramedullary fixation of forearm fractures is due to the mistaken belief that the nail should rigidly immobilize the fragments. Immobilization is not needed; quite to the contrary, it encourages nonunion. In the early 1980s Steve Ross, a member of our faculty at USC, attempted to develop a thin, flexible intramedullary nail that did not immobilize the fractured fragments and maintained their alignment. Unfortunately, he abandoned the project.

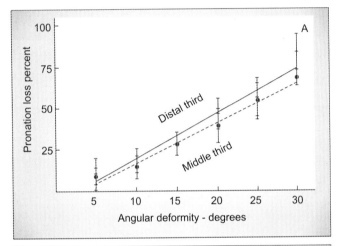

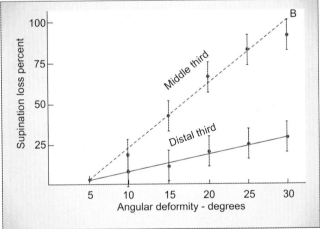

Fig. 58.6: Loss of movement with angular deformity

REPRESENTATIVE EXAMPLES

Some of representative examples illustrating fractures examples illustrating fractures of both bone are shown from Figures 58.7 to 58.17.

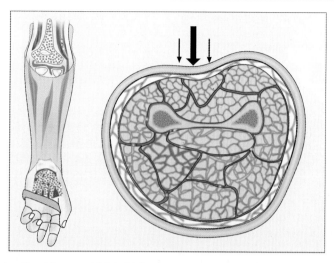

Fig. 58.7: Drawings depicting the functional brace, which hold the forearm in a relaxed position of supination, the elbow and wrist free, but a firm contact of the proximal wings of the cast (or brace) over the distal upper arm. This construction, which we have called a Munster–like configuration permits slightly limited flexion and extension of the elbow, while preventing pronosupination.

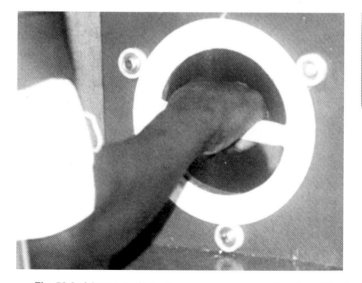
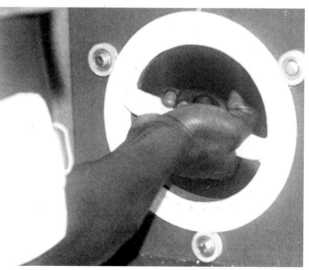

Fig. 58.8: A home-made system to measure range of motion of the forearm. The apparatus prevents shoulder rotation and records the degrees of pronosupination.

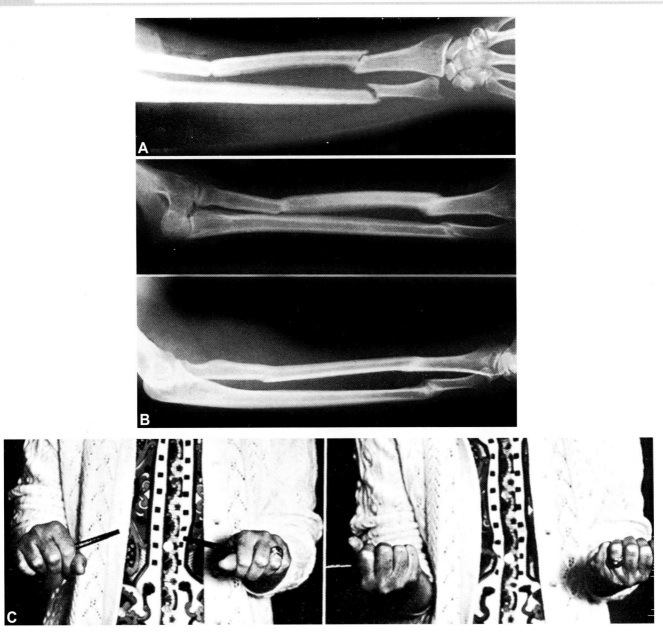

Figs 58.9A to C: (A) Initial radiograph of fracture of both bones of the forearm. The radial fracture is segmental. The patient refused surgery. (B) The fractures were treated with a functional cast and healed with a deformity that, nonetheless, was not associated with severe limitation of motion. (C) Patient demonstrates the loss of the last few degrees of pronation.

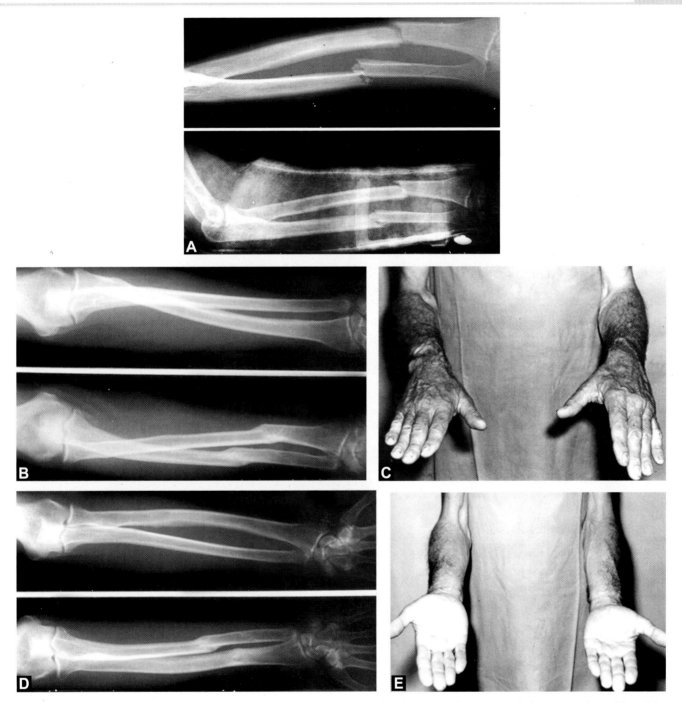

Figs 58.10A to E: (A) Radiograph illustrating the initial fracture of both bones of the forearm, and the accepted alignment and overriding of the fragments in a functional Munster-like brace. (B and C) Radiological and clinical illustrations of the degree of supination of the forearm. Final supination of the forearm. (D and E) Radiological and clinical illustrations of the final degree of supination.

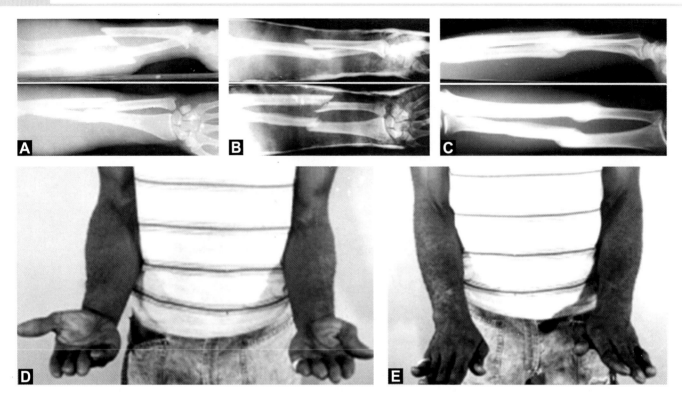

Figs 58.11A to E: Oblique fractures of both bones of the forearm treated with functional brace. Functional result was satisfactory. Sequential radiographs of fractures of both bones of the forearm treated with a functional cast that freed the elbow and wrist joints but prevented prono-supination. The fracture healed uneventfully and the function of the forearm and elbow was very acceptable.

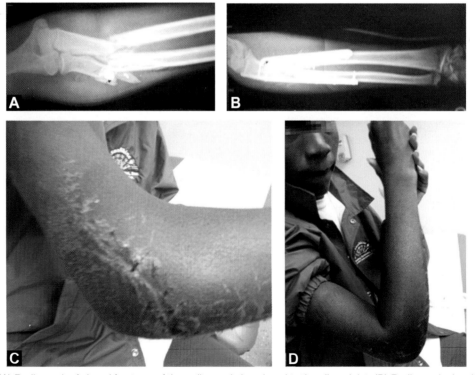

Figs 58.12A to D: (A) Radiograph of closed fractures of the radius and ulna closed to the elbow joint. (B) Radiograph showing the plated both bones. (C and D) Patient demonstrates the severe limitation of motion of the elbow. Prono-supination was completely lost.

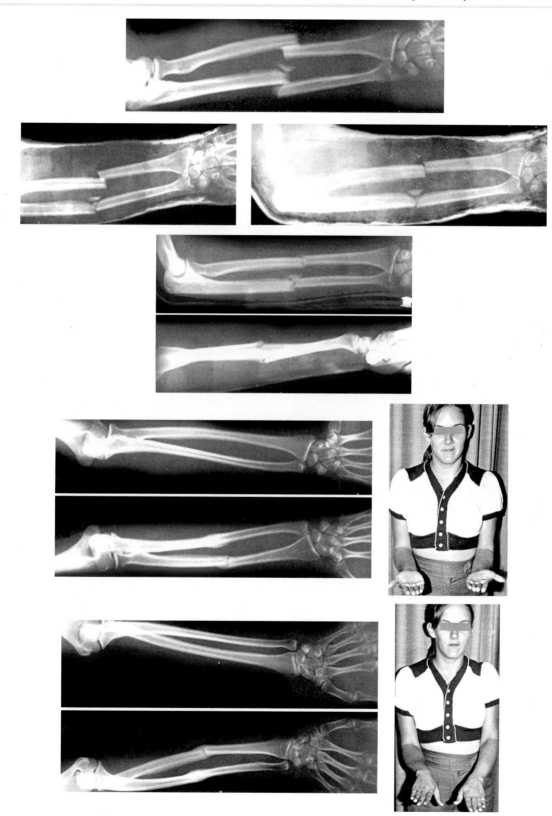

Fig. 58.13: Radiographs of closed fractures of both bones of the forearm. The initial reduction was not satisfactory, requiring a second manipulation using finger-traps suspension and reapplication of a cast. The final function was satisfactory as demonstrated in the radiological and clinical photographs.

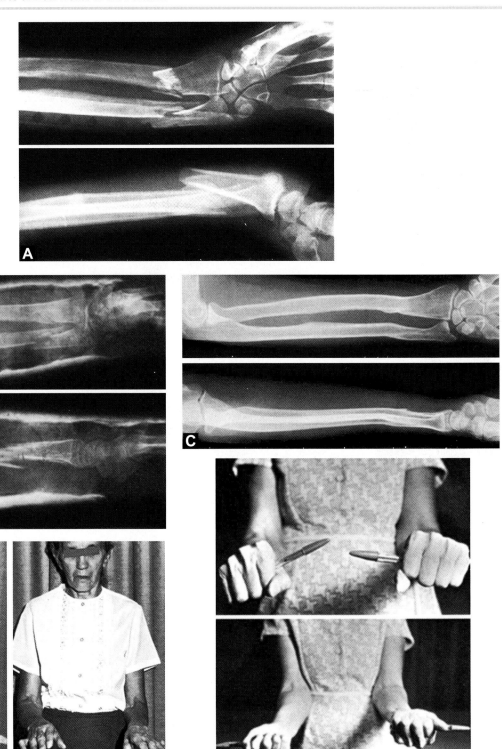

Figs 58.14A to E: (A) Radiograph of fracture of both bones of the forearm with major displacement of the fragments. (B) Radiograph obtained after manual reduction of the fracture. (C) Radiograph demonstrating the healed fracture with good alignment. (D) Patient demonstrates the range of pronosupination of her forearms shortly after completion of healing. Notice the limitation of pronation. (E) Patient demonstrates the range of motion present a few months later. The limitation of pronation is minimal.

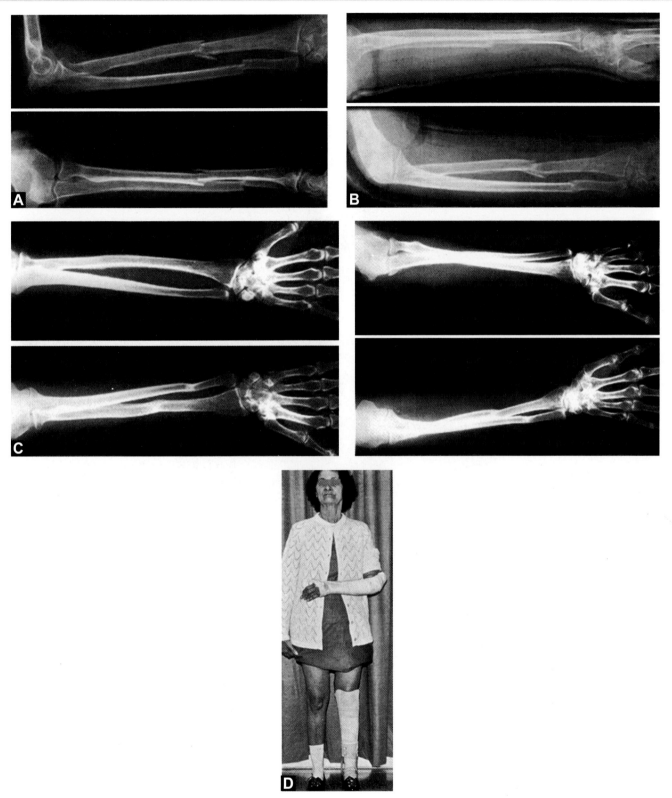

Figs 58.15A to D: (A) Radiograph of fractures of both bones of the forearm. (B) Radiographs obtained after application of a functional brace. (C) Radiographs of supination and pronation of both bones of the forearm identified after completion of healing. (D) Patient had an associated fracture of the tibia which was treated with a below-the-knee functional brace.

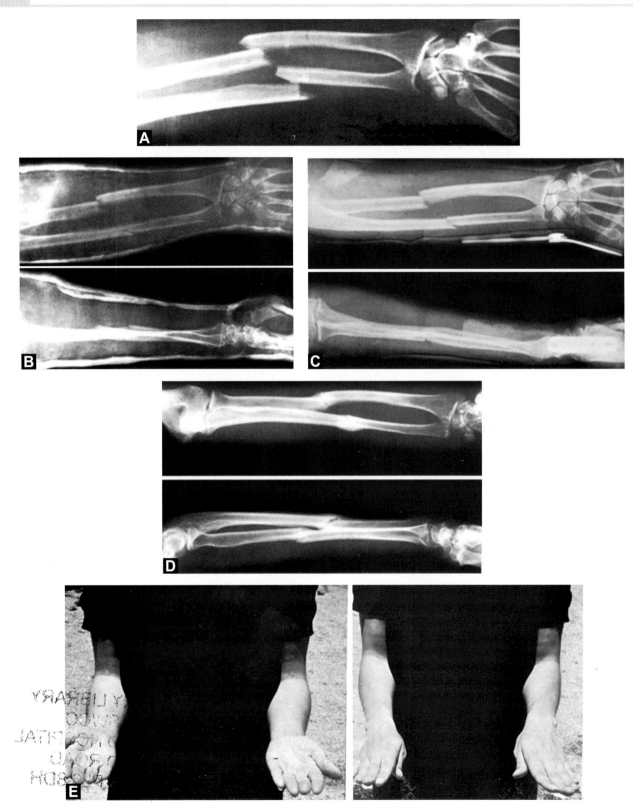

Figs 58.16A to E: (A) Radiograph of fractures of both bones of the forearm. (B) Radiograph obtained after reduction of the fracture. (C) Radiograph taken after the application of the functional plastic brace. (D) Antero-posterior and lateral radiographs of the healed fractures. (E) Patient demonstrates the final range of motion of her fractured forearm.

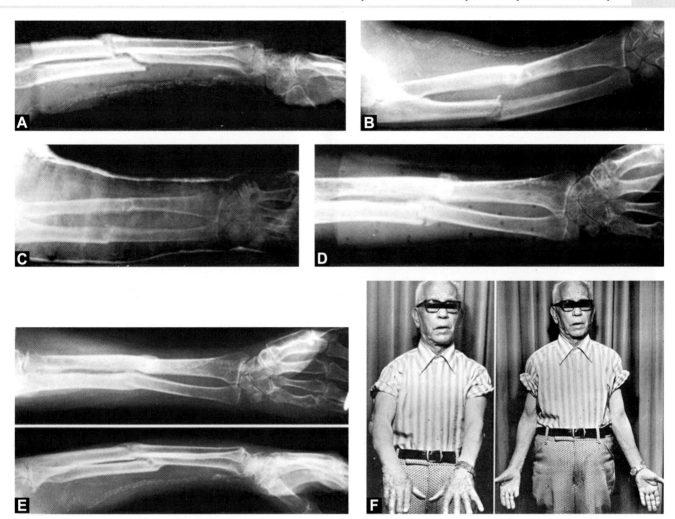

Figs 58.17A to F: (A and B) Radiographs of fractures of both bones of the forearm showing the angulated fragments. (C) Radiograph obtained after reduction and stabilization in an above-the-elbow cast. (D) Radiograph showing callus bridging the fragments. (E) Final radiograph illustrating healing with mild-to-moderate deformity. (F) Patient demonstrates the function of his forearms. A residual limitation of pronation is being compensated very inconspicuously by shoulder rotations.

Isolated Radial Shaft Fractures

59

Rationale, Indications, Technique and Representative Examples

The indications for functional bracing of isolated radial shaft fractures are relatively few due to the fact that many of these fractures are the result of falls on the outstretched hand associated with subluxation or complete dislocation of the distal radio-ulnar joint. This pathology is a serious one, in which a closed reduction is usually unsuccessful. Open reduction of the fractured radius and surgical repair of the damaged ligament are essential for a successful clinical result. Failure to take care of the distal pathology leaves, in many instances, an unstable situation associated with chronic pain.[1-3]

On the other hand, radial shaft fractures, the result of a direct blow, do not damage the distal radio-ulnar joint unless severe displacement of the fragment has occurred, as in the case of open fractures with major soft tissue damage. Simple, uncomplicated fractures with minimal angular deformity can be successfully taken care of by nonsurgical functional means

in a similar way isolated ulnar shaft fractures are managed. The loss of the bowing of radius, which according to popular practices is considered a very critical feature, should not be taken to unreasonable extremes. We have documented that a mild loss of the radial bowing is tolerated very well and without easily recognizable loss of motion.

We are of the impression that plate fixation of radial fracture located in the proximal-fourth of the shaft are much too often associated with permanent loss of pronosupination (Figure 59.1A and B). Sometimes this is due to the formation of a synostosis bony bridge between the radius and the ulna. Other times, without the bony bridge, a permanent limitation of motion is the result. This fact must be kept in consideration when determining the most appropriate treatment. In addition, refractures following removal of the plate are not uncommon due to the thus far unavoidable atrophy of the cortex under the plate.

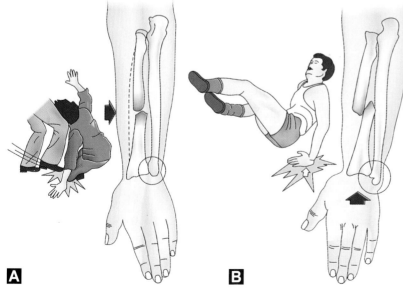

A   **B**

Figs 59.1A and B: Illustration of the two mechanisms leading to the production of a radial fracture. (A) The fracture is produced from a direct blow over the radius. In this instance the distal radio-ulnar joint is not damaged. (B) When the fracture is the result of a fall on the stretched hand, the distal radio-ulnar joint experiences subluxation or frankly dislocates from the ulna after damaging the annular ligament that connects the two bones. The greater degree of dislocation occurs when the interosseus membrane is ruptured.

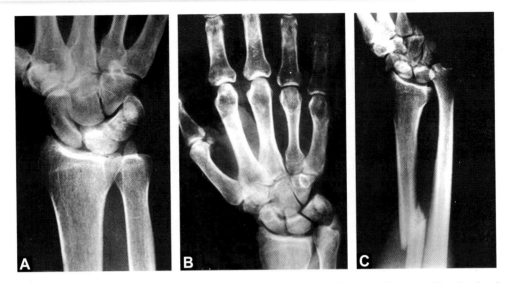

Figs 59.2A to C: (A) Radiograph of a cadaver specimen after the production of a surgically created fracture of the distal radius. The specimen is being subjected to vertical loading. Notice that the force does not result in subluxation of the distal radius–ulnar joint. (B) The same specimen under identical mechanical circumstances, but after the annular radio-ulnar ligament has been severed, an obvious dislocation is visible. (C) Severe dislocation occurs when in addition to the severance of the distal annular ligament, the interosseus membrane is severed.

TECHNIQUE

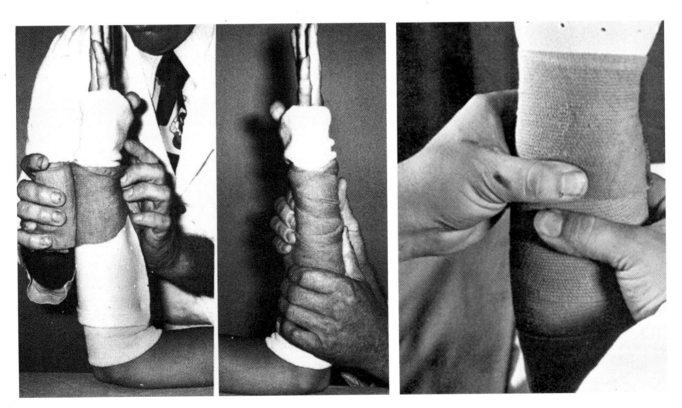

Fig. 59.3

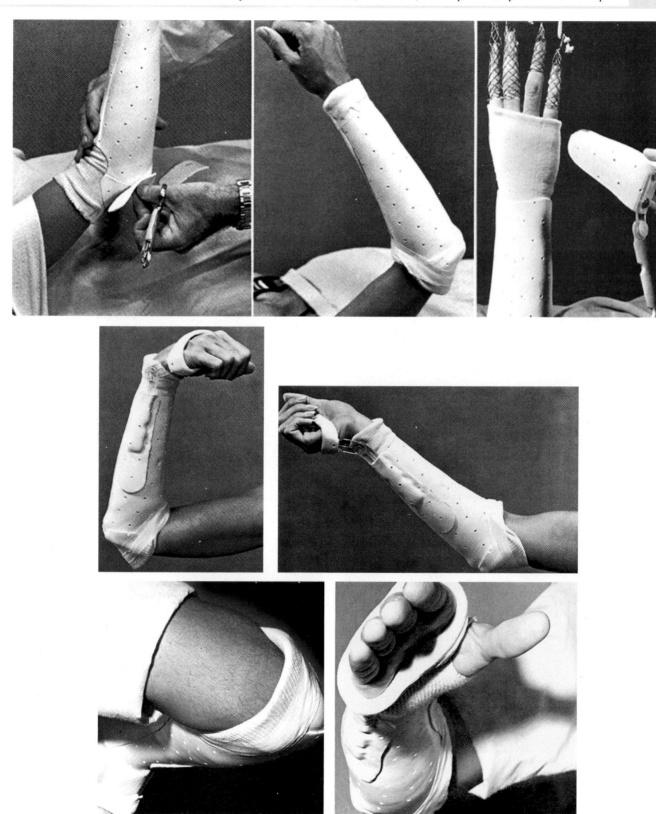

Fig. 59.3: Step-by-step illustration of the application of the Orthoplast Munster-like brace. Notice the freedom of the wrist joint, the proximal extension of the lateral wings over the distal arm in order to prevent the last 25° of extension.

REPRESENTATIVE EXAMPLES

Some of the representative examples illustrating isolated radial shaft fractures are shown in Figures 59.4 to 59.6.

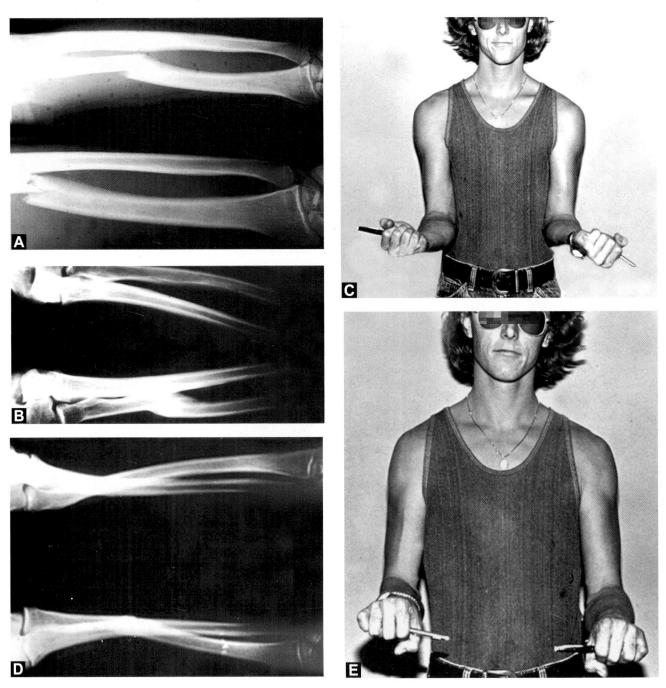

Figs 59.4A to E: (A) Radiograph of isolated fracture of the radial shaft resulting from a direct blow with a baseball bat over the radial shaft. Notice the loss of the radial bow. (B and C) Radiographs and clinical pictures with the forearm in supination. The loss of supination demonstrated by the patient is virtually unnoticeable. Function is normal and asymptomatic. (D and E) Radiograph and clinical photo of the forearm in pronation. The loss of pronation is minimal and readily compensated with shoulder flexion and mild abduction.

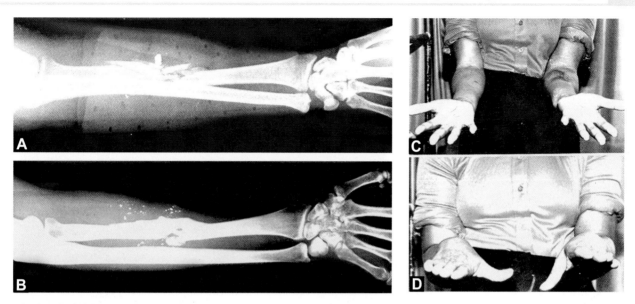

Figs 59.5A to D: (A) Radiograph of isolated fracture of the radial shaft produced by a low-velocity projectile. The alignment of the fragments is acceptable and there is no evidence of distal radio-ulnar pathology. (B) Radiograph obtained after completion of healing. The fracture was treated with a functional brace of the Munster-like type (C and D) Patient demonstrates the range of motion of her forearms.

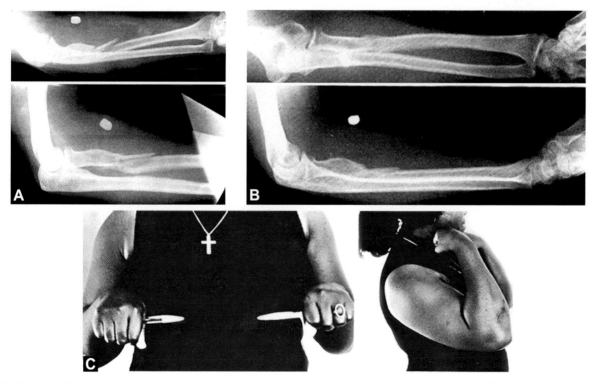

Figs 59.6A to C: (A) Radiograph of isolated fracture of the radial shaft, the result of a low-velocity bullet. (B) Radiograph obtained after completion of healing. The fracture was treated with a Munster-like brace that prevented pronosupination but permitted flexion and extension of the wrist. (C) Patient demonstrates the pronation of her forearm and the flexion of her elbows.

REFERENCES

1. Sarmiento A, Latta LL. The Closed Functional Treatment of Fractures. Springer-Verlag, Heidelberg. 1981.

2. Schneiderman G, Meldrum RD, Bloebaum RD, Tarr R, Sarmiento A. The Interosseous Membrane of the Forearm Structure and Its Role in Galeazzi Fractures. Trauma. 1993 Dec; 35:6.

3. Tarr RR, Garfinkel AI, Sarmiento A. The Effects of Angular and Rotational Deformities of Both Bones of the Forearm: An in vitro Study. J. Bone and Joint Surg. 1984; 66A(1):65-70.

Index